About the Author

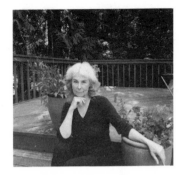

SUSAN MCCUTCHEON is an award-winning science educator, named to the Association of Science-Technology Center's Honor Roll of Teachers for her "exemplary collaboration with the Bishop Museum in Hawaii, to significantly improve the quality of science education."

Her degree is in chemistry. She taught physics and chemistry for ten years in Honolulu and was selected to present a workshop at the National Science Teachers Association Conference on her successful strategies for teaching science. Following that, the editor of *Learning Magazine* engaged Susan to write an article disseminating her ideas to many more teachers around the country.

The governor of Hawaii appointed her to serve a two-year term on the Hawaii State Health Plan Development Committee and then the Hawaii State Regionalization of Perinatal Care Committee.

She is a Certified Childbirth Educator, having studied directly under Dr. Robert Bradley in his very first teacher training, and has been teaching the Bradley Method® for fifty years, teaching thousands of couples, and is a conference speaker and instructor at teacher training workshops across the United States.

She is currently teaching the Bradley Method® in Portland, Maine, and is also an active Certified Doula and has personally supported hundreds of women in labor.

She's had three natural births herself, using what she teaches others: the incredibly effective Bradley Method® techniques.

Acknowledgments

SPECIAL THANKS to my agent, Heide Lange; editor Nina Shield; fellow Bradley instructor Theresa Zawalski; all of whom greatly contributed to the production of this book.

Praise for
Natural Childbirth the Bradley® Way

"The Bradley Method® is the best and the safest approach to childbirth possible. Its high level of success speaks for itself: 80 to 90 percent totally unmedicated, natural birth. This book fills a great unmet need. . . . It will help countless families to have healthier babies."

—David Steward, PhD, executive director, NAPSAC

"Informative and immensely practical . . . an important contribution to the childbearing literature."

—Marian Tompson, cofounder, La Leche League

"On the cutting edge of childbirth reform . . . overall the book is a splendid account of the natural-childbirth process."

—From *Birth Journal*, by Margot Edwards, RN, MA

"Every pregnant couple should study this book!"

—Tom Brewer, MD, chairman, Nutrition Action Group, coauthor,
Brewer Medical Diet for Normal and High-Risk Pregnancy

"I highly recommend this book for preparing couples for totally natural, unmedicated birth by the Bradley Method®."

—Robert A. Bradley, MD

Susan McCutcheon

Natural Childbirth
the Bradley® Way

Illustrated by

Erick Ingraham and Robin Yoko Burningham

PLUME

PLUME
An imprint of Penguin Random House LLC
375 Hudson Street
New York, New York 10014

Originally published in a Dutton paperback edition.
First Plume Printing, 1984
First Plume Printing, revised edition, May 1996
First Plume Printing, revised edition, June 2017
Copyright © 1984 Susan McCutcheon-Rosegg and Peter Rosegg. Copyright © 1996
Susan McCutcheon. Copyright © 2017 Susan McCutcheon.

REGISTERED TRADEMARK—MARCA REGISTRADA
PLUME

ISBN: 9780525537991
(Previously published under the ISBN 9780452276598)

Printed in the United States of America
10 9 8 7 6 5 4 3 2 1

Illustrations by Erick Ingraham and Robin Yoko Burningham

THE BRADLEY METHOD® is the trademark of the American Academy of
Husband-Coached Childbirth and is registered in the United States Patent Office.
Only those teachers currently affiliated with the Academy may teach the Bradley
Method® or use the term Bradley® in connection with childbirth education.

THIS BOOK IS DEDICATED TO MY CHILDREN,
BRIAN, ROBIN, AND POLLY.

TO BRIAN, *whose labor taught me patience and the depths of concentration attainable during a hard first labor.*

TO ROBIN, *whose birth taught me the sweetness of an easy labor and the power and rewards of selecting a supportive environment.*

TO POLLY, *whose hard labor taught me not to anticipate what any labor will be like (each is a new experience and takes its own pattern and shape), and whose birth at home made this, although my hardest labor, my best birth.*

IT IS ALSO
DEDICATED:

TO DR. WES SOKOLOSKY, *who, bringing along his best smile, kindly attended my home birth of Polly, and who had the uncommon wisdom to do nothing when nothing was called for.*

TO THE THOUSANDS OF COUPLES
I HAVE HAD THE PRIVILEGE TO TEACH,
many of whom allowed me to be present during their labors and births and who in turn taught me through the generous sharing of their experiences.

AND FINALLY TO WOMEN WHO HAVE HAD THE COURAGE
TO SPEAK OUT AND PRESS FOR CHANGES IN CHILDBIRTH:
Lester Hazell, Doris Haire, Suzanne Arms,
Nancy Wainer Cohen, Lois J. Estner, Gail Sforza
Brewer, Marjie Hathaway, Ina Mae Gaskin, and, of
course, all the Bradley teachers.

—SUSAN McCUTCHEON

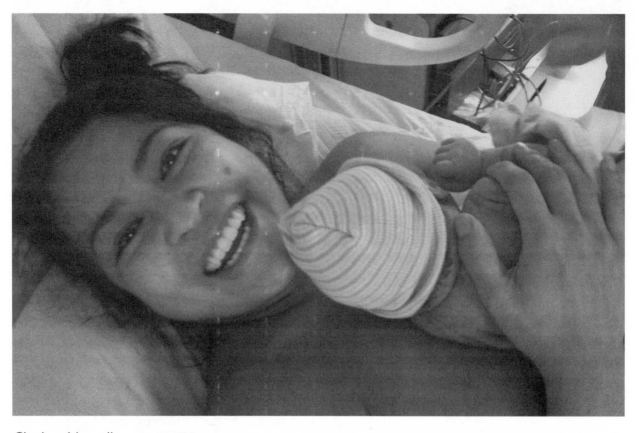

Charlene Maxwell, nurse-practitioner

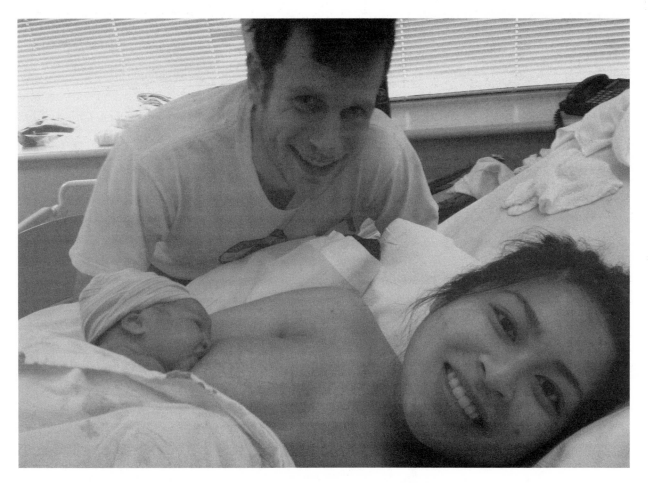

Charles and Charlene Maxwell, nurse-practitioner, and Baby Matilda. First baby.

"We had a beautiful baby girl, who arrived on her due date. I was so happy to do the whole thing unmedicated and felt really in control."
—Charlene

Contents

Preface by
Robert A. Bradley, MD

I HIGHLY RECOMMEND THIS BOOK for preparing couples for totally unmedicated births by the Bradley Method® of true natural childbirth. Mrs. McCutcheon was a student in our very first Bradley class many years ago and has given unmedicated births herself. She is well-read and knowledgeable in her subject.

The preparation and focus of *Natural Childbirth the Bradley® Way* follows the natural instinctual behavior of all mammals in bearing their young. I first described and stressed the importance of this human imitation of instinctual behavior in 1947 while in obstetrical training at the Mayo Foundation in Minnesota. At that time, I observed a group of pregnant nurses who volunteered to try my ideas after seeing them work so well with a small number of clinic patients. This first experiment in true natural childbirth without medication or drugs was interrupted by Navy duty in the Korean War, but was reported and illustrated by the *Minneapolis Tribune* in a full-page article, "Better Start for Babies," in 1949.

In 1962 I published an analysis of my first four thousand cases following these principles in private practice, entitled "Fathers' Presence in Delivery Rooms" (*Psychosomatics* 3, no. 6). Over ten thousand copies of this article were requested from all over the world.

The Bradley Method® was preceded only by the late Dr. Grantly Dick-Read's *Childbirth Without Fear* in 1944. I met Dr. Read in Chicago in 1948, and he accepted my invitation to visit with me later in Denver. We had a wonderful visit, but I did have a bit of trouble with some of his theories related to fear and with his assertion that "a little gas or medication wouldn't hurt anything." From the very first, I felt we should use no drugs of any nature in pregnancy, labor, or birth unless dire complications warranted them.

Also, from the very first I had included husbands in the birth team as coaches and minimized the role of the physician to resemble that of a lifeguard, who, when watching swimmers, did nothing as long as everything was going along all right. I put the husband where Dr. Read sat, at the head of the bed, to capitalize on the lover relationship and found it worked marvelously.

The Lamaze method came along later, using female "monitrices" as coaches. I tried this and found it most ineffective, as reflected in a low percentage of unmedicated births. With husbands coaching in our method, we have over 90 percent totally unmedicated births. No other approach comes anywhere near that figure.

Inevitable conflicts arose between advocates of the Bradley Method® and the Lamaze method, and as I am an Irishman, I'm guilty of not smoothing but stirring the troubled waters. I was ridiculed for my no-drugs approach, as they continued to claim "a little medication wouldn't hurt anything." Also, I was mocked with the label "Barnyard Bradley" for my insistence on imitating animals and for the term "natural childbirth," which I still prefer to "psychoprophylaxis."

Recent new research on the effects of maternal medication on the fetus and infant verifies the assumptions I first made in 1947: drugs are all bad during pregnancy. Also, the meddlesome interference with nature's instinctual conduct and plans (induction of labor, silly "due dates," routine IVs, monitoring, etc.) are very well covered in this book.

Our large American Academy of Husband-Coached Childbirth®, located near Hollywood, California, continues to train and affiliate childbirth educators of the Bradley Method®. It is the safest method of having a baby. Regardless of where you have your baby, or whom you choose to have in attendance, do not deviate from nature's great principles.

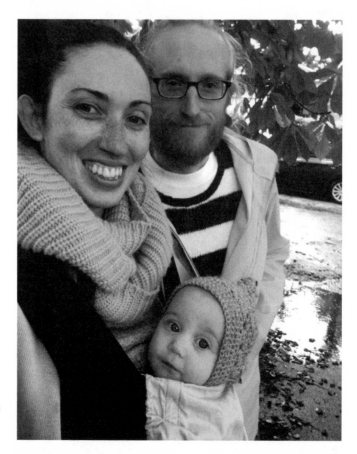

Laura and John Roberts with their baby, Hannah

PART I

GETTING READY

CHAPTER ONE

An Introduction

IN 1968, I STARTED teaching childbirth to a few friends, and in the next year I completed my first teacher-training course at the American Institute of Family Relations. That course was described as "Lamaze plus." I had really just started my career as a childbirth educator, but very soon I felt that there had to be something better. There was. I was fortunate to be in on the first formal teacher-training workshop in the Bradley Method®, taught by Dr. Robert A. Bradley himself in 1970.

Dr. Bradley was a pioneer in getting husbands into the delivery room and has led the movement to return to natural, drug-free techniques in childbirth. Although I was already a certified childbirth teacher, I found in Dr. Bradley's course the real foundation for the next fifty years as I began teaching what I believe to be the most successful natural childbirth method available today. Since then I have taught over three thousand couples, coached hundreds of women in labor, and been present at many more births.

Many people mistakenly believe that natural childbirth is already quite common—that "everybody" is doing it. This is just not true. Most births today are still medicated, forceps, or vacuum-extractor deliveries or cesarean surgery or induced labors—*not* natural, drug-free, normal childbirth. Instead of natural births, most people who take "prepared" childbirth classes are being prepared for cesarean surgery, or for deliveries with drugs and mechanical interventions that unfortunately are used routinely in almost all births.

In fact, so few women have a natural (meaning, no drugs) childbirth, that *many* of my students come back to class telling stories of how everybody crowded into their hospital room to see this.

One told of a doctor who was so amazed he hugged

the nurse (who happened to be his wife), and they congratulated each other as enthusiastically as if they were the ones who had just given birth!

Another had visits from different hospital staff members, nurses, and residents who wanted to ask her how she did this, as word got around about a natural birth, and with a first-time mom.

Yet another first-time mom was told by the medical staff she was the poster child for natural birth, as the mom was so vibrantly and enthusiastically welcoming her child, scooping him up herself, whooping with joy, as he was emerging from her body.

Rachel Angleton-Walker and Jim Walker had this to say:

> We had an incredible journey that will forever be a part of our partnership and we learned how great a team we can be. We even had an L&D nurse send us a card after to tell us how much of a joy it was to witness our journey and what an impression our techniques made on her . . . pretty cool from someone who does this every day for their job.

Linda Thompson and Joe wrote:

> Thank you again so much for all of your instruction! Our doula, Rebecca, was brought to tears by our birth experience and said that she has never seen a couple work so well together. I couldn't have done this sixty-three-hour labor without your class, or Joe's coaching! He never left my side (except when Rebecca thankfully made him go eat).

This book is for pregnant women who are looking for the real thing, birthing normally and naturally without the routine use of drugs or unnecessary interventions—in short, the Bradley Method®.

SUSAN McCUTCHEON
2017

TO THE COACH

Today, there are fewer men who think their part in the whole process of birth was finished nine months before and that the nurses and doctors will take care of everything. (And, oh yes, aren't there drugs for all this birth stuff?)

In fact, the nurses have their hands full, and most people are amazed to find out that doctors rarely even show up until the last few minutes of birth. And as for drugs, the reality is that drugs come with risks to the mother and the baby. They can affect the mother's heart (causing cardiac arrest) or the muscles she uses to push the baby out, and this can slow down labor, making intervention a necessity. The myth is that the medicated labor is painless. But it is the medicated mother who later talks most about pain (and the earlier you have them, the more likely you are to have complications). She may have thought drugs would see her through labor, so she didn't take the opportunity to get her mind and body ready.

In contrast, the trained, natural-childbirth mother talks primarily of hard work—because she knows what to do in labor. Her body is ready and she knows how to keep herself comfortable and relaxed.

A Bradley-trained mother in labor is incredibly different from the woman in agony you may have imagined from novels, television, or the movies.

But the natural-childbirth mother cannot do it alone. Human birth has never been the completely solitary experience that is common among animals. It is an awesome, beautiful moment that should be shared by people who care about each other.

It is hard to imagine a woman laboring and birthing without knowing how to help herself and without a trained coach to support her, though sadly, this happens all the time. First of all, there are physical needs and sensations—like a backache—that can be alleviated with the help of a caring person. Then, there is a mood to create; a relaxed, warm, loving environment that is only possible with another person whose full attention is on the laboring woman.

Finally, there is a joy to be shared and celebrated, a once-in-a-lifetime moment of happiness, excitement, relief, closeness, and love.

For all these special things, are you going to depend on the doctors or the nurses? Hardly. A busy obstetrician may have one or two *dozen* births a month. He could not spend hours with each laboring woman and still run a practice, even if he wanted to. And what about the nurses? Well, they are essentially trouble-spotters for the doctors. They have little time for a mother with a normal, uncomplicated labor. By now you see the bottle that has been spinning is coming around to stop in front of you.

For some men the question may come down to a simple "Who else?" But for most it is a more positive decision than that. Are you going to leave this responsibility to your partner for someone else and miss this chance for a once-in-a-lifetime experience?

More and more men now actively want to be part of the birth experience of their babies and to support their partners in this hard work they have started together. It is one of the most authentic things you may ever do in your life. A lot of people these days are preoccupied with trying to recapture simple values through meaningful human contacts and true-life experiences. This happens at the most fundamental level in birth.

Many men are actively defying the degrading caricatures of the brainless father standing uselessly by the mother's side, with nothing more to offer her than a hand to squeeze. They know it is no longer outlandish to be caring, active husbands and fathers. Our classes are filled with men eager to accept their responsibilities. They look forward to helping their wives in labor and to sharing the rewards of birth.

In the following chapters, the two of you will learn that labor is really a simple process. The mother will learn how to work with her body and let it fulfill its task unimpeded by tension, fear, or drugs. Don't think you get off without some hard physical work, though. Birth is very much a team effort. Like any other coach, you must get involved right at the start of training. Don't wait until just before the big event. Get started right now.

—SUSAN McCUTCHEON AND PETER ROSEGG

NOT ALONE

Women who do not have a male partner, whether by circumstance or by design, will be glad to know that a best friend, a sister, a mother, or a significant other can also acquire the Bradley coaching skills and do an excellent job of supporting you in birth. I do think that your first-choice person should be someone who loves you. Be sure you choose someone you have a good relationship with and who you can count on to drop everything and stay with you through the entire labor.

Here's another option: Call your nearest Bradley teacher for help. Bradley teachers, besides being certified doulas themselves, will be able to direct you to other doulas who are familiar with the Bradley Method®.

CHAPTER TWO

How Is the Bradley Method® Unique?

"If a mother truly wants a natural childbirth and
wants to deliver in the hospital, Bradley classes give
her the best odds of achieving the birth she wants."

THAT QUOTE COMES FROM *The Birth Book*, by William
Sears, MD, and Martha Sears, RN.

They aren't the only ones to notice that more mothers
using the Bradley Method® actually *do* get to a natural
birth.

Dr. Silvia Feldman, whose book *Choices in Childbirth*
looks at just about every method available, says: "If you're the
kind of person who likes to do your own thing and can count
(a great deal) on your husband to help you do it, then I recommend the Bradley Method® to you. For those with enough
self-confidence, it may be the most rewarding
natural-childbirth method available in the United States."[1]

A new class begins and students introduce themselves as we go around the room. And here's what one of
them recently said:

"I told my doctor I really wanted to have a natural
childbirth, as long as I was birthing normally. I let him
know this was important to me." And her doctor replied:
"In that case, you should probably skip the hospital classes
and get into a Bradley class."

It's not the first time I've heard this. The surprising
rate of success with the simple but effective Bradley techniques is the most unique part of this method. Drugs are
not withheld from Bradley-trained mothers. It's just that

the techniques are so effective that most Bradley-trained mothers don't feel a need to ask for them.

There are many personal stories for you to read in this book. And I tell many mini stories throughout. When I do that, I'm not just babbling. Real stories are important. Toni Morrison, who won the Nobel Prize for Literature, said in her acceptance speech that we learn best from narrative, from story. So, with the permission of the parents whose accounts I sprinkle in here and there, you will learn much from other mothers, which is the way it should be: mothers teaching mothers.

CHAPTER THREE

How to Choose Your Childbirth Teacher

WHEN SHOULD YOU CHOOSE your childbirth educator? Ideally, before you choose your doctor. An independent, natural-childbirth educator will know who is practicing in your area and can suggest those doctors (or other birth attendants) who will meet your desires. (However, don't shy away from a Bradley Method® instructor just because you have already chosen a doctor.) The independent natural-birth educator will also have the scoop on local hospitals and birthing centers.

A natural-childbirth teacher will use the word "natural" with no apology, because the goals of her class will reflect her experience with successful techniques. In fact, she should be happy to talk statistics with you.

A teacher who avoids the word "natural" and uses the word "prepared" childbirth does so because most of her students will have "prepared" but medicated deliveries. The limited effectiveness of the techniques she is using are reflected in her limited goals.

Because they are preparing a woman for what will happen to her in birth, rather than teaching what she needs to have the kind of birth she wants, prepared-childbirth teachers often take it upon themselves to withhold information about the risks of drugs or the hazards of procedures that might be used. This is done in "misguided kindness." It stems from the mistaken idea that few women are able to have totally unmedicated labor and birth anyway, so why tell a woman about things that might be avoided if it will just make her feel guilty and unhappy afterward? Advocates of "prepared" childbirth education will often warn expectant couples against natural childbirth, saying, "That will just make you feel guilty if you end up needing medication or forceps, as most women do . . ." But the problem with this approach is that it then becomes a self-fulfilling prophecy: Because instructors don't tell students the facts about avoidable procedures, chances are far greater that their students will undergo those very procedures.

The logic of "prepared" childbirth is based on a faulty premise. The average woman *is* able to labor and give birth without drugs or unneeded routine interventions *if* she is trained and supported throughout labor. But when information is withheld, future parents are denied the opportunity to make responsible decisions. How much better to teach an expectant woman that drugs and interventions have risks; that she can learn to give birth without them if she wishes, except in the rare cases in which medical help is indeed necessary.

Once you understand the differences between "prepared" and "natural" birth education, you need to analyze a teacher's ties. Is she an independent teacher, a hospital's teacher, or a doctor's teacher? Let's take a look at each.

THE DOCTOR'S TEACHER

The doctor's teacher is exactly that: She works for the doctor. If the doctor pays her salary (or sends her all his patients), she can easily be influenced by him and be limited in her point of view and reluctant to explore up-to-date information (which tends to make a doctor who does not keep current uncomfortable).

I tell you this from personal experience since I've worked for half a dozen doctors. Some have been excellent. They have sincerely supported the woman's desire to have a natural childbirth using the Bradley Method®. Others have asked me to omit information on the protective function of the bag of waters, because it was their routine to always break it; or not to explain the value of delayed cord-cutting. I have been asked by doctors to "sell" women on the fetal monitor; forceps delivery to shorten the pushing stage; lying flat on their back in delivery; routine use of IVs; and the three-day hospital stay (with the explanation, to me only, that the hospital needed the beds filled for increased income).

The doctor's teacher may offer a good class, but you will never know how much she didn't get to tell you.

THE HOSPITAL'S TEACHER

Most hospital classes are set up as a defensive response to the "irritation" caused by independent classes. You will usually find that a good deal of time in these classes is spent on justifications for staying in the hospital three days, and submitting to IVs and fetal monitoring. You are certainly not likely to learn about unnecessary procedures that increase risks to you and your baby.

"Part of the instructor's job, as a hospital employee, is to prepare mothers to fit nicely into hospital routines and delivery procedures," says Dr. Silvia Feldman in *Choices in*

Childbirth. "A Lamaze educator at one hospital told me proudly, 'Few couples who have been through our classes here in the hospital object to the rules and regulations.'"[1]

In general in these classes, the woman is taught passive acceptance of all procedures used in a particular hospital. As might be expected, this reassurance *drastically reduces consumer demands for change and updating of services offered. You don't have to think too hard to realize just whom this class serves.*

You should, of course, take advantage of all tours offered by a hospital that you plan to use. You will want the chance to see the facilities.

THE INDEPENDENT TEACHER

You have probably figured out by now that the independent teacher is the one who works for *you.* She has no financial ties to anyone else and therefore cannot be motivated to omit information you should have. She is not motivated to "sell" you on any procedures that current research shows to be harmful. She is able to supply you with any information that may be pertinent to your decisions about birth. The independent teacher is the expectant couple's teacher.

ASKING THE RIGHT QUESTIONS

Choosing a childbirth educator is obviously very important. Here are some of the questions to ask a prospective teacher.

Are you an independent teacher? Listen to the answers carefully. A teacher who says she's "independent" but teaches in a hospital is not an independent instructor. She bases her claim to independence on the mere fact that *you* will be paying her fee and she is not on the hospital's payroll, but she will be under the same pressures to tailor her teaching as the hospital-salaried instructor would be—that is, if she wants to continue using the hospital's facilities and drawing her students from among its patients.

Where did you get your teacher training? AAHCC (American Academy of Husband-Coached Childbirth®) does Bradley teacher training. I would ask this even before I asked what method she is teaching. The reason for this will become clear with the next question.

What method are you teaching? Since more and more people are seeking out Bradley classes, teachers with dwindling classes are prone to say, "Oh, I teach a combination of Lamaze and Bradley and whatever else is out there." This sounds like a car salesman: "Whatever you want, I've got it." Beware. It is just not possible, for example, to combine the normal abdominal Bradley breathing with altered breathing techniques or distraction techniques with the Bradley relaxation response. This is why asking a teacher where she got her training is a most important question. Having picked the method you want to use, you will want to be certain you've picked a teacher who knows how to teach it.

Altered breathing techniques are sometimes called patterned-paced breathing, which is no more than a name change.

If totally natural, coached childbirth is what you're after, why not take a class from a Bradley teacher who is trained in a proven method and has been teaching it all along? That way you avoid the problem of not really knowing what you are getting.

Have you been to any births recently? Going often to births is important. After fifty years of teaching I gain some new insights from every single birthing couple I work with, and that benefits my students.

Have you had any children using this method? You would not want a teacher who hasn't had a good birth herself.

How many of your students are experiencing unmedicated natural childbirth? You might also ask for the names of some recently birthed couples.

Finally, ask if she is a nurse. The "real" careers of nurses are too often jeopardized if they get into some of the controversial issues of childbearing. For example, if many of her students change from certain doctors with high cesarean surgery rates, she has made a powerful "career" enemy at the hospital where she may already work or desire to work at some time in the future.

The nurse-midwife is no exception. She is not independent of the hospital or the physicians working there and is subjected to a great many pressures. If she is teaching the hospital's classes, she must take great care not to antagonize the "traditional physician" or to cast doubt upon the way he practices even if he has a 50 percent cesarean surgery rate. She may still be a good birth attendant and not do these things to her own clients, but as a teacher she is often walking a tightrope. There will inevitably be issues on which her tongue is tied.

The non-nurse educator's career is birthing. She can expect to do well *only* if your needs are met completely and safely. *Changing current maternity care to safely suit the needs of women and babies rather than perpetuating routines that are more familiar or convenient for the hospital staff is her business.*

These are important questions to sort out before you attend a class. Once you've asked them, ask if you can come to the first class and then decide whether or not this teacher is right for you. Remember, your time is limited in pregnancy. You don't want to complete a series of classes and then realize that you feel uncomfortable with your instructor or that you haven't really been taught how to have a baby naturally. You probably won't have enough time left to start over in another class.

To locate the nearest Bradley teachers in your area, go to www.bradleybirth.com.

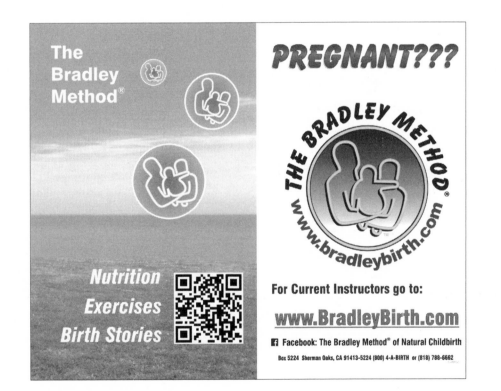

CHAPTER FOUR

Choosing Your Doctor or Your Midwife

IN THE FIRST AND SECOND EDITIONS of this book, after informing women about the important questions in birth, I encouraged them to evaluate their choice of a physician and change physicians (or midwives) if they didn't measure up. It seemed simple. Just go find another doctor or midwife who supported natural childbirth in actual practice.

Today that doesn't work as well: The homogenizing effect of litigation has resulted in a loss of autonomy for many obstetricians and midwives, as hospital administrators, advised by hospital lawyers and insurance companies, demand *conformity to current practices, even when they fly in the face of evidence-based medicine.*

So today, changing to another obstetrician is like going to a shopping mall and finding the same clothes in most of the stores. Choices are contracting, not expanding, contrary to popular belief. So a new strategy has emerged to help women have control over their bodies and their births. It is a strategy that leads to safer, healthier birthing.

This strategy is explained in detail in the chapters of this book. You will find a section that helps you learn about different kinds of evidence. You'll learn how to start getting that evidence when you need it. There is also a chapter called "The Mother's Dilemma and the Doctor's Dilemma," where you will see how to apply information. And you will read about the doctor's dilemma, which will help you to understand what is happening in birthing right now.

Even so, there are things you should know right here in this chapter that haven't changed.

It is one of the word games of obstetrics to say that the physician is responsible until your baby is born. Responsibility belongs to those who will ultimately live with the consequences of the decisions made during birthing—the parents.

Once you have chosen a childbirth instructor, get the lowdown from her on the doctors and facilities available to the birthing couple in your area. It is best not to call a teacher, even one you've heard good things about, and announce, "I'm going to Doctor So-and-so." If you make it obvious you are not shopping for a doctor, even if your choice is the worst in town, a teacher may not be inclined to say so—especially over the phone to a stranger.

However, if you discuss doctors with an independent childbirth teacher before you make up your mind, she will be best able to give you the names of two or three doctors, and perhaps some midwives, who are known to be supportive of natural childbirth couples. It is a better starting point (if still not perfect, due to those homogenizing effects mentioned above).

The risk of brain damage is greatly reduced by choosing a physician who does not interfere with normal labor and birth. The risk of a depressed infant is greatly reduced by choosing a physician who shies away from routine use of anesthetics and analgesics. The risk of toxemia is greatly reduced by choosing a physician who is up-to-date on maternal health and weight gain during pregnancy.

Even your risk of cesarean surgery can be greatly reduced by your choice of a doctor.

Some doctors do cesarean surgery 7 percent of the time, while others do cesareans 70 percent of the time! For that 7 percent, am I talking about fifty years ago, when I first started teaching? No! Lead researcher Katy Kozhimannil looked at almost six hundred hospitals across the U.S. for the year 2009 and discovered this huge gap.[1]

When they looked only at low-risk mothers, the differences were even more striking. Some doctors do cesareans 2.4 percent of the time on low-risk mothers, and others, 36.5 percent of the time.

The same researchers debunked all the popular excuses for the higher rate. It had nothing to do with hospital size, geographic location, teaching status, or obesity.

And you set your risk the day you pick your birth attendant. What's your birth attendant's cesarean rate? At this time, you cannot find out. It's a secret. But independent teachers have students going to many different doctors, and they will have a good idea who is doing the most cesareans and who is doing the best job of working hard to reduce the number of unnecessary cesareans. If you want to maximize your starting point for a natural childbirth, find out who your independent childbirth teacher recommends. And if you don't get to choose your doctor in your health plan, don't despair; the new strategies you will learn in later chapters will help make a difference for you!

Some doctors think of forceps or vacuum-extraction deliveries as "controlled" and preferable to natural childbirth. Others are alarmed at the risks to the baby when forceps and vacuum extractors are used instead of the mother's own pushing. If you have picked a birth attendant who sees little natural birth and usually uses forceps or the vacuum extractor, then chances are good that you will not have a natural birth. It will be "taking too long," or you will "need a little help."

Sometimes people mistakenly think that if they pick a hospital that has an alternative birthing room they will get to have a labor-bed birth. The mere presence of a room doesn't mean a thing. Some doctors have the bed broken down into a typical delivery table with stirrups.

Still, many people think that regardless of how their obstetrician "normally" practices, they will be able to just talk to her and tell her how they want things to go. We have couples in our training classes who go to physicians who use the common practices of fetal monitoring, routine IVs, pudendal blocks for birth, and forceps or vacuum-extractor deliveries. They describe the natural birth they would like to have and get the doctor's reluctant agreement. Then, in labor, they are frequently told, "Sorry, it looks like you will need all those things after all." What is the couple going to do? Play doctor? Decide for themselves on the spot that they don't need something even when the doctor says they do? Ignore the critical attitude of the doctor and hospital staff?

So whenever you can, choose a doctor who supports natural childbirth wholeheartedly and whose actions reflect his words. And whether you get to choose your doctor, you will find many useful strategies in this book to help you navigate to a safer, heathier birth.

CONSIDER A CERTIFIED NURSE-MIDWIFE

If you are lucky enough to have a nurse-midwife working in your area, she may well be the first person you will want to interview for your birthing. (She can make a good *birth attendant* but not a good teacher. *Your teacher should always be independent of your birth attendant and the institution you are birthing in.*) A nurse-midwife can provide top-quality maternity care and often has a much broader background and understanding of the variations of *normal* labor than the average disease-oriented physician.

Study after study has shown that the quality of care by the certified nurse-midwife is superior to the average doctor's care. The CNM is a registered nurse (RN) who has continued her education to study nurse-midwifery. When she finishes her training (if it included home births) she has more experience than most obstetricians in normal childbirth. An obstetrician's training focuses on abnormal childbirth that requires intervention. In their training, many obstetricians (OBs) never see a woman give birth naturally—that is, without an episiotomy, the use of forceps or a vacuum extractor, or cesarean surgery.

A midwife will be particularly prepared if she has attended a number of home births. Whether you're looking for a home birth, this is your guarantee that she will understand the range of *normality* in birthing. She will be highly skilled in helping women birth without a tear, and do a much better job of providing the means for relaxed, unstressful, low-tech birthing. She may catch your baby for you in a hospital, but that home-birth background of hers will eliminate the high-tech midwife.

If a midwife's training and her experience are all hospital-based, then she has been limited to the same high-tech focus on abnormality that most obstetricians have had. The hospital-trained nurse-midwife may turn out to be a junior OB you would rather avoid.

A midwife generally has the time to offer more information on nutrition and give better support to the woman throughout her pregnancy than the average doctor. But she is also trained to recognize complications, and when she sees them, she refers the expectant mother to her physician backup for care.

In fact, during labor a midwife can often spot problems more quickly than the OB. This is simply because the midwife in a freestanding birth center spends hours with the laboring woman, while the average busy OB may manage your labor over the telephone, checking with the labor-and-delivery nurse to see how you are doing. The ordinary RN on duty has less training than the nurse-midwife in spotting problems.

We know that many obstetricians leave standing orders with the nurses not to call them to attend a birth until the baby's head is showing. Then the woman often has to wait for the doctor to get there before she is allowed to push. This makes for an unnecessarily hard pushing stage. The nurse-midwife, however, is there all along, waiting to take her cue from the mother. Delaying birth is definitely not in the interest of the infant's health or the mother's.

A first-rate certified nurse-midwife is usually much more tuned in to the needs of the natural-childbirth couple.

THE LAY MIDWIFE

As it happens, the best birth attendant I know is a lay midwife. She received her basic training in one of the several states that license lay midwives. She has attended many births and is fully competent to do prenatal care, to attend a normal birth, and to spot any complications developing. In many ways her experience with normal birthing is superior to most physicians'. For example, she recently attended a couple from one of our classes birthing at home. Their baby was born with the cord looped three times around its neck—unusual, but not out of the range of normal. The lay midwife calmly slipped the loops one by one over the baby's head in a matter of seconds and the body was born with the next contraction. She had listened to the fetal heart tones frequently and knew the baby had been in no danger. Later, at the hospital birth of another of our couples, the baby's head emerged with the cord looped once around the neck—something quite common. The baby was having no problems, but the physician attending was shouting at the mother (whose control was perfect) not to push. The doctor then pulled out a bit of the loop, clamped it, and cut the cord before the body was born. That meant the baby *had* to breathe immediately since the lifeline supplying it with oxygen had been severed. Fortunately, it did. Neither baby had any problems at birth, but the hospital baby had been put at greater risk.

HOW TO FIND YOUR BIRTH ATTENDANT

The most important starting point in your search for the right birth attendant is to ask your teacher, "Whom do you recommend?" She will probably respond with her own well-considered list: "Drs. Jones, Smith, or Casey; or nurse-midwife Coleman; or lay midwife Mills." Stick to that list. Remember, *your teacher sees and talks to women who have birthed with every attendant in town. She knows which ones help women have natural births time after time and which ones always seem to have a problem that justifies a forceps delivery or another cesarean surgery. If a doctor's name is not on her recommended list, there is probably a good reason.*

Talk to a few suitable-sounding candidates from her list. Call for an appointment, but make it clear you do *not* want an exam, that you and your husband want to discuss a few things first. Ask if they charge for this kind of visit. Some do, some don't. If they do, you will want to know how much, so you'll have no surprises later.

IF YOU ALREADY HAVE A DOCTOR

If you already have a doctor, ask him questions now and make sure the two of you are not on a collision course. If you don't like his answers, try not to get upset. I get calls from women who have reached this collision point (they're usually halfway through my classes and down to their last month or so). It's always possible to change, but the longer you wait, the harder it becomes. Get your teacher's recommended list *now* if the doctor you've been going to is no longer acceptable to you. Then consider your options carefully.

Don't burn any bridges behind you yet. Start by making appointments to just talk to a couple of the people on your teacher's list. After talking to other physicians who practice in a manner that better suits you, it may suddenly seem far less threatening and traumatic to change doctors and leave the nonsupportive one behind.

If so, *change*. Don't stay with a doctor if you're unhappy. Don't give your birth away. Do not be afraid of hurting her feelings. Believe me, she won't remember the details of your birth even one year later, while you will remember this experience all your life. If you stay with someone you're worried about, someone you worry will not help you give birth normally, then you will carry fear and tension with you into labor. You will be tensed and ready to argue, and you cannot argue when you are in labor. You cannot possibly use relaxation techniques if you are anxious. Get yourself to a birth attendant you feel will help, not hinder you. Then your energies will be freed to focus on the work of labor.

If you are in a medical plan that does not let you choose your own doctor or you are using a military hospital, I cannot mince words: You are in a poor situation for birthing. You get potluck in labor—whoever is on duty. All your well-laid plans could go awry. You may try to talk to three or four different doctors, describing what you want and getting agreements about your birth, but then in labor you may end up with someone you never have met before, or worse, someone who was hostile to your requests. The doctor on duty is not obligated to honor the agreements you made with another doctor. The tension a woman experiences as she enters the hospital in labor wondering if she will get a doctor who will help or hinder her is not helpful for the work ahead. So I urge you, if you have the option, switch to a health-care plan that allows you to pick your doctor or other birth attendant.

If this is not an option for you, maximize your chances of having a good birth by following these instructions:

1. Make a detailed list of what you want and don't want in birth, in the order that is important to you.
2. The coach should go along on every prenatal medical visit possible.
3. Try to see a different doctor on each visit. Discuss your requests with each doctor. (Don't bring in your written list; memorize it. Doctors hate to be questioned by someone with a list in hand.) Have the first doctor write what you want on your chart. The doctor is more likely to remember you if he plays an active part in getting your requests down.
4. On later visits ask each doctor to read what the previous ones wrote so you can see if there is anything else to go

over. This confirms previous agreements and gets the new doctor actively involved in seeing that your birth turns out the way you want. It also allows you to keep expressing your preferences. (By the way, if you get a hostile reaction from an occasional doctor, be glad you got to see it before labor so you are forewarned.)

5. About three weeks before your birth, you should hand over your written list and see that it is attached to your chart.

6. Have three copies of your list to take with you to the hospital just in case your original was "misplaced" and is not with your chart.

7. Take a supportive person, in addition to your coach, with you to the hospital when the big day comes. This person's function is not so much to intercede on your behalf as to simply be there for moral support as you deal with any situations that might come up. Ask your Bradley teacher. She may have a "graduate" student whom she can recommend as just the right kind of person.

8. The corollary to informed consent is *dissent*. This is necessary if the concept of informed consent is to have any meaning at all. So you may need to be ready to decline a procedure that is objectionable to you.

WHAT ARE THE QUESTIONS TO ASK?

You can hardly know what to ask and why a particular point is important until you have a good idea of what birthing normally is all about, which you will learn in the pages ahead. Then, in Part Four, when you have more background, we will go over a list of specific questions to ask your doctor. At that point, you will have a complete understanding of why those questions are important and what impact the answers will have on your birth.

CHAPTER FIVE

Nutrition: How Does Your Garden Grow?

MOST OF US PUT more thought and effort into growing a garden than we put into growing a baby. A pregnant woman's diet is often sorely neglected in spite of the fruit she is about to bring forth.

DOES IT REALLY MATTER WHAT A PREGNANT WOMAN EATS?

Yes, studies have shown that women on poor diets actually have harder labors[1] and that their babies run a higher statistical incidence of infections in the first year of life.[2] Animal experiments have shown that low-protein diets lead to a reduced number of brain cells in offspring.[3]

Most important, **toxemia,** the most dreaded disease of pregnancy, can often be avoided through proper nutrition.[4] Ironically, one of the reasons doctors were originally afraid of women gaining weight was that women who developed toxemia had sudden weight gains. For a time, it was thought that sudden weight gain was a *cause* of toxemia.

In fact, a women becomes ill with toxemia as her body cannot throw off toxic substances stored in its cells. She swells up with retained fluids. She has severe headaches, blurry vision, high blood pressure, and protein showing up in her urine. This is all very dangerous for the woman and for her unborn baby. She can go into convulsions and a coma (called eclampsia), but before her condition goes that far the woman usually ends up with an induction or cesarean surgery. Dr. Tom Brewer's research has shown that weight gain is not the cause of toxemia at all, but merely a symptom of the problem. Instead, a diet *deficient* in protein and other nutrients can be a primary cause of toxemia. Dr. Brewer condemned the practice of restricting weight gain, since it restricts the mother's access to the good food she needs.

Still, a woman often comes out of her doctor's office with little or no information about nutrition. Worse, having been scolded by a doctor or a nurse for gaining perhaps five to seven pounds in one month, she may have resolved to diet to avoid gaining "too much weight." She immediately starts cutting calories and skipping lunch, which leaves her irritable and without energy. Some women will actually starve themselves completely the day or two before their visits to the doctor's office just to keep their weight a pound or two lower on the scales.

So the question of what to eat often becomes academic when all the attention is focused on not eating. The woman who gets on the scales and discovers she has gained more than "allowed" never gets to question what she *should* have been eating.

In the second edition of this book I wrote the following: Fortunately, ideas on weight gain have changed and are still changing dramatically. The up-to-date doctor is more likely to encourage you not to worry about weight gain on good, natural foods. This is called positive weight gain.

Well, here we are in the third edition of this book, and weight gain is a big issue once again. While the nation is concerned with increasing obesity, does pregnancy seem like a good time to go on a diet? Do fads come and go in medicine? Apparently so; what else can it be called when the pendulum swings from restricting weight gain during pregnancy (with the assurance that this is the safest thing for mothers and babies) and the next decade when the pendulum swings back to the importance of *not* restricting weight gain (because this is now the safest thing for mothers and babies) and today, when we are swinging back, yet again, to restricting weight gain (because this is the safest thing for mothers and babies)? What does it take to get this right? Perhaps just common sense! Imagine my surprise to find the following statement in the latest edition (2014) of *Williams Obstetrics:*

> Marked weight gain restriction after midpregnancy should not be encouraged even in obese women.[5]

And yet I currently have women coming into classes proud to announce that they are six months' pregnant and haven't gained a single pound. Some even talk about how much weight they have lost while pregnant! A reducing diet changes your blood chemistry dramatically, altering what is available for the baby. We need to get back to encouraging women to work at a "positive weight gain," which means working to eliminate naked calories, bereft of nutrition, and carefully choosing nutrient-rich food.

There are also more and more women who think that being able to walk out of the hospital in something skin-tight is the goal that trumps getting adequate and optimal nutrition to the baby. I call this the Hollywood Effect, where women are bombarded with images of movie stars flaunting their bone-thin bodies the day after their babies are born. Such shortsightedness ignores something we have known for a long time. The baby's birth weight and brain development are highly correlated, and the lower the birth weight, the higher the risk of cognitive developmental problems.

For example, the human infant has a spurt of brain growth beginning at the last third of pregnancy which continues through the first eighteen months of life. If the child does not get proper nourishment in this critical period, he could have permanent mental disability.[6] And yet, too often in this last important phase of pregnancy some doctors advise women to cut calories severely, often a doctor who has not taken the time to keep up on developments in nutrition science. The result is a restriction of calories, including the good ones, right at a crucial time of the pregnancy.

HOW MUCH WEIGHT SHOULD YOU GAIN?

Rather than looking at weight gain (the outcome of your eating habits), you should concentrate on the habits themselves. The focus should be on protein intake for a pregnant woman of about eighty to one hundred grams daily.

Sometimes, of course, it is not the doctor who stands in the way of good nutrition but the woman herself. If she is concerned about staying super-skinny throughout pregnancy, she may sell herself on the following fallacy: "It doesn't matter what I eat; the baby will just take what it needs from my body anyway." The idea is that the baby can cannibalize the mother's tissues for his own needs. That's possibly true to some extent, but that certainly doesn't mean he's getting *all* the nutrients he needs in the amounts needed. The baby must settle for reduced amounts!

Sure, most babies do survive their mother's diets. But one thing is overlooked here. I'm sure you want more than a baby who survives in spite of your diet. You want one who thrives because of it.

I thought I knew all about good nutrition when I took my first teacher-training course years ago. After all, I knew about the four basic food groups and a balanced diet; but I didn't know enough about protein. Oh, I had heard about it, but I figured if we just ate a balanced diet we would get enough protein.

It was during that training, when I was learning just how important protein really is, that I decided to count my family's protein intake, just to be sure. I discovered we were getting a dismal thirty-five grams of protein a day.

I examined our daily dietary habits and discovered that we unthinkingly ate a great many junk foods. Some meals were so low in protein (for example, just cereal, juice, and toast) that it was no wonder at all that I recognized symptoms of low protein intake in myself and my family.

Protein is not a direct source of energy, but it slows down the absorption of carbohydrates and fats so that you get a sort of time-capsule effect. Protein helps allow your blood sugar to rise steadily over a number of hours so that you have a steady prolonged source of energy rather than ups and downs during the day. Protein is the key to *steady* energy. When you're getting plenty of it, along with a balanced diet, you feel great! Problems seem so much more manageable, and you find it easy to accomplish a great deal and maintain a pleasant disposition.

When your protein intake is low, however, the world doesn't look so good. It seems that little problems are too much to bear. They are so annoying that you think you just can't stand another one. If you switch to eating your highest protein meal (say, forty grams) in the morning you'll be amazed at the energy and enthusiasm you have. Your metabolism gets going great guns and your blood sugar goes up gradually and stays up longer, providing sustained energy for more hours.

If your food intake has been low in protein yet high in calories, you won't be able to just add more food and calories. You would end up rather uncomfortably stuffed. Something needs to be subtracted, and that something needs to be food with low nutritional value: cookies, cake, doughnuts, four-hundred-calorie designer coffees, soda, chips, frozen dinners, candy, etc. You'll want to make room for the good stuff.

The reverse situation is a woman who doesn't eat *enough* calories (even though she may be getting eighty to a hundred grams of protein). If your caloric intake is insufficient, then your body will break down the protein to use for your energy needs and less will be available for growing your baby, your uterus, your placenta, and your blood volume.

AFRAID YOU'LL GROW TOO BIG A BABY?

Consider that question carefully. Are you thinking that you want to deliberately try to grow a small baby, that you might have an easier labor by restricting calories and nutrients? I'm sorry to say that undernourished tissues in your body do not make for an easier labor. Uterine muscles need adequate nutrients to work well in labor, and tissues deprived of needed nutrients do not expand as well.

Recently, a former student called me to share her good news. She was pregnant with her second baby. Her first birth had been an especially happy natural birth. Since she had moved to another state, she wouldn't be able to come back for a refresher series of classes. Her new nurse-midwife told her not to bother getting all that protein; it would just make a too-big baby. I pointed out to my student that her first baby was seven pounds, which is by no means a big baby.

We talked a little longer, and she chatted happily about how glad she was that she didn't have to track her protein intake this time and go to all the hassle of modifying her diet. I knew I was listening to a woman with her mind made up.

Months later, she called again in tears. During that day's prenatal checkup, her nurse-midwife told her that her baby was *too small* for its gestational age, that she was very concerned and she wanted her to go the hospital and start an induction. She was just thirty-six weeks' pregnant.

This was the same midwife who had told her she didn't need to eat all that protein, that it would just make too big a baby. Now she was being induced one month early because her baby was too small. The idea here is that her baby would grow better in the Neonatal Intensive Care Unit since it was "failing to thrive" in her uterus. One month on life support in the NICU and the baby is finally home with mom. The mother plans on counting her protein next time and finding a different nurse-midwife for her next pregnancy.

WHAT IS A GOOD HIGH-PROTEIN BREAKFAST?

Well, it isn't two pieces of bacon, orange juice, and toast (about eight grams of protein). It certainly isn't the packaged cereals that are so anemic they have to have handfuls of vitamins added to them to justify their use at all. Cereals are just about worthless for protein. Those commercials plugging high-protein breakfast cereals are counting the milk you put on the cereal; they could never make those claims counting just the protein in their product.

When I first started working at increasing my protein intake, I mistakenly thought that high-protein food was going to be boring. I thought I would be forever eating cottage cheese to rack up the needed grams for the day. With the threat of monotonous meals looming in the future, I began to think about how to get this protein into my diet and like it. In fact, it only took a little imagination.

One of the most aggravating iatrogenic (that is, doctor-caused) food fads nowadays is skipping eggs for fear of cholesterol. Actually the egg white is loaded with lecithin, a substance that breaks cholesterol cells into teeny particles that can pass easily through the walls of the blood vessels without clogging them. Perhaps cholesterol is a dietary problem, but *not* from the egg, since the lecithin comes already built in for you. (As long as you don't just eat the yolks.) Eggs are cheap compared to other sources of protein. They pack a goodly amount of protein in a yummy package that can be served in many different ways: souffléed, scrambled, fried, in omelettes, boiled for snacks or chopped into sandwiches or salads, and added to lots of foods you happen to be cooking, just for the extra protein. Beyond protein, the egg is similar to milk in that this tiny oval wonder has so many of the other vitamins and elements you need for good health. You would have to munch your way through quite a variety of items to touch as many of the nutrients as come all together in the egg, or in a glass of milk.

Here's a tip. What you bring into the house is what you will consume. Face it, if food is there you will eat it. So at the market put the cookies, frozen dinners, potato chips, rolls, and so on back on the shelves. Bring home protein-rich foods like cheese, meat, chicken, fish, yogurt, cottage cheese, milk, and eggs. Then balance the diet with vegetables, fruits, and whole grains. Salt your food to taste. Salt is an essential ingredient.

Pregnancy is a good time to try whole wheat bread. It will give you some of the B vitamins you need. Beware of breads that are called "wheat" but are not whole wheat. You will be tipped off to such phonies by the list of ingredients, which usually reads "caramel dye and wheat flour." They often charge the same price you pay for the real thing.

Yogurt is a fantastic food. If you enjoy it, then indulge yourself, especially during pregnancy. Yogurt lines your intestines with lactic acid and turns them into a B-vitamin factory for you. In the U.S., it is common for women to have "pregnancy mask," a brown freckling across the forehead and the bridge of the nose, extending out toward the cheeks. In fact, this is so common it is considered a normal occurrence of pregnancy. In countries where women usually eat more dark breads and yogurt, however, this is not common and is not considered normal. It is treated as a B-vitamin deficiency.

Liver is a great food. Try it out and see if you can work it into your diet. It is high in protein and B vitamins.

Count your protein intake and make sure you're getting the recommended amount. You should also get some carbohydrate and fat with each meal for a steady and prolonged rise in blood sugar. Most of us reverse this and have large carbohydrate meals with only a little protein. Eating such meals will certainly shoot your blood-sugar level up, but it zooms down fast, too.

TWINS

I've saved the best for last. When mothers with twins ramp up the protein, the outcome is amazing. Mothers of twins are almost always told that twins come early and often need special care in the NICU (neonatal intensive care unit). But many Bradley moms carrying twins have surprised their doctors by carrying their babies to term, and instead of producing low-birth-weight babies with special needs, they grow healthy babies who bypass the NICU experience and go home when Mom does. For more twin stories, check out www.bradleybirth.com.

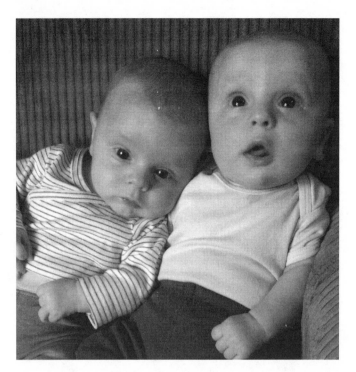

Kate Piper and Kyle Piper-Smyer: First pregnancy; babies Bailey and Gus

"Protein was very important to our twin pregnancy. Kyle's stomach got squeezed so much so early on that there really wasn't much room for food; she never felt hungry and got full quickly. Because of this, Kyle focused on protein content in everything she ate. The best food we found was plain old whole milk. It was full of calories and protein and didn't take up a lot of room in a very full belly. It was great to add a glass between meals. Our boys were each over six pounds when they were born at thirty-eight weeks and one day."

—Kate Piper

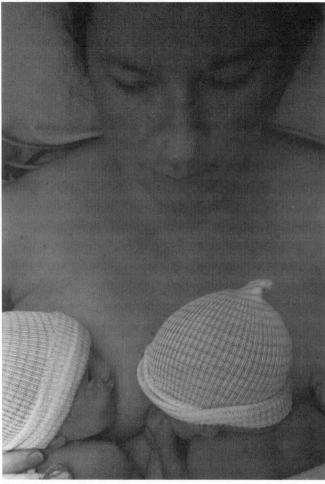

Emily Meisner: First birth

"I always feel so grateful and lucky to have had such an easy pregnancy. I stayed in excellent shape throughout the pregnancy by swimming, walking, and lifting weights. I squatted constantly and followed the Bradley diet as closely as possible. As a vegan, I know some people had concerns about my protein intake. I did start to eat some dairy and occasionally eggs while pregnant and was easily able to meet my protein goals. Lots of nuts, beans, and lentils. I tried to shoot for over one hundred grams per day. Our boys were born one day shy of thirty-eight weeks and were 7 pounds and 5.8 pounds. They went straight to the breast, had no NICU time, and came home with us the next day."

—Emily Meisner

CHAPTER SIX

Drugs During Pregnancy

THINKING ABOUT TAKING A drug during your pregnancy? How about just something for that early-pregnancy nausea? It's such a nuisance, isn't it? Or an aspirin for that headache? And there's always that inevitable cold that you're bound to have during the course of nine months, so how about an antihistamine for that troublesome stuffy nose? STOP. LOOK AT THIS NEWS STORY.

ANTI-NAUSEA DRUG, BIRTH DEFECT LINKED.

NEW HAVEN, CONN. (AP) Women who took a form of the popular anti-nausea drug Bendectin in early pregnancy may have quadrupled the chances that their infants would suffer a potentially fatal stomach ailment, two Yale epidemiologists report.[1]

Wouldn't you rather put up with a little nausea? Oh, but that headache. Now there's something you really must have an aspirin for, right? Did you know that the use of aspirin has been shown to prolong pregnancy?[2] Really, nine months is enough, don't you think? You will by the end of your pregnancy. Perhaps you stay pregnant longer because your baby's development has been interfered with and now he needs more time to finish growing. And remember, there are more than a hundred common medications available over the counter that contain aspirin, including Alka-Seltzer, Bufferin, Empirin, Anacin, and Four-Way Cold Tablets.[3]

Wouldn't you rather tune into your body and try to listen to its cues when you have a headache? Your body may be trying to tell you to eat a meal if your blood sugar has dropped to the headache-producing level. Or perhaps you need to slow down for a while. Instead of masking the warnings your body is giving you with medications, be good to yourself and your baby. The two of you deserve it.

Does this mean that you have to put up with a stuffy nose the next time you catch a cold? I'll leave that for you to decide. Nose drops can shrink the placental bed (the site where the placenta is attached to the uterus).[4] The placenta spreads out as far as needed to get access to enough oxygen and nutrients for your baby. (In fact, women who live permanently at high altitudes grow larger placentas to meet the baby's oxygen needs.) Shrinking the placental bed reduces the baby's access to the things he needs. If you take nose drops, the placenta cannot suddenly expand to keep food and oxygen flowing to your baby in optimal amounts during the hours those drops are working. (In addition, some nose drops contain antihistamines, which are also associated with an increased incidence of malformed babies.)[5]

Look at it this way. Most drug dosages are determined by body weight. You would not give your two-year-old an adult aspirin; the dose would be inappropriate to his weight. So what's a safe dose for your child of no years, still in your uterus, yet to be born? *Any drug you take, designed to affect your adult size body, may be approximately twenty times too much for your unborn baby's body.* Alarming, isn't it? How about cutting down the dosage so it won't have an effect on the baby? In that case, it would be a dose too low to have an effect on your body, either, so what's the point in taking the drug?

Dr. Bradley is fond of saying, "Don't pollute the bloodstream." But when you find yourself putting up with a stuffy nose during your pregnancy it really wouldn't be fair to blame it all on Dr. Bradley. Warnings about drugs during pregnancy are currently coming from many sources. You should know that the Committee on Drugs of the American Academy of Pediatrics addresses this problem head-on! They have clearly laid it out for pregnant women, stating that "there is no drug, whether over-the-counter remedy or prescription, which, when taken by the childbearing woman, has been proven safe for the unborn child."[6]

Would you want to take a drug not proven safe for your baby? No, of course not, not unless your obstetrician prescribed it for you—then it must be safe, right? Look again at the statement by the Committee on Drugs. It does not absolve prescription drugs. They are included in the warning.

Nowadays, most people have already heard that the placenta is not a barrier between your baby and drugs, but few realize that *the prescription pad is also not a barrier!* I'll bet you've read the warning, *Don't take drugs during pregnancy* somewhere else, or perhaps you've heard it on the radio, but the small print that is always tacked on is the last line *unless prescribed by your doctor.* This is the number-one loophole through which millions of pregnant women get drugs. It's time for women and their doctors to change this qualifier to something like *Don't take drugs during pregnancy unless necessary to your continued life and health*. A diabetic will need drugs during pregnancy, and so will other women with serious life- and health-threatening problems, but this is not what most drugs are prescribed for in pregnancy.

Does this mean your doctor might write an unnecessary prescription for you that could harm your unborn baby? I'll let you be the judge. Let's take Bendectin, the anti-nausea drug. The *New York Times* reported on June 19, 1983, that "according to manufacturer estimates, in the 27 years during which Bendectin has been sold, more than 33 million pregnant women throughout the world have used it to curb their nausea and vomiting."[7]

In the United States, according to the Yale study I cited earlier, Bendectin was used by about 25 percent of pregnant women. That, those doctors added, "suggests a considerable amount of overprescribing."

Overprescribing is an understatement. If 25 percent of all pregnant women had this drug prescribed for them by their doctors, it was clearly being given for the ordinary harmless nausea that many women experience in early pregnancy and not reserved for the persistent, continuous vomiting that can occasionally require medical help, but certainly does not occur in one out of four pregnancies.

If obstetricians and pregnant women had been following a line of thinking like *Don't take drugs during pregnancy unless necessary to your continued life and health*, the nausea drug would never have been prescribed for women in those numbers. "If there is a lesson to be learned from the Bendectin story," said Dr. Hugh R. K. Barber, director of obstetrics and gynecology at Lenox Hill Hospital in New York, "it is that no drug or drug-like substance—even vitamins—can be assumed to be completely safe during pregnancy."[8]

You can't expect doctors to step forward to be held accountable for the later-discovered aftereffects of drugs they prescribed for you. That would open wide the door of liability. The drug company will not be quick to even admit there *might* be a problem with a drug they have produced until forced to do so, much less to admit responsibility or accountability.

But let's be fair. Let's not heap all the blame upon doctors. They do not practice in a vacuum. If you call a doctor when you have an ordinary cold and the sniffles, then you must realize this is a statement that you are *not* willing to cope with the symptoms. If you were, you would not be calling about it, because he doesn't have any chicken soup to put on the stove for you; his cupboard contains only drugs.

By calling, you indicate that you want him to *do something* and the only something he can do is *prescribe*. If your intention is to just check out the symptoms, be sure to say clearly that you prefer to avoid drugs during your pregnancy and are willing to put up with the symptoms.

Speaking to a conference on developmental disabilities, Dr. Sanford Cohen of New York University had some good advice. He said that if a pregnant woman's doctor prescribes a medicine, she should ask if it is "absolutely essential" for her health or the baby's. If the answer is no, Cohen said, then she should forget it.[9]

So far, unfortunately, little more than lip service has been given to the idea that pregnant women should not take drugs. I, for one, believe the warnings. And it is time to change the *unless prescribed* rider that effectively cancels the caution to *unless necessary to continued life and health.*

And those nonprescription items you buy at the drugstore, are they really drugs? You know, Maalox for heartburn, Rolaids, Tylenol, and ninety-nine other over-the-counter remedies? Yes, they are real drugs! Even concerned women taking classes for totally unmedicated childbirth often don't realize this. Do you have a blind spot? Are you currently taking an over-the-counter drug?

Occasionally a woman comes up to me after a class and says, "I'm taking such-and-such, is that okay?" If the American Academy of Pediatrics Committee on Drugs cannot absolve any over-the-counter or prescription drugs,

then who am I to absolve a few? False reassurances, however, are often given to women by people who know better (teachers, doctors, nurses) because it is more comfortable for the giver and receiver of the reassurances.

Drugs are not investigated to determine safety during pregnancy for the unborn child. Is this shocking? Not really. Think about it. What is a drug company going to do? Advertise in a local newspaper for a volunteer to test out a new drug—to see if it will deform or otherwise harm her baby? You see the dilemma. But the consequence of this dilemma is even more frightening. Drugs do go on the market without this kind of testing, and that means that *you are the unknowing volunteer* when you take a drug not proven safe for the unborn child.

A drug salesman once told us that when a new drug comes out it's 120 percent safe. By the end of the first year, as side effects are reported back, it's 99 percent safe. Give it a few more years and it falls to 85 percent safe. But by then there will be a replacement drug for it, and this new drug will be 120 percent safe.

This "after the fact" approach has caused and will continue to cause damage to mothers and their babies. For example, at a time when we were feeling rather smug in this country about avoiding the thalidomide disaster (in which babies in Europe were born without arms and legs due to a drug given to pregnant women), the DES (diethylstilbestrol) time bomb was ticking away in the bodies of thousands of children.

It has taken decades for the cancers caused by the use of the drug DES (given originally to avoid miscarriage and premature birth) to reveal themselves. The daughters of the millions of women who were given this drug have a much higher rate of cancer than the rest of the population; male offspring are not free from this, either, and the story gets worse as we learn that the mothers themselves are experiencing higher cancer rates.

Years ago I read the story of a woman whose teenage daughter died of the vaginal cancer she developed as a result of her mother taking DES. The mother was asked if she felt guilty. She replied that she did not because her doctor had prescribed it for her and she was doing what she thought was the best thing, following her doctor's advice, with no questions asked. I would not wish guilt on this mother or any mother who took DES, but the fact is that if a lesson is to be learned from DES, it is that *questions should always be asked before taking a drug during pregnancy*. Your consent should at least be *informed consent*. Ask what the known side effects of the drug are, and if it has been tested for long-term side effects. You are the only one who can decide what risks you are willing to accept for which benefits. No one else can decide for you which risks are acceptable to *you*, and which risks are not.

There is no restitution for the physical and emotional agony caused by DES. There is no way to give those affected back healthy, undamaged bodies or to remove the fearful threat of cancer that hangs over them. There is no satisfaction in suing those "responsible"—drug companies, institutions like hospitals, and doctors who used this drug. The sheer numbers of those involved, well into the millions, make the likelihood of meaningful financial settlement a dim prospect.

With the lesson of DES in mind, we realize that it is a word game to say that drug safety during pregnancy is the responsibility of the Food and Drug Administration, drug companies, or the medical establishment. None of these institutions will feel the devastating impact of tragedy as you will.

Each woman must realize that she is the final guardian of her unborn child. She is the last decision-maker when it comes to putting a drug into her body or undergoing an untested procedure, like a sonogram. It is clear where the buck stops, whether we like it or not. It stops at our own consent. The best thing you can do is simply take no chances. Avoid all drugs during pregnancy except those essential to maintaining life and health.

Pregnant or not, it's just good sense to always know the score about any drug you *do* bring into your home for whatever reason. Always ask the druggist for the "package insert" whenever you buy a drug. Read it for known side effects. (Unfortunately the Food and Drug Administration has lost its mandated patient package-insert program and we must now rely on a *volunteer* effort funded by the Ciba-Geigy drug company.)

One of my students had a vaginal infection and her doctor prescribed a drug for her. She looked it up and discovered that it should never be used by anyone with a history of kidney infections. She had a history of kidney infections! She let her doctor know this and they dealt with the problem another way. Another student looked up a prescribed drug and decided that she could not accept the risk of the *known* side effects. She felt the problem she was given the prescription for was minor while the risks of this particular drug were major. She discussed this with her doctor and they both agreed that since it was a minor problem that often disappears in later pregnancy, she could do without the drug.

ULTRASOUND

Could ultrasound be like the 120-percent-safe drug? Will we be reading about it as a health hazard in a few years? (It's already suspect and being investigated.) If so, we're in real trouble because I can tell you that many women are getting three to four ultrasound exams in one pregnancy.

Some are getting serial ultrasound exams (every three to four days) in their final weeks of pregnancy.

Ultrasound takes a picture of your baby by bouncing high-frequency sound waves off him and translating the echo into a picture. We don't know what the long-term side effects of these sound vibrations ("anywhere from 20,000 to millions of vibrations per second") might be. We do know that, in the short term, cells behave abnormally after just one diagnostic ultrasound exposure. Their shape changes temporarily and their movement becomes frenetic.

There are studies today casting doubts on ultrasound.

In 2006, researchers discovered that ultrasound prevents neurons in the brain from migrating to their final destinations. The study was conducted with mice.[10]

In 2010, researchers concluded that scanning the fetus without a medical indication should be avoided.[11]

Remember what the FDA doesn't do for us. Remember the statement of the Committee on Drugs of the American Academy of Pediatrics: "There is no drug, whether over-the-counter remedy or prescription drug, which when taken by the child-bearing woman, has been proven safe for the unborn child." And remember, the same applies to diagnostic procedures like ultrasound.

CHAPTER SEVEN

Weighing Evidence

ISN'T THE NEWS FRUSTRATING? One year you read the headline: EATING EGGS WILL LEAD TO HIGH CHOLESTEROL AND HEART ATTACKS. And a few years later, NO NEED TO LIMIT YOUR EGG INTAKE: STUDY SHOWS NO INCREASE IN HEART PROBLEMS IN PEOPLE WHO EAT TWO EGGS A DAY.[1,2,3]

In the meantime, you've given up eggs and substituted cholesterol-loaded pastry for your breakfast. You don't know what to think or who to believe and end up deciding that you can't trust studies, so you stop paying attention.

Here are some tools to help end that frustration.

There are many different kinds of "studies," and they are not of equal value. The different kinds of studies are just like different coins: pennies, nickels, dimes, quarters, and fifty-cent pieces. One of those coins has fifty times the power of the penny, just as a certain kind of study has much more power (value in terms of reliability) than other kinds of studies. When you finish this chapter you will be able to quickly distinguish a featherweight study from a sledgehammer study.

The gold standard of studies is the **Randomized Controlled Trial**. This is the preferred and most powerful study, called RCT for short. When you need evidence to inform your decision making, this is the study you want. This is the heavyweight champion. In an RCT, researchers use the scientific method: a matched control group and an experimental group, looking at one variable only. Size matters. (Ten people won't do; these are usually done with a couple hundred people or more.) Ideally, the researchers involved should have no preconceived bias about the outcome, and no vested interest in obtaining one outcome or another.

And the real hallmark of the scientific method is *repeatability*. That means different researchers halfway around the world could repeat an RCT and expect to get similar results. *Repeatability, repeatability, repeatability* (oops, I should stop repeating myself).

Here is something that many people don't understand. An RCT is not invalidated by the mere passage of time. It doesn't suddenly become invalid the day it turns ten years old, or twenty years old or thirty years old. The only thing that can invalidate a randomized control trial is a lack of repeatability. If other researchers cannot get similar results in an RCT of the same size or larger, then something is wrong; and that lack of repeatability is the only thing that can invalidate an RCT.

So now you know, if someone says to you, "Well, that RCT is ten years old so it isn't valid anymore," then that someone doesn't understand the randomized controlled trial and the scientific method. The mere passage of time does not invalidate a randomized controlled trial. There is no "Goldilocks-just-right" age for an RCT. An RCT stands unless and until other researchers are unable to repeat it and get the same results.

Another powerful study is called a **literature search**. Imagine this. You're a billionaire with a burning need for information about a particular health question. Your doctor wants you to take a certain diagnostic test. You don't relish the idea because you're not having any particular problem, nothing appears to be wrong, and you feel quite healthy, but your doctor does this test routinely with all his patients.

Well, since money is no problem, you hire a team of experts, perhaps a perinatologist, a research scientist, a consumer advocate, a statistical analyst, and set them the task of finding every published piece of research in the literature about this diagnostic test. In other words, they don't do an experiment; they do a study of studies.

Your team pulls everything they can find. They throw out junk science and studies that are too small to provide reliable evidence. They give more weight to RCTs over other kinds of studies. After narrowing the pool of evidence, they look at the researchers involved and check for bias or vested interest. Finally, they look at the collective data, analyze that collectively, and come up with the conclusion. Let's say they conclude that this is not only an unreliable test but it often leads to unnecessary interventions, and those interventions have risks. (Not an uncommon finding at all, by the way.) They conclude that when there is no indication that anything is wrong in the first place, the test provides no benefit to you, while increasing risk to you. Now you have the information you need to make the best decision you can.

Wow, don't you wish you were a billionaire and could do this? Well, here's the good news. You don't have to be a billionaire. That's exactly what the Cochrane Collaboration is all about. They get teams of experts to do this kind of literature search for you and publish the results in the Cochrane Reviews. Now, not everything in the world has been studied, but you would be surprised at how much is available. This information is there for doctors, nurse-midwives, and *you*, the consumer.

Does it take a medical degree to understand the results? No; remember, this information is being provided specifically for you, the consumer, too, to help inform your choices. When you look up a review, it always begins with an abstract, a paragraph or two that tells you what question was studied and what the investigators concluded. Abstracts are clear and easy to read. While I like to read the entire report and look up many of the individual studies included in the analysis, most of my students are happy to read the bottom line, and that's the abstract. I suggest you also go to the end of the report and read the conclusion paragraph.

The Cochrane Collaboration is a global network of researchers, scientists, health policymakers, and consumer advocates. More than 28,000 people in 120 countries provide their time and expertise. This is a highly respected, internationally recognized source. If you find it difficult to navigate the Cochrane Reviews, ask your birth attendant to pull one up on the particular test, drug, or treatment being proposed. So what do you do with the information acquired? The least you can do is to use it to have a discussion with your birth attendant.

How powerful is a literature search? If there are no RCTs to examine and there are only weaker studies available, then the resulting conclusion can still be useful. You will be able to comprehend that the procedure, drug, or diagnostic test is experimental, rather than backed by scientific evidence.

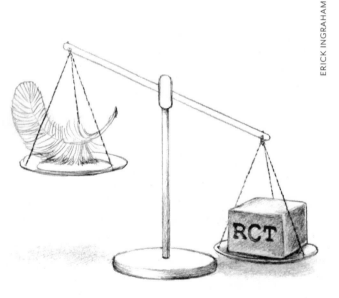

ERICK INGRAHAM

And it is most powerful when there are RCTs to examine; then, that literature search is another hammer.

What other kinds of studies are there?

Some are simply **observational studies**. By observation alone, a conclusion is drawn. Some obstetricians feel that their "clinical experience" trumps scientific studies, like RCTs, but clinical experience alone is just another term for observation. This is closer to an opinion. It is not a scientific study, and any trial lawyer will tell you that eyewitness observations are often unreliable. Compared to an RCT, clinical experience is a featherweight.

Another type of "study" is the **questionnaire**. Its best use is in collecting hard facts, such as "Have you been diagnosed with diabetes?" It's kind of a black-and-white answer. It can provide clues to tell us what needs further investigation.

Then there are **data-mining studies,** or **looking-backward studies,** where you go back through records, say, over the past twenty years, and try to determine something that way. But these may be way off the mark. For example, at one point many obstetricians were claiming that, yes, the C-section rate was rising, but that was a good thing, because they were saving more babies by doing more C-sections.

And doing a data-mining study confirmed that over a period of twenty years (during which the C-section rate dramatically increased), more babies were indeed surviving. But later, it was determined that while we were saving more babies during that time period, *it had nothing to do with subjecting young mothers to more and more C-sections.* NICUs (neonatal intensive care nurseries) had come online across the country during the same time period, and the NICUs were saving more babies—and mostly one group in particular: severely premature babies. Many more were now surviving. Nearly all the improvement that occurred was reflected in this one group. Neonatologists and NICUs made the difference; not obstetricians doing more cesarean surgeries. Unfortunately, it took a while for this reality to emerge, and in the meantime this seriously wrong belief fueled a drive for more and more major cesarean surgeries, with the justification that it was okay, even though it increased risk to the mother and prolonged pain and recovery for her, because it was saving more babies.

In the end, obstetricians could not take credit for the improvement made by perinatologists and neonatologists and NICUs. And that's the problem with a data-mining or looking-backward kind of study. You could have proposed a hypothesis that because more people eat kale, more babies survive, and by mining the data you could say, "Aha, it must be true, because more babies are surviving."

So why bother with anything other than an RCT and a literature review? Well, not everything has been studied in a randomized controlled trial; RCTs are expensive. These other studies are starting points to thinking and help point us in the direction of what should be subjected to an RCT.

You now have the tools to help you evaluate the quality of evidence. Keep them in your mental toolbox!

Now, I'll bet you can ace the following quiz. (Stop! Take the time. Reading and believing are only one level of learning. Recalling and reiterating are a higher level of learning and will serve you better.)

Which is the gold standard type of study applying rigorous scientific methodology, with a control group and experimental group?

Retrospective studies (looking-backward and mining-data) have serious limitations and can often lead to flawed conclusions. Can you recall the example given? (Hint: It has something to do with a claim that escalated the incidence of C-sections.)

Is there an expiration date on a randomized controlled trial?

What does it take to invalidate a randomized controlled trial?

CHAPTER EIGHT

Sexuality and Birthing

To BEGIN TO UNDERSTAND what happens in birth, you must know how your birth organs work. Of course, they happen to be your sexual organs also, so I don't think you'll be too surprised to discover some similarities between sexual responsiveness and the mechanics of labor and birth.

Take a look at picture 1 (on page 41), a cross-section of a woman's body. The thing shaped a bit like a horseshoe in this picture is the **uterus**. (Dr. Bradley calls it "the baby box." He loves simple terms and clear mental pictures, so we'll interchange his picture words with more technical language and soon you'll have all the right mental images with the correct terminology.) You'll notice the uterus is at somewhat of a right angle to the **vagina**, or the birth canal. You will push your baby out of the uterus and down this birth canal when you give birth.

During intercourse, the penis goes into the vagina only. It does not go up into the uterus, where the baby is growing, so you do not have to worry about hurting the baby during intercourse. The uterus and the vagina are two separate compartments.

Now, notice the nice neat little funnel toward the front of the picture. This is the bladder from which you urinate. In the middle, of course, is the vagina or birth canal and toward the back is the rectum.

If you look for a little thing shaped like a peanut you will find the clitoris. It's loaded with nerve endings capable of receiving lots of stimulation. In fact, it used to be thought that the clitoris is where a woman experiences a climax. Now it is known that it doesn't happen quite that way.

A climax is experienced as a series of muscular contractions or squeezing in the muscles around the vagina and the muscles in the uterus. The muscles squeeze and relax, squeeze and relax, alternately. A climax is just muscles, squeezing and relaxing from about four to twenty times.

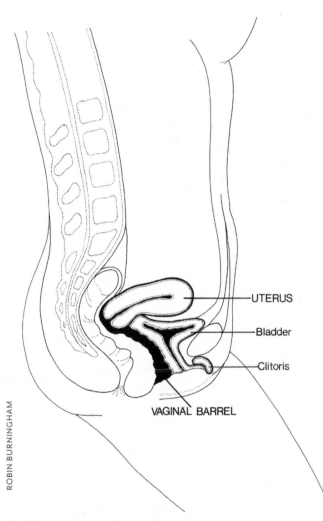

ROBIN BURNINGHAM

UTERUS

Bladder

Clitoris

VAGINAL BARREL

01. The woman in this example is not pregnant.

By the way, during your second or third pregnancy you may notice your tummy (actually your uterus) hardening and relaxing repeatedly after climaxes during intercourse. Don't worry, you haven't triggered labor. This is very common and normal and it's probably beneficial; those muscles have a chance to rehearse a little.

The clitoris is thought of as a kind of passion trigger, but because it is loaded with nerve endings, direct or prolonged stimulation can often be irritating instead of exciting. In other words, in order for stimulation to be a turn-on instead of a turn-off, a couple needs to communicate. A husband should find out what his wife likes and how much of it.

A woman's nipples are much the same as the clitoris, loaded with nerve endings capable of receiving stimulation. But again, prolonged stimulation can have the opposite effect. It can be irritating. Which is why a woman may say, "Oh, I like that," one minute and the very next minute she'll say, "Don't do that, it doesn't feel good anymore."

Let's take a few minutes here to see what happens inside a woman's body when she's sexually excited. First, her vagina does not merely stretch as the penis enters. If she is sexually excited, the vagina barrels outward, expanding to two or three times its nonexcited size. When the vaginal barrel expands outward, it bumps the bladder

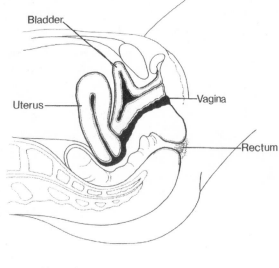

Bladder

Uterus

Vagina

Rectum

02. The vaginal barrel

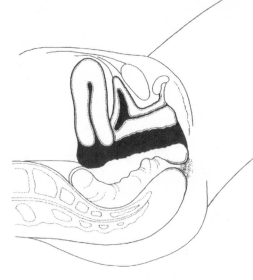

ROBIN BURNINGHAM

The vaginal barrel in the excited state

upward and out of the way of the thrusting penis, protecting the bladder from being bruised. The rectal wall is also shoved back for protection.

While the vagina is barreling outward, it elongates by about an inch at each end, and the outer lips of the vaginal barrel stiffen outward somewhat, preventing friction or a dragging sensation as the penis enters.

While this is occurring in the vaginal barrel, the uterus responds, too. It balloons forward and upward toward the navel, pulling the bottom part of the uterus out

of the birth canal, preventing it from being battered or thumped during intercourse.

How does all this expansion happen? It occurs the same way a man achieves an erection, by engorgement. During an erection more blood goes to the blood vessels than goes out, which has the effect of making the penis stand erect and elongated. The same kind of engorgement occurs in the vagina and uterus when a woman is excited, making the vaginal barrel stand outward and elongate. If you climax during intercourse, the engorgement rapidly disappears, but when you do not climax it can remain for quite a while, sometimes causing backache, a pelvic dragging sensation, and general crabbiness. So it's a good idea to have a climax—and it's fun!

There is one other time when these same responses occur. Can you guess? Yes, it is when you are pushing your baby out. Here, again, your vagina does not merely stretch as your baby comes down and out. Your vagina *expands*, somewhat like an accordion, to accommodate the size of the passenger. The next time you hear of a woman opting for a C-section to save her vagina for sex, to prevent it from being all stretched out, don't laugh. Share this information with her about expansion. It is amazing, but in a way logical, that the same responses that occur when you are sexually excited also occur when you are having your baby. In fact, some women have a birth climax when they have a baby.

THE BIRTH CLIMAX

Now, I've had three babies and never had a birth climax. Darn! (I'm kidding; I had wonderful births. You don't need a birth climax to have a great birth. I've taught more than three thousand women, and only four or five of them have had a birth climax—so it's not very common, but it is real.)

I happened to be in the hospital taking pictures of one of my couples when a doctor, who knew what I taught, came in and asked me to go down the hall and see if I could help out the lady in Room 3. She was a second-time mother and had been in the pushing part of labor for hours, but no one could get her to push and nothing was happening. There was talk of doing a cesarean. Well, I must tell you, it is not my favorite thing to be with a mother who has taken no responsibility whatsoever to learn anything about how to give birth, but it has been noted more than once that I can be a marshmallow.

So I went down to Room 3 and introduced myself. I told Angela that I knew some techniques that might help her out, if she would like me to work with her. She said, "Oh, *yes*, please." So I told her that the next time she felt her uterus begin to work, I would coach her to calmly take two deep breaths, then while taking the third, which she would hold, she could pull her legs back and push to the point of comfort.

She said, "There's one now." She did the work; I gently talked her through it, suddenly she made a startled sound. I thought, "Oh, I know that startled sound," and asked if I could pull down the sheet. She said yes, and when I looked, there was the baby's head appearing at the vaginal outlet. One push! The C-section was off. I ended up going into the delivery room with her; well, honestly, she wouldn't let go of my hand. At this point, things were going so quickly that no one had a chance to medicate her. As it turned out, she appreciated this since she had had a birth climax.

But this woman had never heard of it and didn't know what it was. She said, "Whew, those last few pains were great!" I was astonished. I asked her what kind of a pain feels great, and she replied, "Well, you know, it's kind of like during intercourse only a *lot* stronger." I was amazed. Here was this woman who'd learned nothing at all about birth, and *she* had a birth climax. Not fair! No, really, I was glad for her. I asked her if it had been painful at all, and she said, "No, it just felt good."

Yet it was interesting that this mother was so culturally conditioned to equate childbirth with pain that she used that word *pain* automatically, even though she was describing a sensation that she thought was wonderful.

Remember, the birth climax is real, but very few women get to experience it. If you have one, I hope you will write to me and tell me what you think the trick is, and I'll pass it on.

OVULATION

In picture 3, you can see just the uterus and the fallopian tubes. The vagina is left out of this picture.

The little sacs on each side (called ovaries) are full of eggs. You can see tubes that extend out of the uterus to these egg sacs (the fallopian tubes).

One month an egg will erupt from your right ovary and the next month an egg will erupt from your left ovary. An egg has just erupted in this picture. It will now journey down the tube to the uterus, and if it meets with sperm at the beginning of its journey then you find yourself needing this book. When it doesn't meet the sperm it just falls

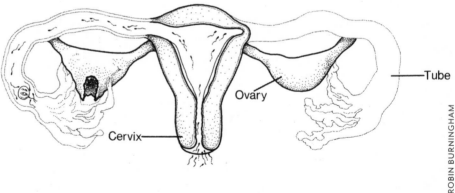

Tube

Ovary

Cervix

ROBIN BURNINGHAM

03. Ovulation

apart, and you have a regular period at the end of your monthly cycle.

Sometimes more than one egg will shoot off. If both eggs are fertilized (this would take two different sperm), then you really have your hands full at the end of nine months. Your twins would not be look-alikes, however, since they came from two different eggs and two different sperm. Sometimes an egg will split soon after fertilization, and then you would have identical twins.

The actual eruption of the egg from the ovary is called ovulation. It occurs on about the tenth to fourteenth day of each menstrual cycle (ten to fourteen days after your last period). We start off with the ovaries looking smooth like almonds; eventually, after all those monthly eruptions, they look pitted and wrinkled like prunes.

If you know what to look for, you can easily recognize when ovulation occurs. When you have ovulated, your vaginal discharge is somewhat heavier, the consistency of egg white. There is quite a lot of it. Your vagina is well lubricated whether you are excited or not.

This is important to understand. Men often mistakenly think that if the vagina is wet, the woman is ready for intercourse. In fact, if she is ovulating she will be wet even if she is not the least bit excited. She could be thinking of what color to paint the walls and still be wet at this time.

But several days later the man could approach her and think that because she is not as wet, she is not interested in making love. Indeed, she may be very interested. To understand each other and to enhance communication, it helps to realize how the body works.

While you are ovulating you may be aware of an aching or burning sensation to the right or left side, depending on where the egg came from, and a slight backache on the same side. It's not all that noticeable until you get into bed. Then you find you are more aware of the sensation and you may be a little restless.

THE UTERUS

Next in picture 4 (page 46) you can see the uterus of a woman seven months' pregnant. That large round organ in the upper two-thirds of the uterus is called the **placenta**, or the afterbirth, because it comes out after the baby. The side of the placenta facing the baby is smooth and shiny but the side facing the uterus is rooty or clumpy-looking where it implants into the uterine wall. You can ask your doctor to show it to you after birth. It looks like a fat piece of liver.

Notice the umbilical cord in this picture. It's usually about twenty to twenty-two inches long, but sometimes

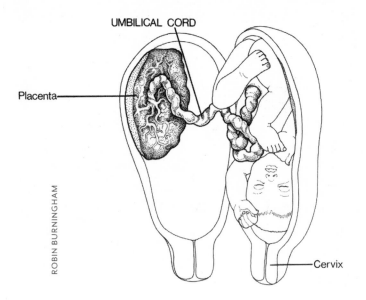

UMBILICAL CORD

Placenta

ROBIN BURNINGHAM

Cervix

04. Placenta and umbilical cord

You could say the mother's lungs act in place of the baby's, but the mother's lungs are an organ that belong to the mother, so it is the placenta that acts as the baby's lungs. Since the placenta is an organ that belongs to the baby, it grows specifically for and with the baby and is the site of immediate transfer of carbon dioxide and oxygen for the baby.

longer. The longest cord I've ever seen was five feet long. You could have skipped rope with it. We were all amazed as foot after foot of brilliant blue cord followed the baby out. The cord is a lovely turquoise blue at birth for a minute or two after the baby is born. The blue is from the three blood vessels inside the cord. One large vein carries oxygen and nutrients to the baby and two smaller arteries carry away carbon dioxide and waste products.

If you look closely, you can see the blood vessels from the umbilical cord branching out into the placenta. They get smaller and smaller as they branch out deeper into the interior of the placenta. There is no direct hookup between the mother's bloodstream and the baby's. Instead, these small vessels branching out through the placenta run close to the mother's own blood vessels. The nutrients and oxygen the baby needs pass out of the mother's blood vessels and into the tiny capillary veins leading back toward the cord and baby.

The whole thing works in reverse to get rid of waste the baby no longer needs. That waste is passed back into the mother's veins and carried off to her kidneys for her to eliminate with her urine. This is one reason you run to the bathroom more frequently when you're pregnant. You are handling the baby's disposals as well as your own.

The cord itself is amazing. It is like a fire hose with

water running through it forcefully, which keeps it from kinking. It might reassure you to know that if you just must have your baby in a taxicab or an elevator, you don't have to worry about doing something with the cord. Most of the blood in the placenta and cord will pump into the baby's body, whether you hold it low or put it to the breast. (This process takes a few minutes or more.) There is no hurry about cutting the cord. The blood will not back up. The vessels inside the cord are surrounded by a jellylike substance that expands rapidly at birth, pinching the blood vessels in the cord to close them off.

In the past, milking the cord (pinching it between two fingers and running them from one end to the other repeatedly as though milking a cow) was a common practice at birth. The purpose was simply to hurry things up. Recent research, however, is putting this procedure in a bad light. Such milking may be setting up future heart problems for the child by forcing his heart muscle and blood vessels to accept the blood at a faster rate and volume than nature planned. This could put a strain on the heart and blood vessels. Since it only takes a little while to let nature take its course, that seems the wiser thing to do. On the other hand, cutting the cord *before* allowing the cord blood to go to the baby deprives him of as much as one-quarter of his blood volume and is suspected of causing anemia during the first year of life.[1] Perhaps even more important, the cord contains a good deal of oxygenated blood and can prevent anoxia (lack of oxygen) in the new-born infant. [2,3,4,5]

When your baby is born, it can take a few seconds or sometimes minutes before he takes his first breath. Nature gives him some time to dillydally a bit. How's that? Well, the oxygenated blood in the placenta is now draining down through the unclamped and uncut cord, into his body, still supplying him with the oxygen he needs, for a little while longer, even though he is outside of you now! The bright blue cord color and the pulsating of the cord assures you of this continuing supply; but as the cord begins to turn whitish and deflate a bit and stop pulsating, then it's "showtime."

If your baby isn't already breathing, now *is* the time for him to start running the breathing program. For the baby who dillydallies a bit before jump-starting that program, thank goodness you chose a birth attendant who does not clamp or cut that cord just a minute after he was born. Evidence-based research has shown again and again that it is really not a good idea at all to cut the cord too soon. Researchers have determined that waiting three to five minutes, or longer, is best.[6] Think of it as a reserve tank of oxygen to tide the baby over in case he needs just a little more time to get going.

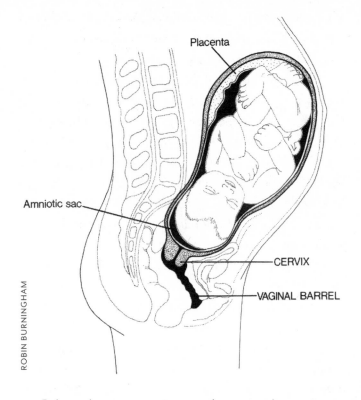

Placenta

Amniotic sac

CERVIX

VAGINAL BARREL

05. Baby in the uterus at nine months; notice the cervix.

In picture 5 you see the baby in the uterus, nine months along.

Did you know your baby is floating in a bag of water? In this illustration you can see the thin line indicating the bag called the amniotic sac. This tough little bag holds approximately one quart of liquid. Your body actually changes this water eight times every twenty-four hours. No wonder pregnant women naturally retain water. You may have noticed your wedding ring feels a little tighter as a result. Your blood volume also increases by almost a third. A certain amount of water retention is not only normal but probably quite beneficial.

It was at one time a common belief–based practice to give diuretics to pregnant women. Fortunately, most doctors wouldn't consider this, because diuretics can be dangerous. They actually decrease your blood volume at this critical time. They can also reduce the volume of blood circulating in the fetus, making it more difficult to get oxygen to the baby's brain.[7]

The bag of water, or the amniotic sac, is a marvelous thing. If you were punched in the tummy you might feel pain, but your baby would not experience the punch as a direct blow to his body. Instead, the force would be spread throughout the water so the baby felt a much gentler, equalized sensation all over. In fact, this is how your baby will feel labor as long as the bag of water is intact: as a gentle, equalized pressure. It's somewhat like a hug and a squeeze each time the uterus works during labor.

Your baby swims around in this sac while he's small enough, and he urinates in it a little. He may swallow the water, but he won't choke because there is no air in his lungs, just water. He even practices breathing by inhaling some of this fluid in and then moving it out of his lungs. He receives his oxygen via the cord. The sac is a comfortable, secure home for your baby until he is ready to be born.

Now here's something you will want to remember. If you put your hands on your hips you can feel your pelvis like a girdle of bones within you. Until about the eighth month, most babies are floating around just above the pelvis. That's why you can feel him kicking you in the ribs.

As you enter your ninth month, things begin to get extra crowded in there, so the baby will settle down lower into the pelvis. You will then have a little more room to breathe but you will find yourself running to the bathroom more frequently, if that is possible. This is because of the increased pressure on the bladder.

This settling-in is called "engaging." Your mother-in-law may call it "dropping." Sometime in your ninth month it is quite possible the doctor will tell you the baby is engaged. By the way, what do you think this tells you about when your labor is going to start? *Engagement tells you nothing at all about when labor will begin.*

My first baby couldn't be bothered to engage until I was pushing him out! Yet another of my babies was well engaged two months before birth. It is important for your peace of mind to remember that there is no way to accurately predict the week, or the day, or the hour your baby will be born.

CHAPTER NINE

The Mechanics of Labor and Birthing

AT LAST, WE COME to what will actually happen when you are having a baby. This chapter will help you understand the birth process so later you can learn to work with it effectively.

The first thing most couples want to know is: How long does labor take? Well, the textbook says one thing, but that is not always what happens. The book says your *first* baby will take about twelve to fourteen hours of labor. Second and later babies come a little faster, after eight to ten hours of labor.

But after years of teaching, we see everything from the *speedster*, to the *textbook* laborer to the *putterer*.

The speedster gives birth after a fast five or seven hours of hard work. That's really fast, particularly for a first baby. The textbook laborer has the ten-to-fourteen-hour labor, and then there is the putterer. The putterer has extremely easy, light labor for several hours or more. Her uterus works perhaps for thirty seconds, maybe every seven to ten minutes. She is not working hard. In fact, she is usually at home continuing her daily activities.

Finally, after a number of hours, her uterus stops playing around and gets down to work. In the long run her labor may last twenty hours or more, but that isn't bad at all when you realize that she really isn't working hard all those hours.

So you have already learned a most important thing about having a baby. Every woman will produce a baby at her own speed, and, in a normal labor, her own speed is the best speed.

THE FIRST STAGE OF LABOR

We will divide labor into three stages. It is just a convenient way to describe things. Your doctor will talk of labor in these same stages, so it is good to know their names.

This is important. Look back at picture 5 and take particular note of the *cervix*, the bottom part of the uterus that hangs down a little into the birth canal.

The cervix looks like the neck of a turtleneck sweater. Here it doesn't look like that because this picture is cut in half, making the cervix look like two ends hanging down. But use your imagination and in your mind put the two halves of the uterus and cervix together.

Dr. Bradley calls the cervix the "door" to the uterus, simply because this has to open before you can push your baby down and out the canal. If you think of the cervix as the door to the uterus, you will always know its function during labor.

Let's suppose a woman is having a textbook labor of fourteen hours with her first baby. The only thing that is happening for about twelve of those hours is that the cervix is opening. Once it is open, she has just one canal, instead of her two separate compartments of the uterus and the vagina, so she can push her baby out. *So the real work of labor, the long work that takes most of those hours, is just getting this door open. The opening of the cervix is called first stage.*

The cervix is pulled open and pulled back over the baby's head, like pulling a turtleneck sweater over your own head. It doesn't just flap aside as the baby moves down the canal. The cervix is pulled back closely over his head. It seems to disappear.

Where does the cervix go? It is drawn into the upper body of the uterus. This upper part of the uterus actually gets a little thicker, which is great because once the cervix is open the thicker, upper uterus acts like a piston to boot the baby out.

So what will pull the cervix back and over the baby's head? *Contractions.* You have probably heard them called "pains." In this book we'll use the accurate term and call them what they really are—contractions.

But what exactly is a contraction? Well, flex the bicep in your arm. That's a contraction. A muscle flexing or shortening is all a contraction is. And that is all labor is—muscles working.

Look at picture 6. It simply shows the uterus, not cut in half, but the way it really is. It is just a big bag of muscles. In fact, this muscular bag is made up of three layers of muscle tissue. A contraction is just this bag of muscles flexing for you.

A woman's muscles may flex for thirty seconds at a time when she begins labor. She may rest for five to seven or possibly even ten minutes at first. After a while this muscular bag will begin flexing for forty-five seconds at a time and she may rest for five minutes or less. After more

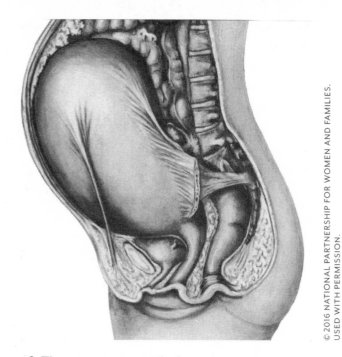

06. The uterus is a muscular bag.

gathering strength, and keep on flexing until she gets a good stretching and pulling sensation at the cervix, to open the door a bit. Then they relax. The muscles gradually stop their efforts for several minutes. They not only *contract* but they also *retract*, or stay somewhat shortened, after each flex. This is what draws the cervix up and over the baby's head.

After a rest the muscles will flex again. Starting at the top, the muscles build up to their work. They keep shortening, sweeping her along to the peak of their strength as they contract all the way down toward the cervix to give her a *good, strong, stretching and pulling sensation,* which opens the door a bit more. Then the sensation gradually diminishes. Her muscles get to rest and so does she.

Finally, at the end of first stage the uterus may be flexing for ninety seconds and her rest periods may be one-and-a-half to two minutes long. But nature is very kind. This is a lot of work, but she always gets a rest between contractions all the way through labor. Now, look at the cervix in picture 7.

You can see that the two-inch neck of the cervix has been pulled flat. It is not open; it has just flattened out along the baby's head, much as if you had just started to put on that sweater, pulling the neck down flat onto your head but not actually pulling it open and over your head yet.

time goes by, her uterine muscles will contract for sixty to seventy seconds and her rest periods will be about three minutes or less. Her uterus has long muscles that go from the top down toward the cervix. A contraction starts at the top as these long muscles begin to flex. They contract and shorten and continue to contract,

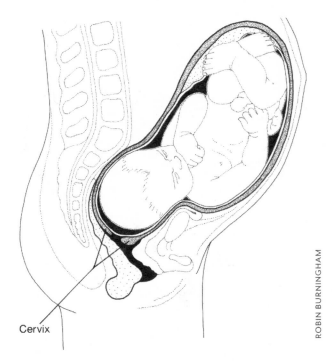

Cervix

ROBIN BURNINGHAM

07. Cervix effaced: The cervix is pulled down flat onto the baby's head.

This flattening of the cervix is called **effacement**. If, most likely in your ninth month, your doctor mentions that your cervix is beginning to efface, you will know what he is talking about. By the way, what do you think this tells you about when your labor is going to start? You are probably on to us by now.

Effacement tells you nothing at all about when labor will begin. You cannot predict the hour or the day. A wise doctor never burdens an expectant mother with unreliable predictions, which only build up her expectations and then let her down. To predict "this weekend, for sure," or "next week, definitely," starts the woman on an emotional roller coaster.

With one of my pregnancies I was examined early in the day and told not to expect anything to happen soon since I was not the least bit effaced. I gave birth later that evening. With another pregnancy I was completely effaced (and the cervix was even slightly open) two months before I went into labor. So, while effacement tells you nothing about the day and hour of your birth, it is nice to know what the doctor means if he says, "Hmm you're effacing."

Now let's look at the cervix in picture 8.

You will see that the door is really beginning to open.

The mother reaches the end of the first stage when her cervix is completely open. It is as if that turtleneck sweater has been pulled down onto the head and the neck of the sweater is stretched open. In picture 9 the cervix is completely open. This is called ten centimeters (or, sometimes, "five fingers") dilated. *Through the first stage her cervix opens, or dilates, gradually until she is "complete," meaning completely dilated.*

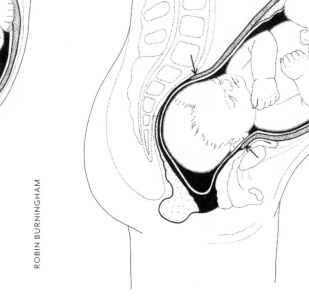

ROBIN BURNINGHAM

ROBIN BURNINGHAM

08. Cervix dilating

09. Completely dilated

Remember, the part that is opening is up inside, so its progress cannot be seen just by looking at the vaginal opening. It can be checked only by inserting two fingers into the vaginal opening far enough to feel the cervix and to estimate the amount of dilation (which takes some

training and experience). Even at this point the number of centimeters tells you very little about precisely when the baby will be born. Some women may dilate at a fairly even pace, perhaps about a centimeter an hour. Others may be measured at four centimeters one hour and jump to ten the next. Yet another woman may seem "stuck" (she really isn't) at three or four centimeters for some hours before opening wider. *So knowing how far dilated you are really tells you nothing about how many more hours or minutes it will be before you give birth.* Vaginal exams can set up the same kind of emotional roller coaster that the news about effacement or engagement did earlier. And they increase the risk of infection and other problems, as we will discuss later.

THE SECOND STAGE

Once the cervix is open, the next thing the mother will do is push the baby out. The second stage begins with her first push. Pushing can be exhilarating after a woman has learned how to work *with* her body. It is the icing on the cake.

In second stage she will still have contractions and rest periods, but now they are pushing contractions. Her uterus now works like a piston to push her baby out. The uterine muscle will apply about thirty-five to forty pounds of force, but that is not enough. She will have to apply additional force to push the baby down and out the birth canal.

When a pushing contraction starts, her uterus begins working to move her baby out. She will push and push and push with it and move her baby down the birth canal. Then her uterus rests and she rests, too. As she rests, the baby slides back a bit. It is not exactly two steps down, one step back—but that is the general idea.

After resting a few minutes, her uterus begins to contract again, and she repeats the performance for a minute or two and then rests again. This is hard and sweaty, but exciting, work. It may take half an hour to two hours or more to push her baby out. Picture 10 shows where she will be at the end of that pushing time. This is still second stage until the baby is all the way out. This is called "crowning" because the vaginal lips look like a crown around the baby's head.

Look again at picture 10. This is just moments before the head emerges. Notice the perineum. It is stretched flat as a pancake, extending all the way up to the fourchette (see the line on the diagram). For comparison, look back to picture 9 where the perineum is a rather thick muscle. It is remarkable the way this muscle stretches so beautifully.

Some doctors will perform a routine episiotomy at this time. That is a surgical incision with a pair of scissors cutting into the perineum. The mother would not feel the cut, because pressure from the baby's head cuts off the circulation to her perineum and makes it numb. This procedure is called a "pressure episiotomy" and no Novocain is necessary since nature's anesthetic works quite nicely. An anesthetic would be injected after the baby is born, while the cut is being sutured.

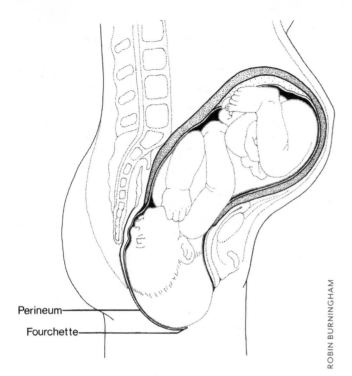

Perineum—

Fourchette—

10. Crowning

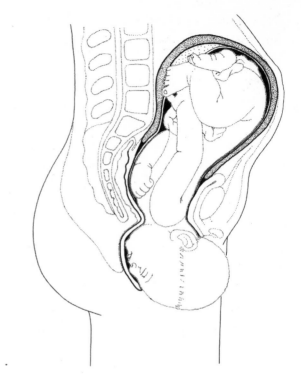

11. Baby's head emerging

But a growing number of women do not believe an episiotomy is necessary or desirable. And we know several doctors who agree and rarely perform episiotomies. These births turn out very well. (In Chapter Twenty-One we will discuss episiotomies in detail.)

In picture 11 the baby's head is emerging and the

perineum is already shrinking back. Contrary to popular belief, this is not the "most agonizing moment." Nature provides its own anesthetic, the same one that makes possible the pressure episiotomy. The baby's head pushing against the perineum cuts off the circulation there. The feeling is similar to when you sit on your leg too long, also cutting off the circulation. When you get up, your leg feels numb and tingly, and this is exactly how your outlet will feel when the baby's head emerges.

Picture 12 shows the baby's head out, but the baby's body is still inside the mother. The work is almost done. The perineum is all the way back to normal and looks like a nice, thick muscle again. In a natural birth, the doctor or birth attendant never needs to pull on the head. The unmedicated mother is quite capable of pushing her baby out.

After a pause, she will give another push and the baby's body will come out quickly, all slippery and wiggly-feeling. This is delightful, and you feel so empty afterward. Once the baby's entire body is out, the second stage is over.

But he is still attached by the umbilical cord to the placenta, which is still attached to the mother. Don't cut that cord yet! All the blood in the placenta belongs to the baby, not the mother. It takes three to five minutes for most of that blood to flow down into the baby's body (this time to stay there), not cycle back into the placenta anymore.

But wait a minute, you say, wasn't that volume of blood always *outside* of his body before? Why does it need to be *inside* his body now? Why can't we just cut the cord immediately and forget the blood that's still in the placenta?

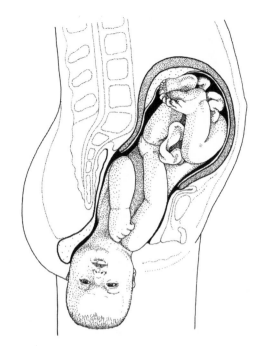

ROBIN BURNINGHAM

12. Birth

Here's why: Previously, just enough blood went to the baby's lungs to nourish the cells of his lungs to keep the lungs, as organs, healthy and well; but now things change dramatically. A trapdoor in the baby's heart muscle snaps open and starts sending, for the very first time, a large volume of blood to the baby's real lungs. This is the route through which the baby will pick up oxygen to circulate to the tissues and cells of his body. The same volume of blood that used to go to the placenta now needs to go to his lungs. If he doesn't get that placental blood for this rerouting, then he has to divert blood already in his circulatory system and needed to support his other tissues and organs.

As much as one-fourth to one-third of a baby's blood volume can be left behind in the placenta by cutting the cord too soon.

Volume is important. Volume affects blood pressure and this pressure facilitates pushing open the trapdoor in the heart; volume dilates the blood vessels going to his lungs, which were not previously filled with blood, and volume perfuses his lungs optimally as he breathes and extracts oxygen from the air on his own.

When you clamp and cut the cord immediately, he is deprived of that increased volume of blood. Your perfectly normal baby is now going to spend energy and nutrients in his first weeks of life to replace that blood supply, which he needs to optimally oxygenate his brain and other organs and cells.

In fact, research has shown again and again that a baby deprived of placental blood can be anemic for up to a year after birth. The first year of a baby's life is a time of incredibly rapid growth, and when the cord is cut in fewer than three to five minutes, some of that energy and nutrition is going to go into catch-up instead of growth takeoff.

THE THIRD STAGE (AND A SUMMARY)

The third stage is easy enough. The mother will simply push out the placenta, or afterbirth. We certainly hope that she gets to nurse her baby right away, even on the delivery table. Nursing immediately at birth makes the uterus contract strongly and prevents bleeding. It stimulates the production of a natural hormone called oxytocin, which contracts the uterus and speeds the birth of the placenta.

Once the baby is out, these final contractions cause the uterus to shrink. The placenta does not shrink with it, so as the uterus contracts underneath, the placenta breaks loose. This can be seen in picture 13. It's like a scab coming off. As the fresh skin under a scab comes together, the surface under the scab shrinks and the scab buckles in the middle, and eventually detaches.

Well, here in third stage, the uterus continues to contract, and with no baby inside, the uterus starts shrinking down with each flex, so the surface under the placenta shrinks and the placenta buckles, and as the surface beneath the placenta continues to shrink, the placenta simply falls off the uterine wall.

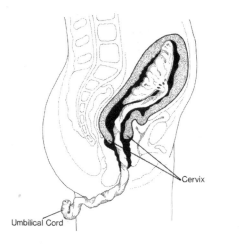

13. Expulsion of placenta

Once detachment has occurred (anywhere from a couple of minutes to thirty or forty, and sometimes longer), it will be easy to push the placenta out. Wait; did I say it would be easy to push the placenta out? That depends. Did you remember to wait to cut the cord so all the blood in the placenta could drain into the baby? If you waited until the cord changed from blue to white and completely ceased to pulsate, then yes, the placenta should come out much more easily. What—that cord cutting story again? Well, yes, we didn't quite finish that story. Not only is it good for the baby to wait to cut the cord, it is good for the mother.

Ask yourself this question: When the blood in the placenta is allowed to drain out into the baby's body, will the placenta get bigger or smaller? It will be smaller, of course. The volume of the placenta will considerably decrease and its texture will be less stiff and more flexible. The smaller size and softer texture make it easier for the placenta to slip out with a small push or two, after it has detached from the lining of the uterus. (It isn't going anywhere until it actually detaches, naturally.) And you know how to help detachment along? Put the baby to the breast. At this point it will be easy to push the placenta out. Often just a push or two does the trick. Letting the placenta break off naturally and pushing it out makes for an efficient, safe third stage for the mother.

To summarize briefly:

First stage is getting the cervix (the door to the uterus) *open.* This is all that happens during most of the hours of labor.

Second stage is pushing the baby out after the door is open. This can take half an hour to two or three hours.

Third stage is expelling the placenta.

It is an incredibly simple process. The door opens, you push your baby out, and then the placenta is pushed out.

THE BABY'S ROLE

Now that you have a clear idea of what happens in the woman's body during labor, let's consider what her baby will be up to. Take a look at picture 14. Most babies are in this position when the mother is ready to begin pushing. They are not quite facing toward the spine, not quite to the side, but somewhere in between to the right or the left. As she is having her baby his face will turn to her back. This is much like a key fitting into a lock. (See picture 15.)

The baby will then move through the pelvis and down the spine, which Dr. Bradley calls "the baby sliding board." As the baby emerges, his head turns to its original position so it is once again comfortably in line with the shoulders. Here there is usually a short pause while the baby's head is outside the mother's body but his body is still inside as in picture 16.

This is a wondrous moment. Quite often (in an unmedicated birth) the baby's eyes are already open. Imagine. There is your child with his body still within you and his head out with eyes open wide. Hardly believing what is happening, you give another push. This part goes quite rapidly. You can feel your child's little body as you push the rest of him out.

At this moment, with your baby's head out and the body just about to emerge from your own, you can look

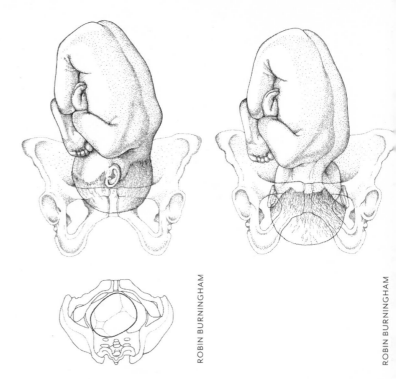

ROBIN BURNINGHAM

ROBIN BURNINGHAM

14. Position of the baby in relation to the pelvis (common position)

15. Like a key fitting into a lock

over your tummy to reach out for your baby. We have seen this spontaneous emotional reaction often and it is beautiful to watch. Very often the baby is the only one in the room with dry eyes. Why should the baby cry when he goes right from the womb to mother's arms with no delay?

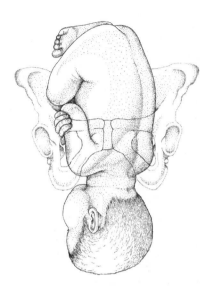

ROBIN BURNINGHAM

16. Head is completely out; body still inside the mother.

From the first moment of birth the baby will continue to hear the same familiar heartbeat and feel the same warmth from the mother's body. No, the baby does not cry, but everyone else in the room does from the sheer, wonderful joy of it.

It is fortunate when parents are able to find a doctor who is tuned in to the new family as a unit. The importance of allowing the parents *immediate touch contact* with the baby cannot be overestimated. Getting to hold or touch the baby five minutes later is not quite the same thing. The intensity of this particular emotional response is diminished with each passing minute.

The baby may actually help himself to get down and out of the birth canal. If you take an unmedicated new-born and press on his feet or hug him snugly, he will push back with his feet. This is recognized as a normal reflex. When the uterine muscles flex, the top of the uterus comes down on the baby's bottom and feet. What do you suppose he does? He pushes back, helping his journey down the canal.

When a mother has not received any drugs during labor and birth, she will find her own pushing efforts to be vigorous and effective. She and her baby will be working together toward the moment of birth.

There is another way the baby is helping to be born. If you put an unmedicated newborn facedown on a blanket, he will pick up his head and turn it to one side. The mechanics of lifting and turning the head are exactly what occurs as he emerges over the perineum.

I'll never forget the doctor's reaction at the birth of one of my children. At this moment, when the head was right at the outlet and turning, the doctor exclaimed with amazement, "Look at that baby spin around!" He was accustomed to the medicated mother and infant and his experience had been limited to manipulating and extracting the infant himself.

When you are in labor yourself, you will want to picture the harmony of the work involved: the baby with built-in reflexes to help in birth, the uterus working in its designed way, and you, the skilled mother, relaxing at the right times and working at the right times with a supportive partner caring for you and coaching you through labor.

Now we're going to go smaller—much smaller—and take an important microscopic view of what is happening in labor.

YOUR BABY AND THE MICROBIOME PROJECT

What's the Human Microbiome Project? Well, instead of life on Mars, more than two hundred scientists on the microbiome project looked at life on man. You have trillions of microbes on your body and in your body, and they're known collectively as your microbiome.

Yuck! Microbes, as in bacteria, fungi, protozoa, all over you! Well, actually, there is no yuck about it. You would be in trouble if you weren't sharing your body with these microbes. You probably grew up thinking all bacteria are bad; while some certainly are, there are thousands more that benefit you, and some are even essential if you are going to be your healthiest self. They help you digest food, enhance and inform your immune system, and help regulate your metabolism. They help you to live; they help you to thrive.

Kind of intriguing, isn't it? You are a walking world for millions of hitchhikers. You are 90 percent bacteria, viruses, and other microorganisms and only 10 percent human cells. More of the DNA in and on your body is actually their DNA. More of what you think of as you is actually them! Thank goodness they're along for the ride, helping you stay healthy! And just as you have your own unique fingerprints, you have your own unique microbial print.

But what does this have to do with birthing? You make a critical microbial hand-off to your baby when he is born through the vagina, picking up three to four hundred species of the vaginal set of microbes. (That vaginal set is not the same as your skin set of microbes.)

Your baby will be inoculated with just the right microbes for a newborn as he passes through your birth canal: microbes that provide protection from infection, microbes that actually teach your baby's immune system, microbes that will help him digest his meals and extract vitamins for him.

Rodney R. Dietert, professor of immunotoxicology at Cornell University, proposes a hypothesis called the Completed Self. Here's what he says:

> The baby comes down the birth canal during vaginal delivery. That is the major seeding event and we know that the gut microbes in particular are absolutely crucial to what happens in the immune system and in the capacity

to break down different nutrients and different environmental chemicals. That's where the action happens, so that is probably the single most important event that is going to chart the course for whether that baby becomes complete and whether that baby experiences a life filled with health or one filled with disease.

But why is it so important that it is the mom's microbiota, and why immediately? After all, your baby *is* going to pick up microbes rapidly; if not yours, then he will pick up microbes from nurses, doctors, the midwife, or whomever else is in the same room at birth. So as long as he picks up microbiota (and he will), why should you care if it's the doctors' or the nurses' or a mixture from several people?

Well, it matters. The microbiota in your vagina actually changes, just before birth, to provide your newborn with exactly what a newborn needs at birth and in his first weeks, months, and early years of life. It is not like the adult microbiome. (It won't be until his third year of life; only then will his microbiome more closely evolve to resemble an adult's.) Your vagina and breasts in particular have rearranged the microbiota for this newborn handoff. Yours is the one he needs. Yours is the designer copy, custom-made for a newborn baby and specifically for your newborn.

Martin J. Blaser, director of the Human Microbiome Project at New York University and author of the book *Missing Microbes*, tells us the main event is at birth where:

> key species gather in breast and vagina. Baby is coated and swallows the founding microbiome for that baby.[1]

And that's why it needs to be your microbiome. There is no one else in that room who has a vagina and breast responding in labor and selecting the key species of microbes and ratios of species to fit the newborn's immediate needs, to jump-start his immune system, to seed his intestines with just the right starter mix of microbes for an infant. You are the leading lady, and your baby is your costar.

Dietert tells us:

> It's a narrow window. If we miss it, the immune system doesn't mature properly.[2]

Now you have a good idea of what your body and your baby will be doing in labor. So let's go on to some important exercises to get you ready for birth.

CHAPTER TEN

Exercises: Getting Your Body Ready for Birthing

EXERCISES ARE A BORE. But to give birth comfortably your body does need some special tuning up. You will find that in preparation for giving birth we are not so interested in building muscles as we are in stretching and limbering them up.

WARNING: Just being in great physical shape is no help to a person who has not learned how to swim and finds herself in the middle of a lake. So, although we will start with exercises, by themselves they will not give you a happy labor and birth. You still need to learn how to labor and to practice the labor and birth techniques you will learn. Also, please note that this book deals with normality, so those who have a medical problem or condition that may be affected by the exercises taught here will want to check with their doctor before undertaking them. It might help to show the doctor this book.

TAILOR SITTING

Here is your first exercise. It is called *tailor sitting* after the way old-time tailors used to work (see picture 17). Actually, it is a posture rather than a conventional exercise, and it is not all that easy. You do have to work at getting your knees as close to the floor as you can. Try touching your knees to the floor in this simple tailor-sitting position while you read the rest of this chapter.

If at first your knees are nowhere near the floor, don't force them. You will have to gradually work up to it at a pace that is suitable for you.

Why are you doing this? When you push your baby out, your legs will be comfortably apart. This is at the end of your labor and may take half an hour to two hours or more. If you have prepared yourself for birth, with lots of tailor sitting, then the muscles on the upper insides of your legs will be stretched and lengthened so you will be comfortable in the pushing position.

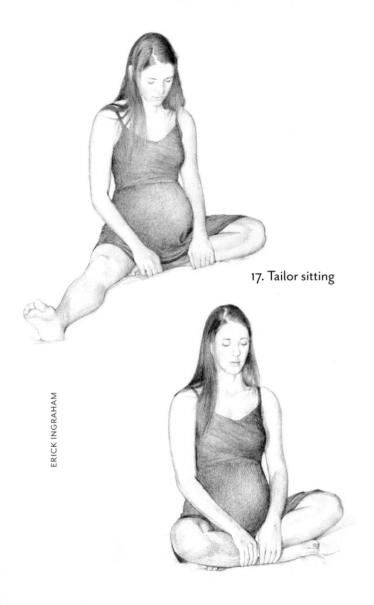

17. Tailor sitting

ERICK INGRAHAM

The untrained mother frequently gets sore legs and even cramps. Can you imagine trying to enjoy the momentous experience of birth with a cramp in your leg? Nothing joyful about that.

TO THE COACH

Keep your wife out of all the soft, cushy chairs at your house. When she sits in a soft chair, her bottom sinks down and her knees come up, so there's no stretch. Start coaching now, by helping her to remember to do her exercises and use these postures. They're easy, and it is not a matter of taking extra time to do them, since they go easily with watching television, reading, or many other activities. If you take the coaching job seriously, your wife's favorite chair will gather dust from now until the birth of your baby.

(If you catch her complaining to friends about how you make her do her exercises, perhaps she's actually bragging about how much she is cared for and about your active part in getting ready for birth.)

SQUATTING

Here's your next exercise, or really just another posture: *squatting*. Simply stand with your feet about a foot or so apart, heels flat on the floor, lean slightly forward, and drop gently down into a squatting position. Leaning forward helps you to keep your balance. Check the illustration.

This usually takes two to do at first or you may find yourself falling over backward. Don't despair if you have trouble keeping your heels flat on the floor. With practice, the tendons at the backs of your ankles will lengthen, and you will soon be able to squat without help and with your heels flat on the floor. Remember to keep your knees wide apart.

And come up *bottom first,* as long as you are not lifting anything, as you unbend your knees. This helps you to deflect the baby forward, out of the pelvic ring. You avoid tamping the baby down into the bony pelvis and impeding circulation to your legs. You can put your hands on your thighs and push to help raise yourself the rest of the way, as you can see in the illustrations.

Why are you squatting? Well, squatting does an even better job than tailor sitting of preparing your leg muscles for a comfortable legs-apart position at birth. But more important, it helps to stretch the perineum, making it more flexible, something you'll really appreciate when your baby's head emerges.

The perineum is the skin and muscle tissue between the vaginal outlet and the anus. It does the most stretching at birth.

Squatting is one of your most important exercises.

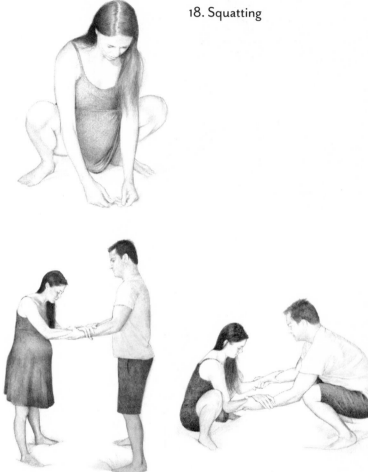

18. Squatting

19. A little help from the coach as you start to practice squatting.

Move hands farther up your thighs to help yourself stand up.

TO THE COACH

To help the mother get started in the squat you should hold her forearms strongly. Be ready to support her weight with a slight pull as she goes down. Try it with her now before going on.

Help her work on the squat until she can do it easily by herself. Don't let her feel discouraged. It takes most women who are not used to squatting a week or two before they are able to do it alone. How much squatting should she do? Lots!

Here is the most important and fascinating reason that squatting is so important:

When you squat, the bottom part of your pelvic bones spread wider apart, making more room for the baby to come out. How much more room? One-and-a-half to three centimeters more room! That is quite a lot of extra room.

How does that happen? Take a look at the illustrations of the pelvis. It's four bones, all connected by joints, *expandable* joints. You can see the sacrum at the back. It's

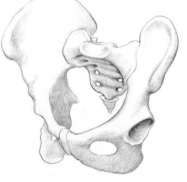

ERICK INGRAHAM

ERICK INGRAHAM

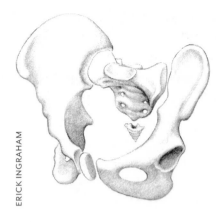

shaped somewhat like your hand. Stand up, let your right arm hang down, put your fingers and your thumb close together. Don't hold your hand stiffly, just let it relax into its normal, slightly curved position. That's a lot like your sacrum. Put your hand, just like that, on your bottom, at the end of your spine. Now sit down, with your hand still in place, and you will feel your sacrum. Try to find the very tip at the end of the sacrum.

At the very tip of the sacrum, you have another bone attached, a tiny triangular one, called the coccyx. It's attached to the sacrum by a *hinge joint*. (The doors in your house are attached to the walls with hinge joints, too.) That hinge joint allows the coccyx to swing back out of the way as the baby's head pushes past. ("Out of my way, I'm coming through.") It's designed to do just that!

Now, the sacrum itself is attached by joints to two larger bones. Put your hands on your hips; that's right, these are the large innominate bones. They make up the sidewalls of the pelvis, one on the right and one on the left.

These side bones are also attached to the sacrum by *expandable* joints (called the sacroiliac joints).

Let's see what the sacroiliac joints enable you to do. Put your hand back on your sacrum. Imagine your hand *is* your sacrum. Stand up. When you begin labor, your baby is just entering the top part of the pelvic ring. Slide your hand up just a bit and tip the heel backward, away from your body; this enlarges the inlet (the upper part) of the pelvis as the baby enters. Now, replace the heel of your hand so once again it rests against your back; slide your hand down your spine a bit. This is how the sacrum moves when you squat. Now press in with the heel of your hand and let your fingers move backward, away from your body. See how squatting makes more room at the outlet (the bottom part of the pelvis)?

There's another entirely different way your sacroiliac joints do wonders when you are having your baby. These joints allow your sacrum to rotate right or left. Stand in front of a chair and raise your right foot to rest on the chair. Your sacrum rotates a bit to the right, making more room on that side of the pelvis than on the other, so a baby can wiggle down and through. Change legs. Now the sacrum has rotated the other way a bit, making more wiggle room on the other side. What a fantastic piece of engineering!

We're not done yet. In the front, those two large sidewall bones, or innominate bones, are connected by a disc joint, the pubic symphysis. (Just like the spongy discs you have in your spine between each vertebra.) This is another expansion joint. So here is yet another point where your expandable pelvis is a marvel of invention.

Here is something else that is important to visualize. Get two salad plates and hold them parallel, about six inches apart (like cymbals). Pretend these are the big sidewall bones. Now move the two plates so that they get closer together at the top (say, just four inches apart). See what happens at the bottom? More room! So, when you are in a squatting position, this is what happens to the innominate bones. They get closer at the top and wider at the bottom. Great for when you see some of the baby's head, which means he's low and on his way out.

Here's how important this knowledge can be for you. I once had a couple giving birth at Castle Hospital in Hawaii and they asked me to join them. When I arrived, the head nurse met me in the hallway (she was everyone's favorite nurse, the one all the natural-birth mothers hoped to get). She told me the doctor was thinking of a cesarean surgery because they had been looking at just a dime's worth of the baby's head for more than an hour. After each push it was still just a dime's worth. I thanked her for putting me in the picture, suggested the mother get out of the bed, squat on the floor on top of a clean sheet and give three pushes in the full squat position. On the third push the baby crowned! No surgery, and the doctor had just enough time to put out a hand and catch.

Take advantage of this when you give birth, because *once the head begins to show,* just getting into a squatting position to push can make the difference between a smooth vaginal birth or hard weeks ahead recovering from major surgery. No, the bed won't do. Your heels sink down, angling your feet at an unnatural angle, potentially causing damage to your feet.

Coach: This really is your job to *remember.* I guarantee after fifteen hours of labor and a couple of hours of pushing it isn't the laboring woman who looks up and says in a perky voice, "Gee, maybe I should get down on the floor and try squatting now." It usually takes a coach, supporting and encouraging her to do this. That's you!

Here's a fascinating fact: Obstetricians used to X-ray women in labor to see if it looked like the pelvis was roomy enough for the baby to pass through. The FDA published a special booklet for obstetricians called *The Pelvimetry Examination,* where they reprinted published research by radiologists trying to explain to obstetricians that you couldn't determine that by X-ray (except in the most extreme cases, where something had occurred to damage the pelvis, like disease or a car accident). Apparently, radiologists had a hard time convincing obstetricians of this. In one of the FDA reprints entitled "X-ray Pelvimetry: Useful Procedure or Medical Nonsense," Dr. J. A. Campbell noted the following:

> For the radiologist to present the limitations of pelvimetry to an obstetrician is like sitting down with your mother-in-law to discuss her faults.

You'll be glad to know that obstetricians won't send you to X-ray to see if your baby will fit through your pelvis now that it is understood how expandable your pelvis is, plus the fact that just *changing your position changes the dimensions of your pelvis.*

Your pelvis is roomier at the top when you stand and roomier at the bottom when you squat. The evidence produced by the radiologists' research finally changed the practice of X-raying women. And no wonder; here's how clearly radiologists stated it:

> The incidence of a truly "small" pelvis in patients selected for pelvimetry is frequently as low as one or two cases in 2,500. In addition, the effects of molding of the fetal head and maternal pelvis during labor may expand these diameters sufficiently (2–3 centimeters) to render them meaningless.[1]

And,

> A simple postural change can increase the sagittal diameter of the outlet by as much as 2 cm and the transverse diameter by 1 cm or an increase of 30% in area.[2]

(What is this radiologist referring to when he mentions sagittal diameter? Think of drawing an arrow from the front of your pelvis to the back of your pelvis and that is the sagittal diameter.)

> So, ladies, practice squatting. You want to be able to squat for three or four minutes at a time. Listening and believing is not enough; you really do have to practice. If you need to use this position when you are pushing your baby out and you haven't practiced, then it's probably not going to happen. So squat a lot!

PELVIC ROCKING

This next exercise is great for the common complaint of backache during pregnancy. It is called *pelvic rocking,* and it is primarily for your comfort.

Simply get down on your hands and knees, with your hands directly under your shoulders and your knees either directly under your hips or a little farther back. (In other words, make a box.) Now start off with a sag of your tummy and a sigh. You'll notice your bottom sticks out more when you do this. The next step is to tuck your bottom under, then relax once again.

The only movement is in your pelvis. Don't get your shoulders going up and down. This should be done at a slow, steady pace. There is nothing particularly beneficial about speed. As you tuck your pelvis under, tighten your abdominal muscles at the same time, and when you return to normal do not sag exceedingly. (There's no need to bounce your tummy off the floor.)

In addition to easing backache, pelvic rocking may help prevent varicose veins. When you get down on all fours, the weight of the baby drops forward, out of the pelvis and off the large blood vessels running along the back of the uterus. This takes pressure off some of the main blood vessels leading down to your legs. So if you have a tendency toward varicose veins, you'll want to use pelvic rocking at brief but frequent intervals throughout the day.

LEGS APART EXERCISE

Here is an active exercise to get you ready for the "legs-apart" position for birth. So far the tailor-sitting and squatting postures you have learned are passive stretching exercises, but the legs-apart exercise will *actively* strengthen the abductor muscles, which you use to open your legs. And this exercise takes teamwork. The pregnant woman

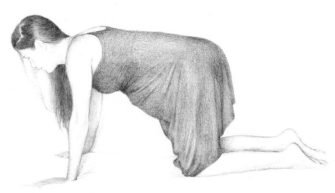
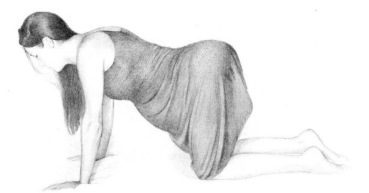

ERICK INGRAHAM

20. Pelvic rocking

sits on the floor, propped up with pillows. Your knees are bent and your feet are pulled back toward your bottom. The coach places his hands on the outside of the pregnant woman's legs at the knee or a little lower on the calf and applies mild pressure as if to hold the knees together while the woman uses her thigh muscles to push them apart. The resistance the coach applies puts the abductor muscles to work. Look at the illustration to see this exercise, which you should do three times a day. Remember, Coach, don't overdo it. This is not a contest of strength. You should allow her to slowly get her knees apart. You are not trying to keep them together, but to see that it takes a little effort.

PRACTICING YOUR EXERCISES

Don't save a certain time of day for your tailor sitting and squatting. Anytime you're sitting down around the house, working, watching television, or reading, tailor sit or squat. When you bend over to pick up something light, squat. Don't bend with your back. You have hinges in your knees, as Dr. Bradley is fond of saying, not in your back.

Pelvic rocking is a good thing to do in the afternoon, say, at two different times, twenty repetitions each. (Dr. Bradley feels pelvic rocking before bed helps restore and improve circulation to the legs after you have been up and around all day.)

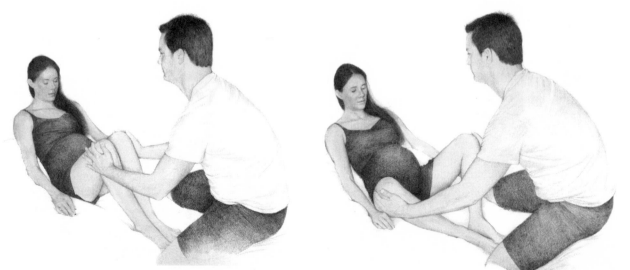

ERICK INGRAHAM

There are other physical exercises you could do, and some women may want to get into a program of prenatal exercise or yoga. But these four movements are easy, simple, and quite specifically geared to getting your body ready to give birth. Whether you do a lot of other exercises, or nothing else at all, you should be sure to do the tailor-sitting, squatting, pelvic-rocking, and legs-apart exercises regularly.

There is one more exercise to learn, one that you will find beneficial for birth and throughout the rest of your life.

THE PC MUSCLE AND YOUR MOST IMPORTANT EXERCISE

Now, you're ready for the best exercise you'll ever learn. Its benefits go beyond birthing. You may have heard of the muscle this exercise strengthens—the pubococcygeal muscle. (There's a mouthful for you.) It's sometimes called the Kegel muscle, after the doctor who invented these exercises. We'll call it the **PC muscle** for short. The PC muscle is a sling or hammock of muscle attached to your pubic bone in front and the tip of the spine in back. It's actually wrapped around the vagina, urethra, and rectum as thick muscular bands.

This sling will hold the inner organs up high *if it is strong enough to do so.* Look at the picture showing a

woman with a nice strong muscle. You can tell by looking at her uterus. It's up high and headed toward the navel. Her vagina is long and narrow, and the rectum is well supported. Her bladder is funnel-shaped.

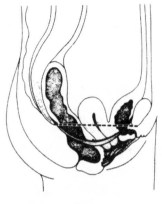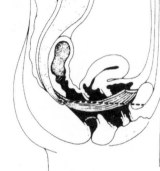

ROBIN BURNINGHAM

The PC muscle:
A weak sling of muscle.   A strong sling of muscle.

Now take a look at the picture, showing a weak PC muscle.

Just look at what happens when this important muscle is weak and saggy. The bladder is not a nice neat funnel; it's collapsed! Every time this woman sneezes or coughs she probably leaks urine, to her embarrassment. Her uterus not only isn't high and toward the navel, it's actually falling down into the vagina. This condition can be so serious that the uterus starts to protrude from the vagina. This is called uterine prolapse, and it can result in a hysterectomy (removal of the uterus).

Intercourse may become quite uncomfortable. When the uterus sags into the vagina like this, a woman is likely to complain of a shallow feeling, as if the penis were thumping into something. It certainly is, it's hitting the cervix; and the vaginal barrel is not the long narrow canal it should be; it's squashed, short, and loose. The vaginal walls are too far apart. They can't possibly come into good contact with the penis, depriving both man and woman of a strong sensation during intercourse.

In fact, look closely at the vaginal barrel in picture 21. Here you do not see the PC muscle, which is wrapped around the vagina. What you do see is the *effect* the muscle has on the vaginal barrel.

The vaginal barrel on the left is well supported by a strong muscle and looks like a squeezed toothpaste tube. The walls are narrow (so they will make good contact with the penis). The vaginal barrel on the right, however, shows the result of little support from a weak muscle. The vagina is too short and wide. The vaginal walls are too far apart to come into good contact with the penis and the vagina is shallow, which will cause the "thumping" sensation during intercourse. Did you know that women have hardly

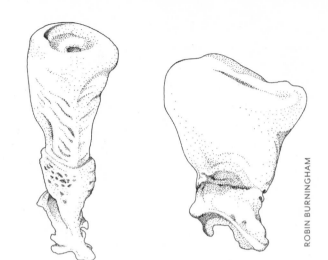

21. The vaginal barrel:
Well-supported   Weakly supported

any tactile nerve endings in the vagina? What feels good during intercourse is the PC muscle.

If the muscle is strong and tight around the vagina, the woman is capable of feeling a great deal of pleasure during intercourse from the deep-touch stimulation of the nerve endings in the PC muscles. If the muscle is weak, all those great nerve endings are wasted. They're too far away to receive sufficient stimulation from the thrusting penis. So, with a good, strong PC muscle you can get more enjoyment from sex.

Dr. Arnold Kegel taught PC exercises to every woman he saw in his gynecological practice. He was concerned with teaching women to flex this muscle to keep the uterus up high and to prevent it from dropping downward with a saggy muscle. Over the years he heard again and again, "Dr. Kegel, since you taught me those exercises I've started climaxing during intercourse. Do you think the exercises had anything to do with it?"

It turned out that Dr. Kegel had accidentally stumbled across the biggest find of the century in female sexual response, and he hadn't even been looking for it! Here was a basic key to female climaxing: having a PC muscle in good tone.

THE PC MUSCLE AND BIRTH

But this is a book about childbirth, so how does this muscle fit into the birth picture?

Simple. The baby is pushed out through the birth canal, of course, and the birth canal is surrounded by the PC muscle. You might think by looking at the pictures that the mother with the short canal would just drop her baby out, while the mother with the long narrow canal would have things harder. *Not so.*

The woman with the wide, loose vaginal barrel will find herself in trouble when she's actually pushing her baby down her saggy birth canal. As her baby passes through her vaginal barrel, the soft unsupported tissue is likely to be pulled forward and dragged downward with the baby's progress. This can result in pinched, torn tissues. This mother is likely to suffer damage to her vagina.

Such damage rarely happens to a trained mother who has learned and practiced the exercise for the PC muscle. She has a strong hammock of muscle surrounding and supporting her vaginal barrel. The tissues are firmly held in place and well supported as the baby passes through.

You now have some great reasons to want to make sure you have a strong, well-exercised muscle: to make love happily; to stay healthy; and to enjoy giving birth to your baby.

HOW TO IDENTIFY THE KEGEL MUSCLE

The next time you are urinating, with your legs apart, stop the flow without putting your knees together. This does not mean you have a strong muscle, but it helps you to be sure you know exactly what muscle we're talking about.

The exercise itself is simple. It is the same squeezing motion you performed to stop the flow of urine, only you can squeeze much stronger and tighter when you are not urinating. We have three ways for you to exercise this muscle.

HOW TO PRACTICE THE KEGEL EXERCISE

The Beginning PC Exercise

Flex the PC muscle tightly. Make it a deep flex. If you are pinching your buttocks together then you are using the wrong set of muscles. A feeling of strain in the lower abdomen would mean the same thing.

If you observe a proper flex closely, what you should feel is the PC muscle tightening first at the back near the rectum and then as you continue to tighten harder you feel it moving foward and toward the clitoris. After a little practice you should be able to flex tightly and deeply just the PC muscle, with abdominal muscles and buttocks uninvolved.

Now, how often should you flex this muscle? Well, let me ask you this. If I asked you for five minutes of actual exercise a day, wouldn't you think that extraordinarily reasonable? Just five minutes? Right. And how many flexes does that make at a quick second or so a flex? Three hundred flexes! But come on now, it's only five minutes of actual exercise, and if you pause to rest for a second or so between contractions, it's still only a ten-minute-a-day exercise program. It was Dr. Kegel himself who recommended contracting the muscle 300 times a day.

Do not stop at just flexing the outer lips of the vaginal opening. This is just a very slight flex. *Concentrate on flexing deeply inside the vagina and way up high.*

TO THE COACH

If you are a husband coaching your wife, remember—she can be a great athlete and still have a saggy PC muscle. Or she could be totally out of shape otherwise and have a strong one. It doesn't relate to her general strength. A husband is the best person to know what condition her muscle is in. Can she squeeze and hold your penis during intercourse? Don't criticize her, but encourage her to exercise regularly.

It is important that you do this beginning PC exercise program each day until you get a good tight flex. It should feel as distinct as clenching your hand. As soon as you get to this point (days for some, a week or two for others), then you will want to move right on to the intermediate PC exercises, which will get you to a very elastic (stretchy), strong muscle (the kind that supports the vaginal barrel and prevents damage). Then go on to the advanced PC exercises, which will give you the ability to consciously release (like opening the hand) to give birth to your baby.

THE INTERMEDIATE PC EXERCISE

When you have achieved the definite flex of the PC and are able to repeat it numerous times, you are ready for this intermediate exercise. Discontinue the 300 flexes.

Here we'll ask you to flex your muscle thirty-six times a day, but when you do, hold it to the count of ten before releasing. Try it now. Flex, two, three, four, five, six, seven, eight, nine, ten, and release. Again, flex, two, three, four, five—*don't let it slip, keep holding it tightly and deeply*—eight, nine, ten, and release. The trick is to hold that flex as strongly on your tenth count as you do on your first.

With this new exercise you are well on your way to achieving a strong, supportive hammock of muscles. We suggest you do this twelve times in the morning, before you get out of bed, twelve times in the afternoon, and twelve times at night before going to sleep.

ADVANCED PC EXERCISE

When you have the ability to hold that flex as in the intermediate exercise, you can discontinue the thirty-six flexes a day, and you are ready for the advanced conscious-release exercises. You will use this releasing ability deliberately when you are pushing your baby out.

Flex just the outer third of the vaginal barrel, now the middle part of the vaginal barrel, and now think of flexing way up high.

Now release up high, release the middle third, and release the lower third of the vaginal barrel.

You can think of it like an elevator going up three floors, stopping momentarily at each floor, and then going down three floors as you let go of this contraction.

At this point you can do about a dozen regular flexes a day to retain the tone you have gained and then do about six one-two-three, release-two-three exercises.

Just a couple of times before the birth of your baby you should try placing your hand on your perineum, and as you are doing a release-two-three exercise, try going beyond that and actively bulge your perineum outward as you release even more. It helps to feel that slight bulging down and out as you release the muscle and direct a small amount of downward pressure toward the vaginal outlet. Don't practice the bulging regularly, just try it out a couple of times before birth so you will be aware of what you are aiming for when you are really pushing your baby out.

TO KEGEL OR NOT TO KEGEL

These important Kegel exercises are under attack. The latest fad is to tell women to stop flexing the Kegel muscle, claiming that it makes it weaker, makes it sag. While the blog promoting this idea was posted some years ago, it seems to just now be going viral. This is a key exercise, an evidence-based exercise, important not just for birthing but for a woman's long-term health, making it essential to address this challenge head-on for your benefit. To start with: *This was a hypothesis.*

Belief should be evidence-based. Science demands evidence to support hypothesis, so let's look first at the "stop Kegeling" hypothesis and then at the evidence. This is a direct quote from the original blog.

> Because the PF [kegel] muscles attach from the coccyx to the pubic bone, the closer these bony attachments get, the more slack in the PF (the PF becomes a hammock).

Now, how do your pelvic bones get closer, making the Kegel sag between them? According to this hypothesis, exercising the Kegel muscle pulls these bones closer together (which it can, yes) and that is supposed to result in the Kegel muscles dangling down between the bones.

However, that is impossible in this scenario. Here's why: A pull is a force; that is basic physics. If the bones are pulled enough to come closer, the Kegel has to *keep up the pull, it has to keep up the force,* so the Kegel muscle cannot then dangle down between the bones, as the bones would *not be pulled* closer together.

Doing Kegel exercises regularly *shortens* the muscles; that is, after all, the goal. To say *tightens* or *strengthens* blurs understanding. Definition is essential to clarity. After doing the exercises regularly, the Kegel muscles attain a greater "resting tension" state. That means, when you aren't even flexing it, its "at rest" state of tension (its shortened state) has been increased, which is exactly why it helps to prevent incontinence as it lifts and supports the bladder.

So here's the bottom line: The Kegel muscle doesn't hang down between these bones when the muscles are shortened by exercising; it can't dangle down *and also* exert a pull between the front and the back of the pelvis. This is basic physics. A pull is a force; a shortened muscle is required in this case in order to exert that force. A sagging muscle exerts no force and wouldn't be pulling those bones together in the first place. And this is exactly what is faulty with this premise. The Kegel cannot both pull on the bones and sag; it can do one or the other, but not both at the same time.

So, we have examined a premise (hypothesis) and found a flaw in the logic. The next most important step is looking at **evidence**.

I quote again from the same original site advocating that women "stop Kegeling":

> But, I've got all of the science backing it up and it makes sense, the Kegel is just such a huge part of our inherited culture information, no one bothered to examine it.

There isn't any evidence in that quote, and it includes the absolutely incorrect statement that no one bothered to examine the efficacy of Kegeling. In fact, Dr. Kegel did just that. *He tested his hypothesis.*

First: He used a perineometer (like a plastic penis attached to a gauge) and *measured, quantified, and verified* the degree of improvement in the Kegel muscle itself. He *defined* improvement as the degree of change in the constant *resting state* of tension in the Kegel muscle (when the woman was not consciously flexing the muscle) as well as the degree of change in the woman's ability to exert conscious pressure while flexing the PC muscle. In science, that is what you are always trying to do: *quantify* results. He was able to document improvement over and over again by quantifying all this before the woman started Kegeling and then after three months. He also made casts of the *result* of Kegeling, casts of the vagina before and after Kegeling, and this provided proof of the connection between Kegeling and the significant improvement in organ support. (Advocates of not Kegeling claim that two or three squats a day will keep the Kegel muscles strong.) *Dr. Kegel didn't teach squatting; he taught only Kegeling to produce these results.*

This is the difference between theory and evidence. Dr. Kegel gave us evidence.

If you want even more, particularly those of you who are health educators, nurse-midwives, yoga teachers, chiropractors, or anyone working with pregnant women, here's a quote that should interest you. It comes from the highly respected Cochrane Reviews.

> The review of trials found that pelvic floor muscle training (muscle-clenching exercises) helps women with all types of incontinence although women with stress incontinence who exercise for three months or more benefit most. [3]

Squatting is, indeed, an important exercise for a number of reasons, and Bradley Childbirth Educators have always taught squatting, but Kegeling is *the* most important exercise for keeping that Kegel muscle in good shape. *Keep on Kegeling!*

A LIFETIME EXERCISE PLAN FOR
AFTER THE BIRTH OF THE BABY

You can begin PC contractions again right after birth. In fact, it restores circulation and helps to promote healing, and since the exercise has such impact on your health, you will undoubtedly want to continue PC exercising to prevent uterine prolapse. Although Kegel exercises are the well-known prophylactic measure to prevent and even correct uterine prolapse, many women are never informed about them. You will want to develop a lifelong exercise habit for these muscles that becomes effortless for you. I do my PC exercises at red lights. Since I manage to hit every one in town, I easily get at least a hundred PC contractions in each day with hardly a thought to it. Find something that you do every day that you can connect your exercises to and make them a lifelong habit for health.

PART II

THE FIRST STAGE

OF BIRTH

CHAPTER ELEVEN

Getting Ready for Labor

As **YOU BEGIN TO** think about your own labor and birth, you are probably already asking yourself: When is this going to happen? Will I know? What are the normal signs? You already know that the flattening of your cervix, known as effacement, is a step toward giving birth, but that it doesn't tell you when birth will happen. And you already know that engagement, or the baby "dropping" lower into your pelvis, is also usually a part of the process, but that doesn't tell you when labor will begin, either.

In fact, early in your pregnancy your doctor probably gave you a "due date," but frankly, that doesn't tell you much about when birth will happen, either.

First of all, unless you are absolutely sure when conception took place, there is no firm date from which to begin counting the gestation period. Counting from the last menstrual period already allows a week or two of leeway on either side of what might be your real due date. But, most important, no two women are alike and neither are any two babies. So it is quite impossible, even if you know the date of conception, to say exactly when a baby will be born.

The best that can be hoped for is to have a good estimate, and that is all that a realistic due date can be. Your doctor would be doing you a real favor if he would tell you to expect your baby "toward the end of August or early September" rather than "August 25" or even "the fourth week in August," when you ask (as you certainly will), "When am I due?" And you would be doing your family and friends a real favor if you would give them that kind of loose estimate about when the baby is due.

There are several reasons for this. First of all, you are going to reach a point when you will be ready to strangle the next person who says to you, "Still pregnant?" It puts a lot of stress on you to know that everyone is watching the calendar as closely as you will be if you have set a specific date in your mind.

Remember, no one has been pregnant forever and the baby knows when it is time to be born. It will happen when the baby and your body are ready.

Furthermore, while you will often hear women say, "My labor began at 3 P.M. on Wednesday," in many cases there is nothing that precise about when labor begins. At that point a series of things will be happening in your body over a period of time that could be as long as a week or more. The uterus may try out a contraction or two and then decide to wait for another day. Or you might have contractions over several hours and get quite excited (naturally), only to have the uterus stop and wait to start again later in the week.

This is often called "false labor," but there is really nothing false about it. It is part of a process that will begin and stop on its own until it is ready to begin in earnest. Who is to say that those early contractions are not really an important part of the whole process of giving birth?

If you count your labor from the first of those tentative contractions of the uterine muscles, you will be able to amaze (and probably frighten) your friends by telling them how long your labor was. But if you wait until labor is definitely under way with good, strong, working contractions that require your complete attention, you may well have a much shorter labor to tell about.

How you count your labor is important to you psychologically. It could make the difference between a birth you will later describe as hard work, to be sure, but a manageable, joyful experience, and a birth you will describe as difficult and exhausting. But it is not just your attitude that is at stake, especially if you are giving birth in a hospital.

The latest trend in obstetrical medicine is to set time limits on birth and to intervene in the process if those limits are not met. For example, in *Active Management of Labour*, by Drs. Kieran O'Driscoll and Declan Meagher (London: W. B. Saunders Co., 1980), obstetricians are urged to put a twelve-hour limit on birth from the start of labor. I know, here it is 2017, but this 1980s book still dominates today's obstetrics! If within a few hours the woman is not on schedule, labor will be "speeded up" with drugs. Though it seems incredible to put a single, hard-and-fast time limit on all women who give birth (even though it should be obvious that women of different sizes, ages, physical conditions, and temperaments will have different birth patterns), it frequently happens.

There are often other time limits imposed on labor, as we will examine later; but for now, it is important for you to realize that birth is a natural process that will occur when your body is ready, with no reference to some imprecise due date, and that once labor begins it will also move forward at its own rate and not on some schedule imposed by others.

Your body knows what to do. It will naturally lead you through the three stages of birth: opening the cervix, pushing out the baby, and expelling the placenta. From the preceding several chapters you have a pretty good idea of what happens within the body during labor. Now it is time to begin to learn the labor techniques. These are the skills that will help you tune in to your body and work *with* your labor.

Relaxation is simple but not easy—at least not until you learn to do it thoroughly and well. That will take more than just learning the theories of relaxation. You must practice until it becomes natural for you.

So be forewarned. You can flip through this book, devouring all the information on controversies in childbirth and making lists of choices for yourself. But if you skip or just skim through this and the following chapters on labor skills, you may as well put your list aside. You will only get to use it by going into labor fully prepared with a lot of practice behind you.

RELAXATION

Your primary concern in labor, above all else, is to relax. Learn to relax as if your life depended upon it. This section will lay the groundwork for the skill of relaxation. If you cannot find a Bradley class in your area, you will want to come back to this section again and again. Master it thoroughly. It is your foundation, and everything else builds upon it.

The purpose of this extreme relaxation response is just to stay out of the way with a limp body and allow the uterus to do its work unimpeded by other bodily tensions. This may sound easy. *It is simple, but not easy.* It takes all of your concentration to keep your whole body really limp and sagging, letting go everywhere as the uterine contraction builds and builds to a peak of strength.

The uterus is just a bag of muscles, but it is the largest collection of muscles you have, and when it flexes you can really feel it as a powerful sensation. You will not eliminate this sensation with what we will teach you, but you will learn to do the right things while that muscular bag is flexing, so that you are working for you and your baby, not against yourself.

Take a look at picture 22. As you recall, you have long muscles that go from the top of the uterus down to the cervix, the muscles that contract or flex to pull the cervix back. Each time they flex or contract during labor, they get a little shorter and stay retracted. They just continue to shorten all through first-stage labor until the cervix is drawn completely back and open. But you can also see the opposite muscle group here, the circular muscles that are most heavily concentrated at the bottom of the uterus near the cervix. These muscles keep the door of the cervix closed while you are pregnant; but in labor, while the long muscles flex and shorten, the circular muscles must lengthen and relax to allow the cervix to be drawn back. These are involuntary muscles. They will work for you in labor no matter what you do, yet you can have an effect on them. Let's see how.

Remember how a contraction starts at the top of the uterus. The long muscles reaching down toward the cervix

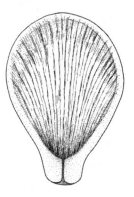 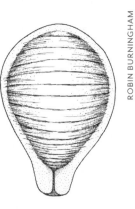

ROBIN BURNINGHAM

LONGITUDINAL MUSCLE FIBERS

CIRCULAR MUSCLE FIBERS

22. Long muscles of the uterus contract or shorten to pull the cervix back for you.

Circular muscles of the uterus relax and lengthen to allow the long muscles to pull the cervix back.

begin to flex. They work a little bit more and continue to shorten. They keep on flexing and shortening until you get a good, strong stretching and pulling sensation at the cervix. Now, what do you think the untrained mother does when she feels a contraction start slowly and work more and even a bit more? You are right, of course, she tenses her body and clenches her teeth to get ready for another one of those contractions. We call this fighting labor.

The woman who fights labor makes contractions last longer. She makes her work much harder by tensing against it. When you are tensed, the uterus has to work harder to get the same amount done with each contraction. It is not accomplishing twice as much, just working twice as hard. So, you must acquire the know-how and concentration to relax. This is a skill that must be acquired through practice, and the untrained mother is not very good at it.

Often when a woman is fighting labor, a well-meaning nurse will say, "Try to relax, honey." The mother bravely tries for a couple of contractions. But does she genuinely relax her body and go limp? No, instead she imitates relaxation by *holding herself still*. She cannot consciously and deliberately let everything go loose and slack. Muscle groups throughout her body are tensed and contracted. She gets no comfort from an imitation of relaxation.

THE BEST POSITION FOR LABOR

Relaxation begins with a comfortable position that makes it easy; it is quite difficult to relax in a position that causes stress or strain. If you could walk through a labor ward in most hospitals, you would find almost all of the untrained mothers lying flat on their backs throughout most of labor. Yet all the current research shows this position to be dangerous to the laboring woman and to her unborn child. Why? The largest blood vessel runs in back of the uterus. If you think of your baby's weight as a bowling ball, you can easily imagine what happens to this large blood vessel when you lie on your back. It is pinched between the pelvic bones and the weight of the baby. And when this circulation is interfered with, your baby's oxygen and nutrient supply is impeded.

A coach should remind the pregnant woman not to lie on her back from about the seventh month of pregnancy through the end of labor. Sounds easy, doesn't it? You think to yourself, "I know it and she knows it, so she won't lie on her back." Yet, when a woman is in labor she is so wrapped up in what is happening inside her body that there is a tendency to remain in whatever position she happens to be in. So if in the hospital, for example, she is examined (for which she must be on her back briefly), she will likely just remain on her back out of inertia. If the coach simply says, "Okay, it is time to get off your back. Let's turn over now," she will readily comply. She just needs some encouragement and help getting started.

Since the pregnant woman cannot lie on her back and she probably won't care to lie on her tummy, that leaves the side as the best lying-down position for labor. (There is an alternate sitting-up position we will go into later.) Picture 23 will show you a comfortable and safe position for labor. It is important, so please study the details carefully. This is a balanced position, worked out by a physical therapist. Each part of the body is equally supported and no part is resting on any other part. There is no lopsided stress or strain on any part.

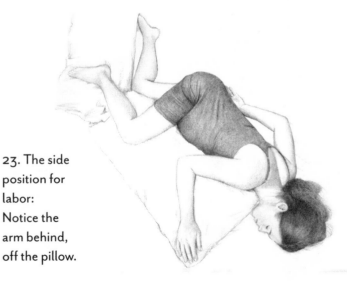

23. The side position for labor: Notice the arm behind, off the pillow.

ERICK INGRAHAM

- Notice the slight curve to the spine and to the whole body.
- The chin should be slightly toward the chest but not on it. Avoid tilting the head back, causing strain on the muscles.
- Elbows and knees should be bent. Keeping them straight creates strain and tension, which you want to avoid completely during labor.
- Use a *flat* pillow under the head. This will keep it level with the neck and in line with the body. Avoid fluffy pillows that prop the head up at an unnatural angle, causing tension. The pillow can be pulled forward and tucked into your chest if this is comfortable.

- The top leg should be extended outward, bent at the knee, and then supported with at least two pillows, one on top of the other. Long pillows that support the entire leg and the foot are best. Having the top leg almost level with the top hip will avoid tension and an aching sensation there.
- Place the bottom shoulder and arm on the bed behind you. Do not rest the shoulder on the pillow. If it is placed on the pillow, the shoulder will feel strained.

Remember, this is a balanced position. It is designed to avoid strain and tension. You will find this most comfortable on a firm mattress (like those on hospital beds) or on a carpeted floor at home. If your bed is too soft it will not be comfortable when you practice, because your body is not given the support it needs. Try this position and have your coach check you out, comparing your position with the illustration and checking all the points.

TO THE COACH

Is your wife grumbling about the arm and shoulder behind her? They are often not very comfortable at first, because she may be stretching muscles and ligaments that haven't been used this way before. Practice is what makes her ready for labor.

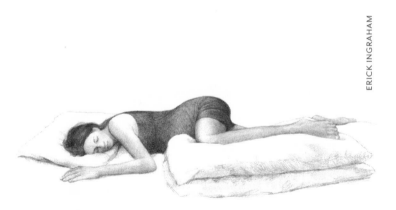

ERICK INGRAHAM

What about pulling her arm under herself, as she may do in sleep? This is a poor substitute for the preferred position because of the pressure on the lower arm. The circulation is cut off quickly in the arm, and discomfort soon sets in. She can get away with sleeping like that for a while, but labor takes intense concentration, and the discomfort from a less-than-perfect position can distract her terribly. This position you have just learned was designed to maximize comfort.

Now ask her to turn over and help her get up in the position on her other side. Be careful to arrange the pillows to support the entire upper leg and foot and to keep that leg even with the hip. In labor you will want to turn her over from her favorite side to her other side every hour or hour and a half to ensure even circulation. She need only stay on her less favorite side for about ten minutes before turning back, if she prefers.

TWO KEYS TO RELAXATION

Once you have mastered this position for labor, there are two keys to skilled relaxation. The first is *observation*. Here is an exercise in observation, *not in relaxation*, for you both to try. Take turns with one of you lying in the side position while the other reads the exercise aloud.

- Tighten up all of your facial muscles, hard. That is extreme tension. It is easy to spot. Now relax.
- Now tighten your shoulders very hard. Just hunch them up. You are very aware of that tension, aren't you. Since you are so aware of it, it is easy to release it now.

But extreme tension is not what you stumble over in labor. The tension you will need to watch for is much more subtle than that. Here are some samples of what you need to look for in labor and to deliberately, consciously release.

- Tighten just a few muscles in your face. Just a slight frown and a few tight facial muscles. You would probably not notice this tension while working around the house or while preoccupied at work. Now, relax your face.

Could you spot that kind of tension in labor? You must be aware of it to release it. *Observation is the first key to relaxation.*

- Now, tighten your shoulders just slightly, hardly enough for anyone else to see. You must be able to recognize the sensation of slight tension in order to concentrate on releasing it. Now relax. You cannot relax to any great depth unless you are skillful at observation.

The ability to relax during contractions directly relates to your degree of comfort during labor.

- Tighten your leg extremely. That is easy to spot. Now release. Tighten just a few muscles in your leg ever so slightly. Imagine that a nurse comes in to check you in the hospital, and when she leaves you are not quite as deeply relaxed as before. Would you notice it? You must be aware of tension, the flexed or shortened muscles in your body, before you can deliberately release them.

You cannot be skillful at relaxation until you are good at deliberately and continuously observing your body. Look for tension, notice it, and let it go.

Now the woman should read this exercise in observation (remember it is not a *relaxation* exercise) to her coach. A coach should be just as familiar with the subtlety of sensations in tension. Try making the same comparisons before going on.

The second key to skillful relaxation is *consciously releasing tension*. (Some birth classes confuse observation exercises with relaxation and never take you on to the next step.) Once you are familiar with the feeling of tension and are able to recognize it, you will be able to *concentrate on deliberately letting it go*.

This is not at all like relaxing to go to sleep. Most of us climb into bed and wait for our bodies to relax. Few of us know how to deliberately release tension from our bodies.

You cannot hold yourself still in labor and wait for your body to relax and sag just because you are in a sleep position. Relaxation will never come. You must practice observing your muscles over and over and then *deliberately releasing tension*. Never be satisfied. You can always let go a little more. Be prepared to spend fifteen to twenty minutes a day in the last months of your pregnancy consciously practicing relaxing your whole body.

RELAXING THROUGH A CONTRACTION

Now it is time to put the relaxation skills you are learning together with the special position and to practice what you will do in a real working contraction of labor. Coach, have your wife lie on her side and check to be sure her body is arranged properly and well supported by pillows (no parts resting on other parts and no dangling hands or feet). Be sure her eyes are closed so she can concentrate. Read the following demonstration aloud at least twice and then put the book down and try it twice on your own. Your goal is to help the laboring woman be totally relaxed for the first stage of labor, which takes practice and skill.

Speaking quietly into her ear with conviction and loving attention, talk her through a contraction as follows, urging her to relax her whole body from head to toe. Pause for a moment between naming each muscle group to let her consciously eliminate the tension before moving on to the next one. This practice contraction should last about one minute:

PRACTICE EXERCISE A:
RELAXING THROUGH A CONTRACTION

- Relax your whole body. Let it sink into the mattress.
- Drop your head down into the pillow; don't hold it up with your neck muscles.
- Relax all the muscles in your face. Really think about them and release.
- Smooth your forehead. Let go with all the tiny muscles around your eyes. Have a relaxed, open throat and let your jaw hang open. Don't try to swallow. (It's even OK to drool on the pillow—that is how relaxed you are, just like you are when you are in deep sleep.)
- Let go of all the tension in your neck. Let it go out of your shoulders. Locate any tightness there and let it flow away. You can always release a little bit more.
- Don't just hold yourself still. Really release and let the tension go. Look for any tightness and deliberately release. Relax as if your life depended upon it.
- Let go with your arms and let any tension go out through your hands and your fingertips. *Have loose, limp fingers.*

- Relax your chest and your abdomen. Think of your tummy sagging and floating out and away from you as it sinks down into the mattress. The stronger the contraction becomes, the more you release and let go with your tummy, sagging extremely. You can always release a little bit more.
- Let go of any tension in your hips and thighs. Let your legs sink down into the mattress and the pillows. Locate any tension in your legs and let it flow out through your feet. Your whole body should be loose and limp.
- Let that big bag of muscles flex *for* you and just concentrate on that powerful sensation of the biggest muscles in your body working and working to open the door to the uterus.
- Let your whole body sag and go limp and get out of the way so that big bag of muscles can do its job. Concentrate on relaxation and release extremely. You can always let go a little bit more.
- *Think* your way up and over this contraction, locating any tension that is left in your body and letting it go, letting it ease out through your hands and feet.

The practice contraction is over. Do not go on until you have read this twice aloud and done it twice without the book, using your own words. You simply start at the head and say what you see: facial muscles, jaw, neck, shoulders, and so on. You don't have to memorize this series exactly as it is written here. But you do have to practice saying it your own way, again and again. Anything you desire to do skillfully requires practice. Repetition is the best way to get it down pat.

TO THE COACH

During labor you have an important part to play in helping the pregnant woman to relax. Indeed, coaching contractions is one of the most important things you are going to be doing during that time. And for this, practice is essential, so that when the day comes the basic coaching skills are second-nature to you.

Don't think for a minute that it is all right to know these things in theory but that you probably will not actually need them. You will need them. These techniques really work and will be much easier to do after a long familiarity through practice.

Though even your wife may think that a lot of practice is unnecessary now, after the birth you both will be happy you took the time to get ready properly. One thing couples in our classes always tell others when they return after their births is, "We are glad we practiced a lot. It really paid off and we think that is the most important advice we can pass on to you."

The first few times you actually coach a contraction can be awkward. It is play-acting, after all, something that most people are not too comfortable with, even in the privacy of home. No one laughs when we coach in class, but there will probably be a lot of giggling the first few times both of you try to coach through a pretend contraction. Laugh together, let the laughing go, and keep at it.

As you practice, don't coach in a monotone or a dull, droning voice. After all, you are not trying to hypnotize her or put her to sleep. The pregnant woman in labor must *think* her way through a contraction. She must use her brain, actively observing her body and concentrating on deliberately releasing tension in her muscles no matter how slight the tension seems, so you want to help her keep mentally alert and thinking. You will need to talk with inflection, thinking yourself about what you are saying, helping her continue with her concentration. Just saying, "Relax your arms, relax your legs, relax your thighs," won't do it. Use different words with an earnest, urgent, actively inflected but calm, soothing voice.

You will find the coaching role in labor similar to the role of a swimming coach. When the swimmer puts it all together, the coach stands by, saying, "Stroke, kick, breathe, reach out farther, keep kicking, etc." The swimming coach is the objective observer and is able to give direction as needed. When the new swimmer is in the middle of the pool and feeling tired or discouraged, the coach offers encouragement and praise. The labor coach is also an objective observer. He (or she) can see how close the laboring woman is to her goal while the woman may be thinking she will never get there. But, like the swimmer, the laboring woman must know her skills and practice them. Then and only then can coaches be of great help.

CHAPTER TWELVE

More on Relaxation: Backaches to Breathing

THERE IS ANOTHER IMPORTANT skill for the coach to learn, and that is how to deal with the backache that the laboring woman frequently experiences. Most women, but not all, have a backache while experiencing strong contractions. The ache begins as a contraction begins, gets stronger as the contraction gets stronger, and goes away as the contraction ends.

Why? The uterus is kept in place by ligaments. If you look back at picture 6 on page 52, you will see one of the two round ligaments in the front, mooring the uterus to the pelvic floor. You may feel these ligaments during pregnancy if you bend over and then stand up too fast. The muscles can sort of buckle under, giving you a sharp pain that quickly disappears. (Remember, there are no sudden, stabbing pains in labor.) Nothing is wrong with you or your baby, and you are not starting labor. What you felt is just a kink from standing up too fast.

You have two ligaments in the back, too, called the uterosacral ligaments. Take another look at picture 6 and you will see them. They look like two thick rubber bands stretching from the uterus to either side of the spine. With each contraction in labor, the uterus pulls forward and puts traction on its anchor point through the uterosacral ligaments, causing the backache that occurs in many labors.

TO THE COACH: THE BACKACHE

Coach, your wife cannot concentrate 100 percent on her task if she is bothered by this uncomfortable backache. So it is your job to clear this obstacle to her concentration. You must take care of the ache. You do this by applying counterpressure in the form of a back rub. It sounds easy, but don't forget, in a "textbook" labor you may be rubbing while contractions occur for fourteen hours. One coach recalled it this way:

"With our first baby I rubbed Sandy's back for twelve hours. My arms were killing me for days after the baby was born. But I couldn't stop, and I couldn't feel sorry for myself. She surely did need that back rub, and I was the only one around who cared enough to give it to her constantly. She labored beautifully, quietly concentrating completely. She says the back rub she received freed her to put all her attention on her relaxation and breathing."

As coach, you need to get this back-rub technique down pat if you expect the laboring woman to do well with labor:

- Be sure to rub exactly where it aches. Obviously, she will be able to tell you just where that is. The spot is not in the small of the back nor all the way down at the tailbone, but usually somewhere in between. You should rub this spot in a small, tight circle. She will tell you just where to rub, and she is the one to please.
- The heel of your hand or the front of your fist usually works best for this back rub. You may find it helpful to wrap your hand in a soft cloth, like an old T-shirt.
- Have your hand in place before the contraction starts. Don't wait for her to tell you the contraction is under way and then try to put your hand on her back. That's sloppy. It is exactly what the untrained husband does when trying to help his wife, and it's exactly why she tells him to leave her alone.

- Rub with a slow, steady rhythm in one direction. If you break the rhythm it distracts her attention immediately and she may snap at you.
- Press your hand firmly into the back and then rotate it in a circular motion. Do not slide your hand over her skin. That is irritating and will soon leave a raw feeling. Press inward—it will require *a lot* of pressure—and let the skin move with your hand in that circular motion. This is a deep massage.

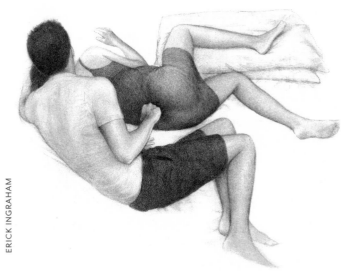

ERICK INGRAHAM

24. Back rub: Do this with great attention to detail, in precisely the right spot for her.

Be forewarned—the most common error is to rub too fast. It must be a slow, steady, deep rub. And don't make the mistake of changing the direction of the rub in the middle of a contraction, even though your arm may feel tired. You will get an instant cranky reaction. The laboring woman is acutely aware of the minutest details (even though she may not seem to be), and a sudden shift in direction is sure to distract her attention from relaxation. Be sure your rubbing motion is steady and rhythmic, with no jerky, uneven movements.

A sloppy back rub may be even more disturbing to the laboring woman than the backache. She senses the coach is tired and not doing a thorough and careful job. She may also feel annoyed because he seems to lack empathy for the intensity of the sensations she is feeling. So to get the back rub right, it will be necessary to practice. It is a little like an isometric exercise, and you may be surprised at how hard she will want you to push. One coach said we should have told him to practice by rubbing a brick wall.

To practice, get the pregnant woman into the side position again and check her out to make sure she has no part resting on any other part and no limbs dangling. The coach needs to find a comfortable position, too, to get good leverage, since a lot of pressure will probably be required. Locate the place where the backache will probably be felt, between the small of the back and the tailbone. Now begin the back rub as you coach some more practice contractions, coaching and rubbing for sixty to ninety seconds and resting for a few minutes in between. Look back at Chapter Eleven if you need a reminder about coaching the muscle groups from head to toe to help her relax.

Even before labor begins, the back rub is quite soothing and you will have little trouble getting her to let you practice it. And once you have learned the back rub, it will serve you well long after the baby comes. The same technique offers great relief for the backache that often accompanies the beginning of a menstrual period. If you can help your wife with that you will earn her eternal gratitude.

ROUND LIGAMENT ACHE

Though less common than the backache, occasionally a woman will have an ache in front in the round ligaments that attach the uterus to the pelvic floor. Like the backache, this ache starts at the beginning of a contraction, gets stronger, and diminishes as the contraction goes away. It is handled much like a backache, except the laboring woman will definitely not want as hard a massage on her tummy as she would on her back. You must talk to her to learn the exact degree of pressure that she desires (it may be very little) and exactly where to rub.

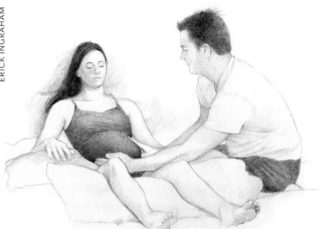

25. For round ligament ache: Rub in two places, using a circular or back-and-forth motion.

As with the back rub, have your hands in place before the contraction begins, massage with a steady, even rhythm, and never switch directions in the middle of a contraction. Use a circular or back-and-forth motion, but now it will be in two places on the front instead of one on the back. And like the back rub, this massage must be done with concentration and concern because the pregnant woman is very sensitive to a sloppy or halfhearted effort.

Do not confuse the round ligament ache with a crampy sensation low in the abdomen. That crampiness can be taken care of by relaxing the tummy extremely. How do you distinguish between the two? Easy. A crampy sensation would be experienced all across the lower part of the abdomen. The round ligament ache would be limited to two areas, perhaps spreading down the legs.

AN ALTERNATE POSITION FOR FIRST STAGE

The massage for round ligament ache is hard to do while the laboring woman is on her side in the position we have taught you for labor, but there is an alternate, called the contour-chair position, which some women find helpful for first stage. I have personally never used this position for first stage because I truly believe that deeper relaxation is possible in the side position. (Although some believe sitting and standing may shorten labor somewhat, I do not consider mere speed a benefit, especially if it is paid for at the price of lessened comfort.)

However, some women are just not comfortable on their sides during labor. If you find that you are one of them, then this contour-chair position is a good second choice. It will still get you up high enough to avoid some of the problems that come from lying flat on the back. Look at picture 26 to see the position. Hospital beds are good for this position because their backs can be rolled up to a forty-five-degree angle (anything less puts too much weight on the vessels bringing blood to the uterus and oxygen and nutrients to the baby), and the bottom can often be cranked up to support the knees. At home a lot of pillows will be needed, or perhaps a large bean-bag chair. Even in the hospital, you will need one or two pillows to support each arm, another for the head, and more still for under the knees if the bed does not crank up. If you cannot get enough pillows, don't bother with this position at all. Arms that just dangle rather than being supported cause strain on muscles and increase tension. Of course, elbows and knees are slightly bent in this position as in the side position to avoid strain and tension. Try this position out now, so that if you need to use it you will be familiar with it.

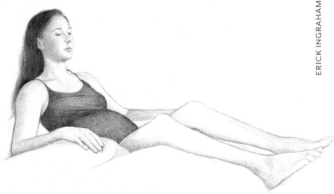

26. Contour-chair position

ERICK INGRAHAM

BREATHING IN LABOR

What about breathing during the contractions? As mentioned earlier, you will learn no altered-breathing states in the Bradley Method®. You have been breathing all your life, and by now you are quite good at it. It is important for both the laboring woman and her baby that her breathing be calm, steady, and normal. All you need to learn is how to *observe* your breathing, so that if it becomes too fast or irregular you can deliberately return it to a calm, steady rhythm. Remember, normal breathing is a reflection of good relaxation, and relaxation is the real key to a successful labor.

Let's return to that poor, untrained mother for a moment. Does she breathe normally during labor? No. Instead, she may breathe in three common patterns: sometimes she panics and breathes in a rapid *pant* (this is actually quite dangerous since it can cause hyperventilation); or she may breathe in irregular gasps; or she may simply stop breathing during a contraction and hold her breath.

All these ways of mishandling breathing spell panic, tension, and discomfort for the mother. The laboring woman needs to keep her breathing simple and normal since her primary aim is complete, skillful relaxation. To ensure that relaxation, the laboring woman should use abdominal breathing, which simply means putting calm, steady breaths deep and low into the abdomen. Therapists in various fields use calm, abdominal breathing to relax excited patients, from asthmatics to the emotionally upset.

The key to abdominal breathing is just to *listen* to the quiet, regular rhythm of your breathing. Think of putting your breath low in the abdomen with an extremely relaxed abdominal wall. The abdomen will naturally expand outward with low abdominal breathing, so you do not need to push the abdomen out or try to hold it there. If you are listening within your body to the calm, quiet, steady rhythm of your breathing, it is impossible to breathe too quickly. If you are concentrating on putting the breath low in the abdomen, it is easy to avoid the chest breathing that can quickly lead to hyperventilation.

When you are practicing, here is the way to check this simple, natural breathing. The coach should sit on the floor with his back to the wall, forming a contour chair for the pregnant woman, who sits between his legs. A thin pillow between the two of you should make this position more comfortable. Reaching around her body, the coach should put his hands on the woman's abdomen, just about at the top of the pubic hair line. Now, the pregnant woman should try abdominal breathing. There will be some movement in the chest, of course, but the real action in this kind of breathing will be felt down low in the abdomen. Do not

tense the abdominal wall or try to push it out; simply put the breath way down low, and the abdomen will expand out and away naturally, and the coach will feel the abdomen rise gently beneath his hand.

There are four main points to coaching the breathing during a contraction. Read them aloud twice and then close the book to make sure you have the four points and can express them in your own words.

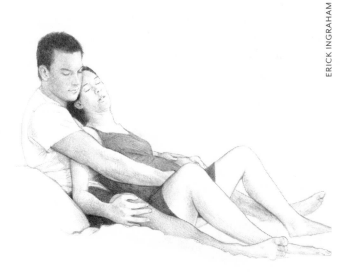

ERICK INGRAHAM

27. This position allows the coach to see and feel your relaxed abdominal breathing. Use this position to start off your practicing and then try it out on your side.

- Listen to the sound of your breathing.
- Hear the quiet, even, steady rhythm.
- Think of putting the air way down low in the abdomen.
- Relax the tummy extremely and let it just expand outward naturally as you breathe in.

Try coaching just the breathing for a while, until both of you are satisfied that it is going well. Now we can put the coaching of the breathing together with coaching head-to-toe relaxation for one more practice contraction so you will see how the whole thing works.

PUTTING IT TOGETHER

Now that you have learned to coach relaxation and breathing separately, practice putting the two together. They go hand in hand. The trick is to coach a little breathing and a lot of concentration on relaxation in each contraction. That is, start out with the four points of the breathing and move right on to head-to-toe relaxation, returning to the breathing very little during the contraction unless the laboring woman seems to need it.

Remember, relaxation for labor is not like relaxing to go to sleep. As long as you keep in mind the purpose of coaching—to help her achieve skillful, deliberate relaxation of muscle groups and breathing in a calm, rhythmic manner low in the abdomen—then you cannot miss. So read the following exercise aloud twice, then close the book, and with the mother in the side position, practice several complete contractions. Don't forget the back rub. Just in the practice sessions, you should also say the things in parentheses.

MASTER EXERCISE I

First-Stage Contractions: Breathing and Relaxation

A contraction begins. You feel it starting to work. Your uterus flexes for you, a little more, and just a little bit more, until you get a good, strong, pulling, stretching sensation around the cervix to open that door.

- Breathe with a steady, even rhythm. Not in the middle of your tummy, but way down low. Listen to the quiet ease of your abdominal breathing.
- Concentrate on relaxing your tummy extremely. Think of it just floating outward and away from you as you breathe in.
- Drop your head into the pillow. Think about it. Don't hold your head up with your neck muscles. Just let it drop down into the pillow.
- Smooth your eyelids, and concentrate on all those facial muscles being loose and slack. Smooth your brow. Let your eyes rest. Let all the tension go from your face. Loosen your jaw and let it sag open. Have a relaxed, open throat. Don't try to swallow.
- Drop your shoulders. Have no tension in them at all. Relax your back and let your tummy relax completely, floating out and away from you. You can always relax your tummy

a little bit more. There is always some leftover tension to ease away.

- Each time you exhale, you let go a little more. Let your whole body sag and relax and get out of the way so that big bag of muscles can open the door for the baby.
- Locate any tension that is left in your shoulders and your arms and let go of it so it eases out through your hands. Let your hands be limp and let your fingers be loose and limp. Everything just sinks down into the pillows and the mattress.
- When you feel that muscle flexing, think your way through the contraction. Your whole body is relaxing to let the uterus do its work.
- Let go of any strain or tension in your chest. Drop your whole body into that bed. Let go. Release everywhere. Relax your tummy extremely. Concentrate on letting go and letting it float out and away from you. Keep your breathing very calm and quiet and steady and way down low in the bottom of your belly.
- Think; drop into the bed, and really let go. Don't just hold yourself still. Keep loose and limp, and let your PC muscle relax completely. Let your vaginal barrel be open.

- Let go as if your life depended on it. Breathe at a nice, normal pace. Observe your body. Look for any tension and skillfully let it go so it just eases out of your body. You can always let go just a little more. Think, observe, release.
- Let your hips be slack and sink down into the bed. Let go of any tension in your thighs. Let it all go out through your legs and feet. Your legs are loose and easy now. Your feet are loose and limp as well.
- That's it. You are doing great. Don't stop thinking about relaxing now. Think your way up and over a contraction. That's what you are practicing right now—concentration. Don't let your mind stray to other things. Keep thinking about relaxation. Look for any tension and deliberately release it away. Sag, go loose and limp.
- Think of your uterus as that big bag of muscles that is opening the door for your baby. It is just a bag of muscles flexing. The more it flexes, the more you relax with it. Stay out of the way with your body. Don't get in the way. The more you relax, the better those muscles work. Think of your baby's head pressing on the cervix as you let go and open, AND OPEN. Let the vaginal barrel be relaxed and open.
- Breathe with a nice, quiet, steady rhythm. Listen to the sound of it, way down low in the bottom of your belly. You can always relax a little more and a bit more. Never be satisfied. Keep thinking. Breathe and sag. Picture what is happening inside you. The bag of muscles flexes to open the door for the baby.
- Think your way up and over a contraction. (And the contraction peaks and ebbs away to the end.)

Practice this Master Exercise every night until it becomes automatic.

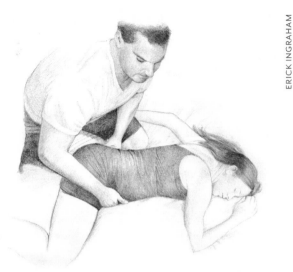

28. During an occasional contraction, put two fingers lightly on the abdomen to check the breathing. You should feel the abdomen move outward as she breathes in.

HOW TO TIME CONTRACTIONS

A contraction is timed from its beginning to the peak of its strength. The laboring woman will let you know when a contraction begins by saying, "There's one," or with a raised finger or a simple grunt. She needs to signal you in the same way when a contraction has reached its peak and begins to subside. This will tell you how long the contraction is.

Why not time the contraction from the beginning to the end? Because it is only really working for her until the peak. Then the uterus is just relaxing and the sensation is fading, so it is hard to know exactly when it does end. So time contractions from the beginning to the peak.

To determine how far apart contractions are, time from the *beginning of one contraction to the beginning of the next*. You do not time from the end of one contraction to the beginning of the next, because it is so hard to say when a contraction ends.

But wait, this is important. When we say, "The contractions are seventy seconds long and three minutes apart," that is not the result of timing just one contraction. The human body is not a machine and it does not work like a clock. Often a good, strong contraction will be followed by a short one, or several long ones and several short ones will alternate. Sometimes a contraction will just fizzle after a few seconds. This is all normal and no cause for alarm. So, in timing contractions, it is important to time and record several—say five or six—and then take a *conservative* average to determine the length and interval of the contractions.

For example, if you timed five contractions and three were forty-five seconds long and two were fifty-five seconds long, what would you say? You would say the contractions were about forty-five seconds long. That is, you would go by three contractions out of the five. Acting on one or two contractions instead of the low average of about a half dozen could give you, the laboring woman, and everyone else, a false idea of where you are in labor.

You have learned a lot in the last two chapters. You now know the best position for labor (and an alternate); how to relax; how to coach relaxation; how to deal with the backache many women have (and the round ligament ache a few have); and how to listen to the breathing to keep it quiet, steady, and normal. In class you would review these things many times, and you should return often to these chapters. There are a few more basic labor skills to learn, but first we will look at another common question: pain.

CHAPTER THIRTEEN

About Pain—and More Relaxation Tools

WHAT ABOUT PAIN? It is something that every pregnant woman certainly wonders about. Is a painless labor possible? Yes, painless labor is indeed possible, *but it is certainly not a promise.* I have experienced painless childbirth, so I am very much aware of the possibility. But what about the women in our classes? We find that about two out of five describe their labors as painless. That is not even half the people we teach.

I can promise you control in labor. All you have to do is want it. If you are motivated to really want an unmedicated childbirth with a labor that is dignified and manageable, you can have it simply by listening to your breathing to ensure it continues in a calm, quiet, relaxed rhythm. The woman who is breathing excitedly or holding her breath is the one who is panicky and out of control.

Personally, I do not consider control enough. So I know you will want to really get into relaxation because it is the key to comfort in labor. How well you skillfully release tension will to a large extent determine your degree of comfort.

How does relaxation affect pain? Does it diminish our response to pain or does it reduce and eliminate the sensation itself? Well, relaxation can do both. If you have pain, then relaxation influences your response to it in a way that eases labor. As you know, tightening up makes labor harder.

But relaxation does more than that. Women who have had painless labors often say that they think it is a matter of doing things right in the first place: not tightening up but going with the strong sensations and looking upon them as "just muscles working." What makes labor painless for them is total relaxation and not fighting to control pain. A deeper, more complex explanation can be found in Dr. Edmund Jacobson's book *How to Relax and Have Your Baby.* His specialty is not babies but relaxation. He has applied what he believes about relaxation to labor quite successfully, though, as he explains,

. . . relaxation proceeds to relieve pain mechanically . . . It requires action of the whole nerve-muscle-brain-nerve-muscle circuit to experience pain. The muscular part of this circuit is under your control and can be relaxed. By relaxing all efforts to perceive the pain and to do something about it, like withdrawing, you can put out of commission the uterine pain circuit.

There are undeniably strong sensations in labor that are felt by every woman, but whether these are described as pain is a subjective matter that depends a lot on expectations and experiences. For example, the childbirth teacher who has experienced hard pain in labor often teaches that this is the only way it can be and almost always has students who have hard pain. The woman who is certainly *not* going to have a painless childbirth is the one who is absolutely convinced that birth must be an agony. She is less apt to *analyze* the physical sensations she feels. Instead, as her powerful uterine muscles flex, she *reacts* automatically with her built-up expectations. Labor will be manageable for her, with good control possible just by listening to the sound of her breathing, but comfort is something lost to her.

Those women who have experienced hard pain sometimes find it difficult to believe that anyone could experience painless childbirth. Occasionally, over the years of

teaching, I have observed a few women who seem to have a real psychological need to deny that painless childbirth is possible. Perhaps this stems from a feeling that if someone else didn't have pain, that somehow invalidates the painful experience of a woman who does have pain.

On the other hand, women who have no pain in labor certainly did feel the uterus contracting very powerfully and they certainly had moments when they felt the emotional booby trap of "I don't think I can do this anymore." Such women understand that labor can be painful with anything less than perfect relaxation, so they have no need to invalidate or deny the pain of those who experienced it. *The reality is that there is such a thing as painless childbirth and such a thing as painful childbirth. It is not necessary to invalidate either experience.*

The pain discussion is a critical part of the class, and I never fail to mention the entire range of experiences possible. I like to have each class hear the story of one couple who had a painless birth; another couple who describe their labor as having no pain or mild cramping at the beginning, going on to moderate pain, and ending up with hard pain for a short time; and finally one couple who had hard pain for most of their labor. This covers the real range of experience, and it is very important for women to hear the whole range. (All these women, by the way, will describe their labors as quite manageable, even those who experienced hard pain most of the way.) Most women in class do listen and hear this range, not "selecting out" any experience, and they come back after birth eager to share how it was for them, because they understand it is acceptable to have had either experience.

Women give many clues about how labor is going to be for them. The woman who has already decided before labor that it definitely will be painful is almost certain to find it so. Like water taking the shape of its container, experiences often take the shape of expectations. And the woman in class who is eager to be reassured that childbirth is painless seems to have a strong chance of having hard pain. What she *wishes* for is a painless birth but it is not what she *expects*, as shown by her anxiety as she tries to get reassurance.

Most women who do experience hard pain tend to do so at the end of the first stage. But remember, there are no sudden, sharp, stabbing pains in labor. Rather, there is a strong building up of sensation with each contraction. In between contractions there is a chance to rest. (The speedster, by the way, rarely experiences painless childbirth. Her contractions are too close. There is not enough time for her to get accustomed to the sensations and to get deeply into relaxation, though she keeps good control with the breathing. The putterer is more likely to have a painless birth since she has lots of time to get used to the sensations and get deeply relaxed.)

The woman in my class who I predict (to myself only) will have a painless birth is the one who is quite comfortable with her body and with *physical strain and sweat*. She will really get into the relaxation techniques, rather than only going for the physical exercises. This woman listens to all the various birth stories and is prepared in a matter-of-fact way for the *backache*, for *powerful sensations*, and for *hard, sweaty work*. She is not looking for any authority figure to reassure her or guarantee her a painless birth. She simply has faith and confidence in the process of labor and birth. I am not talking about religious faith, but about a belief that *birth is normal* and an expectation that her body will function normally as millions of others have done before. *She truly has the idea that labor is nothing more than muscles flexing.*

This is the woman I expect will have a painless or near-painless birth. I am often, but not always, right. This woman usually comes back to the class after birth and tells of her physical sensations in terms of *stretching, pulling, straining, low in the abdomen. She uses words that typically would apply to* working muscles. *Those who report that labor is painless almost always say their favorite technique was picturing what was really happening in their body while they deeply relaxed and let go with it. (This technique, called "mental imagery," or "the bag of muscles technique," will be explained more thoroughly in a moment.)* The woman who said her favorite technique was breathing seldom experienced a painless childbirth.

But let me make it quite clear that women who have experienced both a medicated birth and a trained, natural childbirth are quick to tell you that *medication does not make childbirth painless.* They invariably say their natural childbirth was, by far, the most comfortable of the two. And most women who have had a medicated childbirth, and no other kind, talk about little else but the pain and discomfort.

So let me repeat. I do not promise any woman a painless childbirth. It is a possibility, not a promise. And you do not need a painless childbirth to have a good, natural, unmedicated birth experience, one that you will enjoy remembering.

MENTAL IMAGERY

The Bag of Muscles Technique

This is nothing more than vividly picturing what is happening inside your body each and every time you feel a contraction. A contraction is a powerful sensation. Your uterus is the biggest set of muscles in your body, and when it flexes, you have a strong physical sensation. You

feel as if it could pick you right up off the bed. Do not underestimate labor, for it is the hardest work you will ever do. So you must be prepared for strong sensations. You certainly do not want to tense and tighten up against this contraction sensation. You want to mentally hook up what you are feeling to an accurate image of what is causing it.

You will have to concentrate on going limp, sagging, letting go, and visualizing the long muscles flexing and contracting while the circular muscles lengthen and relax outward in an ever-widening circle, opening the door to the uterus, your cervix. That is why you feel that stretching, pulling, straining sensation low in your abdomen.

"The bag of muscles technique" helps with *perception.* It guides you to think about what you feel and where you feel it; to analyze what you feel instead of just reacting to this powerful sensation. Use it to see if you can perceive a flex of the bag of muscles as just that—muscles flexing, pulling, tightening. It can change the way you perceive this powerful flex. *See if you can apply words that you associate with muscles working for you.*

In this wonderful series of pictures you see the uterus not cut in half but as it really is. You can clearly see that the cervix is not just two ends hanging down into the canal but in fact goes around in a circle just like the neck of a turtleneck sweater.

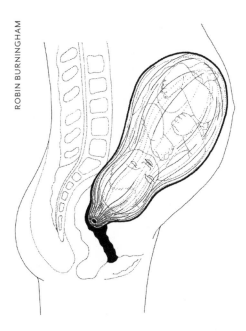

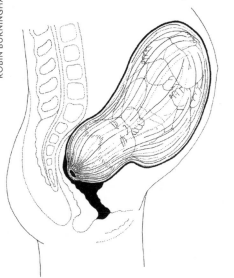

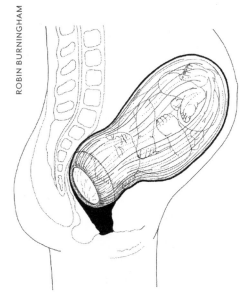

29. In the first picture labor has not started. No effacement has occurred either. The opening you see in the cervix is just the cervical canal.

30. The cervix is effaced, pulled back flat onto the baby's head, but not dilated yet.

31. Here you can see the cervix opening into ever-widening circles as it dilates. The dotted line shows you how the cervix will continue to pull back over the baby's head. Do not confuse this with crowning. This is not at the outlet but up inside where you do not see it opening.

It is not enough to just know this is happening in an abstract way. You have to apply mental imagery, that is, picturing what is happening vividly and deliberately during a contraction. You have something concrete to work with in labor when you *visualize* just *what is happening*. If you do, you will find yourself analyzing what you feel and where you feel it, rather than simply reacting emotionally with fear and tension to a strong sensation. A contraction is not your enemy; as it pulls stronger it is also working better for you. Keep this in mind during a contraction.

And remember, nature is very kind. As your uterine muscles flex and relax, you always get a rest between contractions. Your body works in an intricate and harmonious fashion. There is no onslaught of forces against you, no sharp sudden pains or piercing agony, but there is a definite sensation of a powerful set of muscles working. Visualizing this is as important as the relaxation or breathing during a contraction. If we could give you just one gift with this book it would be the faith in the proper working of your own body and the ability to visualize just what is happening during labor.

Coaching mental imagery, the "bag of muscles technique," is not difficult. Start by taking another look at the picture of the uterus on pages 52 and 109 and hold those pictures in your mind as you read this exercise. You were already introduced to some of the words and phrases in Master Exercise I. Just remind the mother what is happening inside her body.

PRACTICE EXERCISE C: MENTAL IMAGERY

- Stay out of the way with your whole body and let that big bag of muscles do all the work for you, opening the door to the cervix.
- Visualize what is happening inside you. Picture those long muscles flexing and pulling the cervix open. Picture the circular muscles relaxing and lengthening in an ever-widening circle to open the door for the baby.
- The more it works for you, the more you relax with it. The more you relax, the better the uterus works for you as you open and open.
- Concentrate on what is happening inside you. Go loose, limp, sagging while your uterus works for you, *and hook up what you are feeling to the picture of that big bag of muscles working.*

> You certainly have the idea by now. Read over Master Exercise I (the "bag of muscles" technique), read these samples of coaching mental imagery, then put the book aside and coach several practice contractions, using your own words for all the techniques you have learned—breathing, head-to-toe relaxation, and mental imagery.

FLOATING TECHNIQUE

There is just one more technique for the first stage of labor that you may find very helpful toward the end. During the last sprint of the uterine muscles, as the cervix goes from seven to ten centimeters of dilation, contractions will be quite strong soon after they get started. This usually corresponds to the "self-doubt" emotional signpost, which you will learn more about later. You have already learned muscle-grouping, consciously relaxing from head to toe. But when you reach the last part of first stage you will probably find it more helpful to think about relaxing the *whole* body at once. The contractions seem to be coming in bigger waves now, so it is valuable to think of relaxing the whole body and letting it float up to the peak of a contraction's strength so you can just slip over the top.

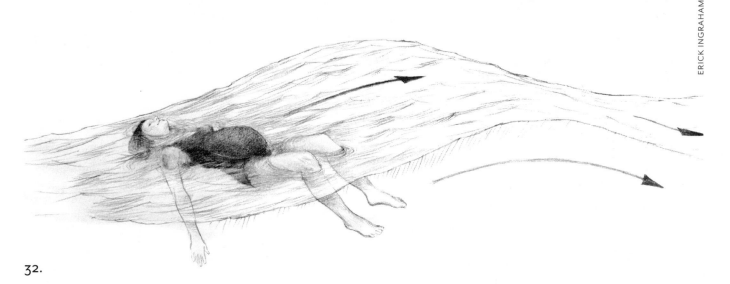

ERICK INGRAHAM

32.

TO THE COACH

The floating technique is simply more relaxation. The only difference is that you are talking about the whole body being loose and limp at once. This will be useful as the laboring woman moves into her hardest and fastest work. When coaching her to float up and over a contraction, do not get off the track with talk about floating on clouds or cotton candy or other such images. The symbolism of the wave is very specific. Contractions seem just like waves, building and building and reaching a peak of strength, just as a wave rolls up to a peak. The laboring woman can relate very well to this idea of staying limp, floating up to the peak of the contraction, and then slipping over the top to the other side.

You coach this technique much as you have done up to now. Start with the breathing, go to full-body relaxation, urge her to think about locating tension and letting go, use mental imagery, and add phrases like these:

**PRACTICE EXERCISE D:
FLOATING**

- Let your whole body sag into the bed and float up and over this contraction. Just keep floating loose and limp.
- Just *a little farther now*, keep floating, the peak of the contraction is just ahead. *Let go and you will slip right up and over the peak and down the other side.*
- Look for the peak. *Look for the end of your work.*

Read this over twice and then do several practice contractions with the book closed, using your own words for all the coaching techniques you have learned. And don't forget the back rub.

CHAPTER FOURTEEN

The Six Needs of a Laboring Woman

IT SHOULD BE CLEAR by now that during the first stage of labor, the pregnant woman's attention is centered on what is happening inside her body. So the labor environment, or what is happening outside the woman's body, is really the responsibility of the coach. Dr. Bradley has identified six needs of the laboring mother. Meeting those needs is really at the heart of the coach's role in the Bradley Method®. As you read through them here, you will realize that you already have learned about many of these needs and how to meet them. But remember, every laboring woman needs someone who has taken the trouble to learn as much as she has learned, someone who can remind her of the goal as she tires and someone to help her help herself. This is why a loving, supportive coach is the very essence of the Bradley Method®.

ONE: **Darkness** and **Solitude.** The laboring woman needs a dark or dimly lit room. Bright lights disturb concen-

tration and she needs 100 percent concentration on relaxation to work properly with labor. Solitude while the two of you are working together is also important. This means no mothers or mothers-in-law. If children are to be present at birth, this is not the time to have them in the room, except for short visits so they can see that Mommy is doing fine. Solitude also means no pregnant neighbor from across the street, despite the temptation to show off a bit.

It is very distracting for most women to have observers in the first stage of labor. The laboring woman finds herself wondering what everyone thinks about how she is doing. The coach, in turn, spends less time thinking about the laboring woman and more time on what the observers think of his coaching. A laboring woman is not performing. She should simply work for herself and her baby. Keeping the room (even a hospital room) dark and keeping observers to a minimum is the coach's responsibility. Whether they are in-laws or hospital personnel, this requires tact, but it should not be left to the laboring woman to deal with. As her work gets serious, she will have other things to think about.

TWO: **Quiet.** It should be obvious to anyone who has ever concentrated on anything, even reading this book, that noise distracts concentration. At home it is usually not difficult to keep noise under control. Hospitals are understandably noisy places, but fortunately, labor rooms do have doors.

THREE: **Physical Comfort.** Be extremely fussy about the laboring woman's comfort. Make sure she has all the pillows she needs, especially a flat one for under her head so her head and neck are properly aligned with her shoulders. Do not allow as much as a toe to go unsupported; if needed, get another pillow for it. Help her to find the perfect position.

Physical comfort also means the laboring woman should not have a dry mouth. In between contractions she can have sips of water. These are things that must be thought of and made available before her labor really gets going. If she says that she is hot but not to worry about it, do worry about it. Get a window open or whatever is required. If she is cold, get her blankets. She is too busy to fuss a lot, so it is up to you to be a perfectionist.

Also, the coach should remind her to turn over every hour or hour and a half. If she has a favorite side, that is okay, but she does need to get off it occasionally to restore circulation. Remind her to go to the bathroom. She will tend to put it off because she is afraid of having a contraction on the way. Usually, though, just because she is worrying about it, if she does have a contraction on the way to the bathroom it will be a light one.

Don't leave physical comfort behind at home. Once you are in the hospital or birth center, start all over to get everything perfect.

FOUR: **Physical Relaxation.** You already know a lot about physical relaxation. It is different from physical comfort, but relaxation depends upon comfort. Remember, it is the subtle, minor degrees of tension that are the hardest to let go of. Help the laboring woman avoid just holding herself still; that is, lying there looking as if she is relaxed but with all her muscles slightly tensed. Don't bark out orders, but in a sincere, concerned voice direct her concentration toward releasing all those slightly flexed muscles everywhere.

FIVE: **Controlled Breathing.** You already know that panting is a symptom of panic. It is so serious that one anesthesiologist considers it a good reason to medicate women in labor, to prevent rapid breathing and avoid the hyperventilation that tends to follow. His concern is specifically aimed at the untrained mother who is panicky and at the Lamaze-trained mother who has been taught faster-than-normal breathing. This doctor's concern is legitimate, even if his solution is excessive. You know that what is needed is to have the laboring woman *listen* to her breathing to ensure the continuation of quiet, rhythmic, abdominal breathing. If the coach is listening to the breathing he will know if she is breathing too fast or holding her breath. The real key is perfect relaxation, because normal breathing is a reflection of good relaxation.

SIX: **Appearance of Sleep and Closed Eyes.** Closed eyes are a guarantee that there will be no visual distractions. The woman who keeps her eyes open is trying to escape from the contraction, rather than go with it. The appearance of sleep is your ultimate goal. Of course, the laboring woman is not sleeping. She is thinking and concentrating on what is happening inside her body. She is mentally alert, and this is reflected in a body that is genuinely limp and relaxed, not just still. But to those who do not know what is happening, the woman laboring with the Bradley Method® appears to be sleeping. Nurses often comment upon it. The appearance of sleep is the ultimate goal, one that can be met when all the other needs of the laboring woman have been attended to.

TO THE COACH

Coach, you know what the laboring woman does during a contraction, and you know that between contractions she rests mentally. You know what you will be doing during contractions—coaching and rubbing her back, if needed—but what do you do between contractions? Unfortunately, you do not fall into a chair and rest. Instead, this time is your opportunity to deal with the six needs or any other problem that comes up.

- Rub her shoulders, if she likes.
- Take care of her dry mouth with frequent sips of water, or ice chips. Remember, she will be breathing through her mouth during the contraction, so she will feel dry.
- Wipe off her face and forehead with a damp cloth. This is sweaty work for her, and the dampness can be uncomfortable.
- Also, use this time for some of the fun things in labor, like taking pictures.

A PRACTICE PLAN

At this point you have a number of very important things to practice, so we have prepared this weekly practice plan.

THE MOTHER'S WEEKLY PRACTICE PLAN

- For fifteen minutes every day, practice skillful relaxation by yourself. This does not mean taking a nap; that isn't practicing anything. Lie down with the idea that for fifteen minutes you are going to push your brain. Remain mentally alert and think. Of what? Dinner? The color of the crib? No, that is drifting, the opposite of concentration.
- You should think of *observing* your muscles over and over from head to toe. Be aware of your body. Seek out slightly contracted muscles. Look for subtle tension. *Then concentrate on deliberately, consciously releasing it.* And remember to listen to your breathing. Normal, abdominal breathing is conducive to deeper relaxation. For fifteen minutes you will observe and release, constantly concentrating on a deliberately and skillfully limp, loose body.

- If you have been doing your PC contractions faithfully, you should now be ready to go on to the Intermediate PC exercise practice plan. Simply change to flexing to the count of ten. When you reach seven or eight, think about tightening even more. Contract your muscle in this manner at least thirty-six times a day—twelve in the morning, twelve in the afternoon, and twelve at night. Remember to flex deeply.
- Continue to squat, tailor sit, pelvic rock, do the legs apart exercise, and continue to count your protein intake to make sure you are getting eighty to a hundred grams a day.

THE COACH'S WEEKLY PRACTICE PLAN

- Practice coaching your wife in relaxation and breathing, doing about five practice contractions a night before going to sleep. Check her labor position, listen to her breathing, and rub her back. In between practice contractions, think about meeting her other needs—rubbing her shoulders, wiping her brow, and so on. Turn back to Chapter Twelve if you need a refresher in coaching, but soon you should be adding your own words and developing your own style. Talk it over with her to find out what words and images work best.

For coaches who are not husbands:

- Be sure to set up times when you can practice together. You may need to think more about developing familiarity and rapport so you will be comfortable as a team with the laboring woman. Touch is important in coaching. If this is a barrier while you are practicing, work toward both of you feeling at ease as you rub her back and shoulders.

REVIEW QUESTIONS FOR BOTH MOTHER AND COACH

Put yourselves through this little test, talking over the answers to the questions and looking back to the associated sections if you are not satisfied with your own answers. When the birth gets close, you will feel a lot more comfortable if you know what is happening and what needs to be done without having to take time to look it up.

1. What are the three stages of labor?
2. Why is it harmful to lie flat on your back during late pregnancy and labor?
3. What is effacement? What is engagement?
4. What does effacement or engagement tell you about when your labor will start?
5. What are the two keys to learning relaxation as a skill?
6. What is the best lying-down position for labor? What is an alternate position?
7. Have you decided where you will labor? Have you set up the pillows to actually see what it will be like?
8. How do you breathe in labor?
9. What are the four points to coaching the breathing?
10. When coaching a contraction, do you emphasize relaxation or breathing?
11. What happens to the untrained mother's contractions when she has not learned skillful contractions and fights labor?
12. What are the six needs of the laboring woman, as defined by Dr. Bradley?

CHAPTER FIFTEEN

The Emotional Map of Labor

Y**OU NOW KNOW ABOUT** the physical side of labor, and how to begin coaching it, but you should also realize that your journey to birth is marked by emotional signposts as well. You should realize from the outset that a natural birth experience is more easily attainable if you learn the emotional signposts that go with labor. That's what this chapter is all about. Before we get to the map of emotions, however, remember that no two labors are alike. And, as discussed before, one of the crucial differences is time. Just as several people may start a journey with the same map, if one walks, one bicycles, and another drives, they will have vastly different experiences. The person in the car may go speeding by some sights so quickly he will barely notice them. The walker may pass these sights so slowly that he doesn't see them as distinct milestones. Meanwhile, the cyclist moves by all the signposts at a speed that allows him to observe each distinctly.

While we will be giving you a very reliable emotional map of the experience of labor that most people have from beginning to end, you will NOT get to choose the speed at which that experience will occur.

The map we will use as our point of reference is of the so-called *textbook* labor—twelve to fourteen hours. The emotional signposts we will discuss are pretty standard, but the time it takes to progress from one to another is *extremely variable*, and the time is not nearly as important as the signposts themselves are. Beware of paying more attention to the time than you do to the signposts along the way.

By the end of this chapter, your goal should be to understand the loose pattern into which the details of your own unique labor experience will fall, so you will be able to tell what is happening along the way.

THE BEGINNING EMOTIONAL SIGNPOST: EXCITEMENT

If you are going by the textbook, your contractions will start off short and easy, with rest periods of five or possibly more minutes. You could have an hour of this or several hours.

The beginning emotional signpost is elation, excitement, a bit of nervousness, feeling, "Oh, my gosh, today's really the day."

Contractions at this point feel like a hardening or tightening sensation, if you start off slowly and easily like our textbook labor. Your uterus pulls forward and hardens somewhat. You probably do not have any backache during these early contractions. During this time your cervix might dilate to about two centimeters or so.

You feel quite happy and excited; you have been waiting for this day for nine months and maybe longer. This is it at last; you feel with some elation. Of course, you may feel a tiny bit of stage fright, too. You feel both eager and anxious.

Self-Help

You really don't have to do much now except keep a relaxed tummy throughout each contraction. Be sure you keep that abdomen hanging loose at all times. This is easiest to do with proper breathing and closed eyes during the contraction, but, for heaven's sake, don't climb right into bed if you start off slow and easy. It can get pretty boring at the other end of twelve or fourteen hours!

When you have a labor that starts slow and easy, enjoy it. This is the fun part. Later on you'll be working hard. Just close your eyes, sag your tummy, and breathe with a rhythm during a contraction. Then go on reading, watching TV, or whatever you were doing before.

TO THE COACH: COACHING THE BEGINNING EMOTIONAL SIGNPOST

In the beginning emotional signpost, the woman is happy, excited, elated, nervous. There's often a smile, and when you see that you know she has a long way to go! The more nervous type does not walk around smiling, but it's obvious that she's not in hard labor.

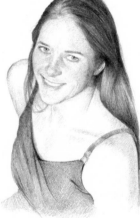

ERICK INGRAHAM

33. First emotional signpost: excitement; today's the day.

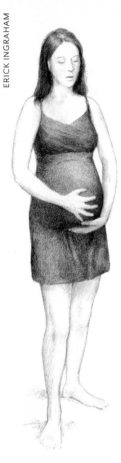

ERICK INGRAHAM

34. Check with your hand. Be sure you are letting your belly relax and expand outward as you breathe in.

What's your coaching job? Well, she's not working hard yet and neither are you. When a contraction starts, she just stops whatever she's doing, sags her tummy, and breathes with a rhythm way down low in the bottom of her abdomen. (Very few women need a back rub when displaying the beginning emotional signpost.)

The coach sets the atmosphere. Encourage her to relax and enjoy this part. A number of couples find they have plenty of time to go out to a favorite restaurant. He has a hearty dinner while she has something light. (Some doctors think light nourishment can be essential to a normal labor and approve of this; others do not.) Go back home and enjoy yourselves. Savor the excitement and help set up an approach, an attitude to this part of labor that you can draw upon later. This is a time to enjoy. Later it will be hard, monotonous work for both of you. This is a time for those silly things. Take a couple of pictures of yourselves. At the time, picture-taking seems so unimportant, but later these may be pictures you'll treasure.

The coach's major job is keeping his wife at home. Don't let her talk you into rushing off to the hospital at this beginning signpost. Most women are convinced that the sooner they get to the hospital the sooner they'll have the baby. This is not true. At this point it can even work the other way around. When she arrives too early, labor has a tendency to disappear on her.

If her labor starts off slow and easy and you dash off to the hospital right away, she may just wind up being hungry, thirsty, poked-at, and interrupted while she labors ten, twelve, or more hours in the hospital. The surest way *not* to have a natural birth is for her to be psychologically beaten down and frustrated by a long stay in a hospital with all its routines and interruptions.

Remember, babies are rarely produced with anything less than hard work. Even speedsters usually work *hard* for at least two or three hours.

Labor is what the word implies: hard work. So please don't go to the hospital when she displays the beginning emotional signpost. Before you even think about the hospital, she should be so wrapped up in her work that she can no longer be bothered flashing a grin at the camera! If she is talking glibly during contractions or in between them, you're not far along.

THE SERIOUS EMOTIONAL SIGNPOST

A few hours pass by. Now your uterus gets down to serious work, and so do you. And that is exactly what the next emotional signpost is. You are serious. Excitement gives way to concentration. Now when you have contractions you definitely feel a *need* to sit down, or even lie down, and get comfortable. You need to concentrate on some real relaxation and to listen to your breathing.

You do this not merely because you are eager to try things out, but because you must work with the contractions. And if you have a backache, you are serious about getting a back rub.

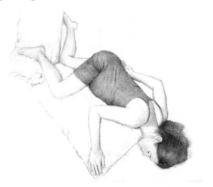

Your physical sensations are definitely stronger. These are good, working contractions, lasting about sixty seconds. (Anything less than forty-five seconds just isn't doing much work at getting the cervix open.)

Self-Help

Now, when you feel a contraction, you fully understand the need for total concentration on a limp, sagging, let-go body. You work diligently because you do not want these contractions to get ahead of you. You can feel the long muscles pulling to open the cervix. Now you are working hard, and you will be for the next several hours or more, if you continue to stick to the textbook.

The serious emotional signpost is total absorption in the work and the need to be undistracted. It is a do-not-disturb and get-to-work attitude.

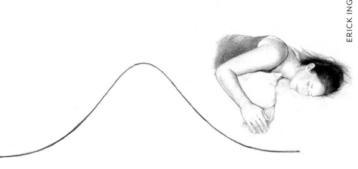

35. Serious emotional signpost: The uterus gets serious and so does she.

TO THE COACH:
SERIOUS EMOTIONAL SIGNPOST

She is in total concentration, dedicated to her work. She snaps at you if you distract her or don't rub her back exactly right.

She won't exactly *jump* from the beginning emotional signpost to the next one. She drifts into it. First, she wants the back rub if she has any backache. Then you notice she definitely needs coaching now. She is serious about working with contractions.

Coach, you should become serious, too. Clear the way for a smooth, steady course. A few hours go by, her uterus gets *more serious*, and she gets *most* serious. It is different now. She is totally absorbed. There is determination you may have never seen in her before as she focuses inward and prepares to greet the next contraction with a totally yielding body. It is this intensity, which often takes hours to establish, that I look for in a woman to know she is now *really* into the serious signpost. She no longer jokes and laughs—she's busy. She wants to be ready for each contraction.

She will be doing this for hours (in the textbook labor), so get a good number of these hours of work behind you at home before going to the hospital. Don't make the mistake of dashing off to the hospital the minute you see the serious signpost.

One wise coach of ours spent three or four hours at home with his wife in the beginning emotional signpost. Contractions were five to seven minutes apart. She didn't need coaching at this point.

When they got down to work, her contractions were mostly five minutes apart and were lasting about fifty-five seconds. She seemed to be showing the serious signpost. The husband coached her for a couple of hours, and then the two of them decided that since they had been in labor for six hours, it was time to get off to the hospital. Contractions were still five minutes apart.

But remember—for four of those six hours they really were not working much. They had been really *working* for only two hours.

Fortunately, they decided to take a picture of her all ready to walk out the door. Looking through the camera lens, the husband saw a confident *smile* and suddenly realized they were not as far along as they had thought.

This excellent coach very gently pointed this out. His wife took her coat off, and they worked at home for four more hours. *Then* they went to the hospital.

By then they were well established in the serious emotional signpost, with contractions four minutes apart and lasting sixty to seventy seconds. So, with four hours of easy labor and *six* hours of working labor behind them, they labored in the hospital for *another six hours before they had their baby.*

The coaching job during the serious emotional signpost is to get to work in earnest the minute she does. The laboring woman sets the pace. Take your cue from her. You match the intensity of your coaching to the work she is doing when she is serious. You should definitely not wait for this signpost to do things like pack the bag or take other children to the babysitter.

Get with the back rub, diligently, if she has a backache. Have a soft cloth ready to do it with. Get the ice chips ready and set up a bowl and a wet washrag. Begin coaching her gently in relaxation; remind her about breathing as well.

Don't wait for her to be desperate to start working with her. You don't suddenly turn into a birth team at the end of labor. So rub her back and talk her over and through contractions, concentrating intently on helping her to really let go and let her body sag. *The primary goal at all times is total relaxation.*

As soon as you start to work, run over Dr. Bradley's six needs of the laboring mother in your mind and be sure that all of them are being met.

THE SELF-DOUBT EMOTIONAL SIGNPOST

Your uterus now shifts into high gear and speeds by the centimeters from seven to ten. You begin to wonder why you haven't reached your destination yet. You wonder if you are going to reach it. Are you really as far along as you thought? You are nearing the end of first-stage labor. *Your emotional response is self-doubt.*

At this point you will be quite absorbed in yourself and your body so that you may not even notice, but your coach sees that you have become uncertain, indecisive. You don't know quite what you want to do, and even when asked you cannot say or explain. At this point, if you are asked any question, the most common reply is, "I don't know." You are not sure that you can do this, and may even say so aloud. This is the self-doubt signpost, and it really means that you are almost done.

Like a runner in a race who saves a burst of effort for the last part when the goal is in sight, the uterus will make a final surge to full dilation of the cervix, from six or seven centimeters to a completely open door. It may have taken you ten or twelve hours to get dilated to seven centimeters, and now you are about to go the last three centimeters in a fast half hour or two hours.

At this time your contractions may last seventy, eighty, or even ninety seconds, and your rest periods are usually one-and-a-half to two minutes. (Most women will still get two minutes' rest.) You feel that the contractions are right on top of one another, but nature always does give you a rest.

If you have had backache, it is stronger now as first stage is ending, but your coach should take care of most, if not all, of that for you with the back rub. Now, when you need it, that rub is fabulous.

What is happening at this point is just more of the same—contractions. But now your uterine muscles are working at their very best to open the door for you. You really feel that big bag of muscles working good and strong for you with a pulling, stretching, or straining sensation around the cervix.

Many women will experience hot and cold flashes during this time and do a lot of burping. A few feel trembly; some actually shake as if they are cold or nervous. This is a physiological reaction that occasionally occurs, and although not seen too often, it is within the range of normal. (Telling the laboring woman to relax does not make the shakes go away, but they usually disappear later as the pushing stage begins.)

A few women feel slightly nauseous; most do not. Very rarely will an unmedicated mother vomit. When she does, it is often just because she had too much to eat too recently.

Do these physical sensations sound unpleasant or frightening? They are not when you really understand what is happening. Imagine yourself in some other kind of intense physical activity, like running a hundred yards at top speed or carrying a very heavy object upstairs without the chance to put it down along the way. When you stop you will probably feel slightly trembly. You might be quite warm with perspiration or slightly cold and clammy. You could feel nauseous.

Many women do not experience any of these physical sensations in labor, even during the last emotional signpost of first stage. Others feel one or two of them. The important thing to know is that they are within the range of normal.

Self-Help

Relax now, really let go. Listen attentively to your breathing. There is a tendency at this time to breathe too fast. Up to now you have mostly only observed your breath without having to control it; now you may have to think to yourself, "Breathe with a quiet, steady rhythm."

Concentrate, really concentrate on a super-limp, relaxed body. You know how. Permit the powerful

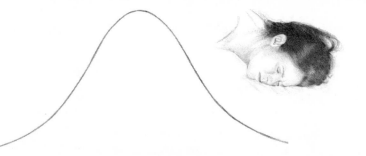

36. Self-doubt signpost, confusion;
completely inward focus.

sensation of the bag of muscles flexing to be there. It cannot "overpower" you because it is part of you, working to give birth to your baby.

You want to float over each contraction. You *think* your way through each contraction. This will be your hardest work, but it will be the shortest part of your labor.

COACHING THE SELF-DOUBT SIGNPOST

In this last emotional signpost, the laboring woman is uncertain; she doesn't know what she wants to do. She experiences self-doubt. Although to you she looks like she is doing a great job and dealing beautifully with the contractions, she may not be sure about that at all. She looks to you for support; she depends upon you for confidence and reassurance.

Remember, the only hurdle here is an emotional one. Physically what is happening is more of the same—contractions—but closer together and longer than they have been before. This is the very last part of the first stage of labor, the last half hour to two hours. It is the hardest part of the work, but the fastest.

My own first labor was a classic example of the self-doubt signpost. With my first baby (a sixteen-hour labor), we had been in the last sprint of first-stage labor for half an hour when I suddenly realized the contractions were quite close. I raised my head and said in a panicky voice, "They're coming right on top of each other. What do I do now?"

I didn't realize that they had been doing this for some time already. My coach, surprised by my concern, said, "You have been having them like this for the last half hour, and you're doing just great with them."

I really didn't believe him. I said, "Are you sure?"

My coach replied, "I'm positive. You've been doing just fine, just keep doing what you've been doing. You're practically done. You are doing just beautifully. Your concentration is great!"

After I was reassured that way, I said, "Oh, okay," put my head right back on the pillow, shut my eyes, and continued as before. In another hour I was completely dilated.

This is the most blundered and mishandled part of labor. The laboring woman who needs emotional support and reassurance seems to frighten her medical attendants. Everyone runs for an epidural or a shot of something—and WHAMMO, the rug is pulled out from under her, *just when she is so close to giving birth after having worked so long and well with labor.* She forgets she has only an hour or two to go.

She often takes the doctor's offer of medication as proof that she must not be doing well and that things are falling apart. Why else would he not praise and encourage her? Also, she can't understand why she feels so wishy-washy, unable to really decide what's best for her.

Here's another example. One of our students had been doing beautifully for ten hours or so. Her doctor came in when she was at eight centimeters (twenty minutes before this mother started pushing) and told her

that if she would like to have something he would have to give it to her now.

The mother looked up and said quietly and calmly, "Gee, I don't know."

Does that sound like a woman in pain or agony who needed to be drugged and delivered? Medication has its uses, but it should *never* take the place of skillful support for the laboring woman. The woman who does not receive skillful support at this point in her labor and ends up with an epidural or a hypo twenty or thirty minutes before she starts pushing may be understandably bitter.

The first time I coached a woman in labor I frankly didn't have the confidence my husband had had when he was coaching me. I had very little experience behind me at the time, and I found myself thinking, "It worked for me, but will it work for other people?"

The woman I was coaching was doing a beautiful job. After she reached seven centimeters she turned to me with a tired look and quietly said, "I can't do this."

I experienced as much of a self-doubt emotional signpost as *she* did. I thought to myself, "Oh, my gosh, it's all over"—I panicked—"what do I do now? Everything's falling apart."

I sort of backed away from her for a few contractions, and then I decided I would have to bluff it and do just as my coach had done for me. I told her she was doing fantastic (and she was), and that she was practically in the birthing room. She sighed and put her head down on the pillow, and continued as well as she had before.

Three contractions later she was pushing. My reaction as her coach was—"Phew! And I almost blew it for her by three measly contractions."

The moral of this story is simple. As a coach you *cannot* also experience a self-doubt emotional signpost. You cannot back away from her. You are the only caring one there who can meet her needs, especially when she is experiencing this self-doubt.

Now, as a more experienced coach, I can hardly wait to see some of the emotions of the self-doubt signpost. I rub my hands together gleefully because then I know we're almost to pushing. I look forward to it!

SPEEDSTERS AND PUTTERERS

Speedsters skip the beginning emotional signpost along with the accompanying easy contractions. Quick birthers frequently get right down to work—no fooling around.

In no time at all, their contractions are three minutes apart and a good sixty seconds long, with a very pronounced serious emotional signpost fast fading into doubt.

Our last fast couple labored about five hours. They started with contractions four minutes apart and forty-five seconds long that went to sixty seconds after just one hour. At the end of three hours the contractions were three minutes apart and eighty seconds, and she was already entering the self-doubt emotional signpost. Her coach wisely decided that things were clicking along faster than the textbook, and they left for the hospital.

She was seven centimeters dilated upon arrival and ready to push after one hour in the hospital. Pushing also took one hour. They were there in plenty of time, because the coach was tuned into the emotional signs as well as into the closeness and duration of the contractions.

The *putterer* has hours of slow, nonserious labor. She is not working hard at all, but can fall into an emotional booby trap if she is hung up on the passing time. She should simply enjoy the slow, nonserious part and not watch the clock.

It is important for the coach to point out to her that she is not really working hard yet. In fact, it is best not to count this as part of labor at all. Keep things light. It is foolish to get uptight when you're not even working hard. Also keep prepared for a possible twelve to fourteen hours of work after you do get down to business.

But some women can get *emotionally* exhausted by this kind of puttering labor before they even get started working. If the couple isn't focusing on the minutes left before going to the hospital, though, it may not become such a strain. Since the mother is not really even working hard, it is foolish to let this happen. RELAX AND ENJOY.

TO THE COACH: SUMMING UP THE FIRST-STAGE COACHING ROLE

During the beginning emotional signpost, take care of whatever is left to get ready. Get your camera set and take pictures. Drop off any other children at the sitter's or in-laws' unless they are invited to be with you at the birth. (In that case you will want to ask your Bradley teacher about the book *Children at Birth* by Marjie and Jay Hathaway.) Now settle back and enjoy the excitement.

Do not dash off to the hospital before she has even started to work hard. *Encourage her not to jump into bed the minute she starts feeling contractions, but to wait until she feels a need to lie down with contractions.* If she starts late in the evening with slow labor, she should go to bed at the usual time to get as much rest as possible.

In the serious emotional signpost, get serious when she does. Coach her in relaxation and breathing. Remind her to go to the bathroom and turn over about every hour and a half. Give a diligent back rub if needed. Have all your props available: soft rubbing rag, wet washrag, ice

chips, and so on. Plan to get as much as possible of the work of labor done at home.

Check Dr. Bradley's list of needs of the laboring mother and make sure you are meeting all of them.

One of the doctors we work for has this well figured out. As long as there is nothing unusual going on—no bleeding, nothing protruding from the vagina—he encourages his first-time mothers who live within a reasonable distance from the hospital to leave home when contractions are two or three minutes apart, lasting at least sixty seconds, with a very serious emotional signpost. Second-timers come in when contractions are four minutes apart and sixty seconds long, with a very serious emotional signpost.

It works out well. Most couples arrive when their labor is well under way and finish out anywhere from five to six hours in the hospital. No long, dragging twelve- and fourteen-or-more-hour stays.

When she experiences **the self-doubt emotional signpost,** you, Coach, cannot. She is not sure she can do this, but you reassure her that she has been doing it all this time, that this is just more of the same thing but closer and longer, and that she is in the home stretch, almost there. Of course, if you are going to a hospital or birthing center, you are there by now.

Continue coaching in relaxation and breathing; rub her back, offer ice chips or sips of water for her dry mouth; and *praise* her for her efforts, give her *encouragement*, and let her know she's making good *progress*.

She's almost done. Never back away from her. Meet her needs!

HOW TO USE THE EMOTIONAL MAP TO KNOW WHERE YOU ARE IN LABOR

The actual amount of dilation is the least reliable guide as to where you are in labor. How far dilated you are is not nearly as important as the emotional signpost, along with how far apart and how long the contractions are. Here's a classic, not at all uncommon example. Ed called me from the hospital at two in the morning. He said, "Susan, look, we've been in labor about fourteen hours, and Sharon is only four centimeters dilated and she says she can't do this anymore. They're about two to three minutes apart. She's really working hard. They're all about seventy seconds."

"Ed," I replied, "I think you'd better get right back there; it sounds like she's almost done."

Ed rushed back to see the baby's face emerging just one half hour later.

It didn't matter that Sharon was only four centimeters dilated. What mattered was *how far apart and how long the contractions were and the very clear self-doubt emotional signpost* she was showing Ed. Sharon was four centimeters, going on crowning. If you look at all three guides, the length and closeness of the contractions together with the emotional signpost, you will know more about where she is than dilation will tell you.

Here's another real example. Judy's contractions were three minutes apart, they were forty-five seconds long, and she was working lightly with them. She went to the hospital right away, thinking that since they were three minutes apart she would be fast. About twelve hours later she gave birth. How could she have known that? By looking at all three guides, not just one. Looking at how close the contractions were she thought she was going to go fast, but if she had also looked at her beginning signpost and the length of the contractions (only forty-five seconds), she would not have been fooled.

Vaginal exams are done to check how far dilated you are, to see how you are progressing. But how far dilated you are doesn't actually tell you how you are progressing. The amount of dilation is the least reliable guide as to where you are in labor, since no one can say, "Oh, you're eight centimeters dilated, so you'll be done with the first stage of labor in an hour or two." You could be done with first-stage labor in the next five minutes or several more hours.

No one can even say, "Oh, you're four centimeters, so you have a long way to go." One of my students was told exactly that when her contractions were two and three minutes apart and sixty to seventy seconds long, and she was in the self-doubt signpost. I'll bet you've already figured out where she was. Yes, close to the end of first-stage labor. In fact, thirty minutes later she was ready to push.

How did you know what the examiner did not? You paid attention to how long the contractions were and how far apart the contractions were and the emotional signpost, as well. When you massage all three together you get a much clearer picture of where you are in labor. You will know she is at the beginning; in the long, boring middle; or in the home stretch of first-stage labor.

Coach, you also have observational continuity since you're with her the whole time, meaning you get to see the difference between the wee hours of the morning contractions that were only thirty seconds long and eight to twelve minutes apart, so you know that you are looking at progress when you move to sixty- and seventy-second contractions, two minutes apart, no matter how far dilated she is at that moment.

Doing an exam just to find out how far dilated you are is also a risky business. The more exams you have, the more likely you are to acquire an infection.[1] The 2014 edition of *Williams Obstetrics* makes it clear that each and every exam increases your risk and your baby's risk of getting an infection. There is no such thing as a sterile exam, only relatively sterile exams. Bacteria from the gums of other people in the same room with you can be found immediately on the examining glove and is introduced into your vagina and cervical canal by that probing finger. Infections lead to temperatures rising, which leads to a need to hurry, using chemicals to force the uterus to work faster, longer, harder; and if that doesn't work to hurry things along, then surgical removal of the baby. That's a pretty high price to pay for a routine exam, particularly since (as reported in the *American Journal of Obstetrics and Gynecology*) researchers have demonstrated that even the most experienced examiners only get it right 19 percent of the time.[2] I know you can do the math—that means examiners get it wrong 81 percent of the time.

But, alas, if you are a first-timer, even knowing all this, if someone offers to do an exam to see how far dilated you are, you will probably say yes. What are you thinking? You're thinking it would be great to hear you're six centimeters or maybe even nine! So you have the exam, and you are told you are two centimeters dilated. You are so let down. You forget everything you learned about the longest, slowest part of labor being from zero to four centimeters, and then second gear is usually between four and seven, and third gear, in a textbook labor, is a fast one half to two hours to the home stretch, completely dilated! If instead you simply focus on the fact that your contractions are longer, stronger, and closer together and you are totally serious, then you have an encouraging picture of progress and you labor better for it. That works whether you have a textbook labor or a putterer labor.

The best birth attendants do exams by exception, when something unusual seems to be going on. They don't do them routinely.

OUR BIRTH STORY: MATT AND TIFFANY PETITMERMET; FIRST BABY

FIRST STAGE OF LABOR
The BEGINNING EMOTIONAL signpost

It all began around 4:30 in the morning on Monday. I felt my first contraction. I continued to be able to fall asleep between each contraction, so I knew it was only the beginning. Around 6:15 a.m. it was getting clear that the contractions were getting more regular, so I began to time them. From the beginning, I tried to be sure that I went into deep relaxation for each contraction. They were between a minute and a minute-and-a-half long, around every twelve minutes. I continued to try to sleep between the contractions.

Four hours later, Matt woke up around 8:30 a.m., and I let him know what was going on. *He got the camera and took a picture.* Matt got me breakfast, and I stayed in bed until 10-ish. Matt also loaded the car with our bags so that when it was time to leave there would not be as much to do.

I spent a lot of the day relaxing, reading, and watching TV. Matt constantly checked to make sure things were going well. He put dinner in the oven and we were thinking that *maybe we would be going to the birth center later in the evening.* We did some walking around the house in the late afternoon. If I had a contraction Matt would have me put my arms around his neck and I let my belly drop as he reminded me to relax.

The SERIOUS EMOTIONAL signpost

At about 5:50 in the evening (about thirteen hours after starting all this), my contractions went from twelve minutes apart to five minutes apart. Matt could see that things had turned serious and began taking over timing contractions and coaching. Up until this point I had been able to stay relaxed without coaching. We continued to labor at home till about 8:00 p.m. (Fifteen hours of work behind us.) He had me use the restroom at some point. He let me lean all my weight on him while I was on the toilet. When we headed to the birth center my contractions were four minutes apart and one-and-a-half to two minutes long. I was hoping that our drive to the birth center would give me a little break. But things sped up to two minutes apart and one minute and twenty seconds long. Matt continued to coach as he drove to the birth center. I had a contraction as Matt opened the car door so I relaxed through that, then another contraction once inside. I collapsed on the stairs and was able to relax through another one. I made it to the room and continued to labor. Matt helped me to the restroom. I had three contractions during this time and lost my mucous plug.

The SELF-DOUBT EMOTIONAL signpost

Matt helped me back to bed, where I continued to labor. I never voiced that I was in doubt, but I was feeling it both physically and emotionally.

SECOND STAGE OF LABOR
PUSHING

Then I had a few contractions that gave me the urge to push, and my water broke. This was both scary and exciting at the same time! These contractions were strong and I would involuntarily push until Matt was able to help me to breathe through the contraction until we knew I should be focusing on pushing.

I originally wanted to birth in the squatting position, but I could barely get turned from my left side to my right, and the pushing contractions had begun to come in full force. I had a few strong contractions and was *looking forward to hopefully starting the emotional signposts over again for the pushing phase. My body had other ideas.* I was able to smile and talk a bit between the first few pushing contractions. (So a very brief beginning emotional signpost.) [Susan's note: You'll learn later in the book that the emotional signposts can reset for the pushing stage.]

RIGHT AWAY INTO THE SERIOUS SIGNPOST: NO TIME FOR A SELF-DOUBT SIGNPOST

Then my contractions sped up so that I would have the contraction, have enough time to take a few breaths, and the next one would begin. Matt did a great job reminding me to breathe before the next contraction began and reminded me to take another deep breath in the middle of the contraction.

The midwife said she could see the baby's head begin to show. She saw her make a 180-degree turn; she was posterior, and a few pushes later she came out. Altogether *about eight good pushes and baby girl was here! I lifted her out and placed her on my tummy!*

I am so happy that there were no drugs and baby girl was able to help so much in her birth. I am also glad we did no cervical checks, and I was allowed to listen to my body!

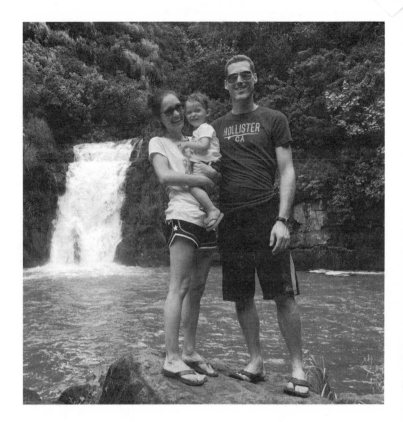

CHAPTER SIXTEEN

First-Stage Labor

THERE ARE TEN DIFFERENT ways the first stage of your labor may begin. We will look at all of them before continuing with a final rehearsal of the whole process.

Opening Scene #1: TEXTBOOK

You start with contractions several minutes apart. They are thirty-five to forty seconds long. You are having a textbook labor and it will last about fourteen hours.

The beginning emotional signpost is obvious to both of you. Your work does not begin for three or four hours and when it does, your excellent coach does not rush you off to the hospital the minute the working part begins, but settles you down for several hours of work at home.

The two of you leave for the hospital after getting a good number of hours of *working* labor behind you at home. You are extremely well established in the serious emotional signpost and have been for a while before leav-ing. You arrive at the hospital and (of course, you don't know this) it will be five hours before you have the baby.

Opening Scene #2: MUCOUS PLUG

You notice the mucous plug coming out, either in little parts at a time or the whole thing at once. There is always an opening in the cervix, not much wider than a pencil, (called the cervical canal) and it is this canal that is stopped up with the mucous plug. It's about one inch long, naturally, since the cervix is about one inch long.

The plug consists of grayish white matter, sometimes slightly blood-tinged. The little amount of blood that may accompany it is from tiny blood vessels on the surface of the cervical canal. These little vessels are delicate and may bleed a bit as the plug comes away. It does not hurt. Parts or all of the plug may come out while you are on the toilet and so you may not notice it.

Please do not get all excited if you see some of the plug. *It is the most unreliable of all the signs.* I passed parts of the plug two weeks before labor with my first child, didn't notice it with the second, and noticed it a few hours after early labor contractions began with the third.

In other words, it's nice to know what it is, but if it puts you on the ceiling with excitement you're apt to be disappointed.

Opening Scene #3: WATER BREAKING

Your bag of waters breaks. Of course, you are in the grocery store with a cart full of groceries, and you hear a distinct pop like a balloon popping. Water, water, everywhere!

Your contractions may start immediately or within several hours. Only rarely will a woman not start contractions soon after her water bag breaks. By the way, you will not have a "dry labor," since you constantly manufacture amniotic fluid. If labor still has not started after twenty-four to forty-eight hours (depending on the individual doctor's views), the doctor will probably induce labor.

Induction means forcing labor to start. This is rarely necessary as long as the woman is close to term and allowed a forty-eight-hour span to start on her own. Unfortunately, one of the latest fads in obstetrics is to insist that a woman have her baby within twelve hours after her water bag breaks. For a more detailed discussion of this see Chapter Twenty-Three. In general, nurse-midwives in freestanding birth centers allow more time.

Opening Scene #4: FALSE ALARM

You start with contractions several minutes apart, as in the textbook labor. They are a mere thirty-five seconds long. You are not really working with them, but you are aware of them. However, instead of getting closer together and stronger, they get farther apart and weaker. Things really never take off.

Real labor starts in a week or so. You are not upset by this because you realize that labor really gets going when you and your baby are ready. You do not bug the doctor by telling him how anxious you are to have the baby.

Opening Scene #5: THE SPEEDSTER

You start labor with contractions sixty seconds long and four minutes apart. You completely skip the beginning emotional signpost because your uterus starts right off to work. You are going to have a five-hour labor!

You stay home for two-and-a-half hours. Your coach has noticed that your contractions are long (sixty to seventy seconds to the peak) and are now three minutes apart.

Your serious emotional signpost is most serious and almost beginning to look a bit like the self-doubt signpost. Your coach knows what's going on or at least strongly suspects, and you go to the hospital. He was right, because you have only two-and-a-half hours to go.

Opening Scene #6: THE PUZZLER

You start with contractions close together, three minutes apart but a mere twenty to thirty seconds long. You think yours may turn into a fast labor at this point, but you don't really know that because, although your contractions are close, they are not hardworking. *Fast labors usually work very hard!*

If you remember that anything less than forty-five seconds is nothing to get excited about, then you won't blow it and dash off to the hospital. You could have a very typical, textbook length of labor if it takes you several hours to work up to good working contractions of sixty seconds.

Opening Scene #7: LEAKING

You start with the bag of water leaking, a little trickle (a teaspoon or two), three or four times a day. Not too much but enough to make you notice and wonder what's going on. (I'm definitely not talking about *gushes* of water, just an occasional slight leaking.)

Doctors have different opinions on what to do about this, and it's important to find out what your doctor says. A doctor who is calm about it and tells the woman to just continue as normal and let him know if anything changes seems to get the best results.

Very often a slight leak will seem to seal over and the pregnancy will continue undisturbed until the baby is ready and you simply go into labor. Women do much better when a slight leak is handled this way, rather than forcing labor to start now with drugs to make the uterus contract. Do not douche, do not insert a tampon, don't put anything into the vagina.

Opening Scene #8: THE PUTTERER

Your labor starts with contractions only thirty to thirty-five seconds long. They are several to ten minutes apart. That's pretty far. Your labor may last about twenty-two hours or more and we hope that you decide to stay home for fifteen of those hours.

You feel confident about staying home, because you saw nothing but the beginning emotional signpost for the first nine hours of labor. It was obvious that you were not hard at work during this time.

You may have been lying down for some of this time, but only because it was late in the evening or you were simply tired of fooling around doing other things, not out of a *need* to work with labor yet.

You and your coach finally see the serious emotional signpost and decide to get as much as possible of the working part of labor behind you at home. You do this for seven hours and arrive at the hospital with contractions sixty seconds long and four to five minutes apart (still on the early side).

You're certainly glad that you didn't come any earlier and that you understood the emotional signposts to guide you, because you find that you have eight hours to go in the hospital.

Opening Scene #9: BACKACHE ONLY

You start with a backache. It gets stronger. It's recurring. It has a peak of strength, after which it drops off and several minutes go by before you experience it again. You start timing, and sure enough this is the real thing. A *few* women experience contractions only as a backache. If it is strong enough to stop your conversation and require that you lie down, plus it comes and goes and gets more frequent and stronger, then you should realize what's happening.

Opening Scene #10: ANY MINUTE NOW

I commonly have students walking around who are four and five centimeters dilated. They are not in labor. Sometimes they are like that for three or four weeks. This is usually discovered on a routine office visit, and invariably the woman is informed that she is going to start labor any minute and certainly won't make it through the weekend.

The woman inevitably goes home emotionally very high and awaits her first contraction. Monday morning rolls around and she is still waiting. The next Monday morning she is still waiting. Weekends come and go and finally she is emotionally frazzled from all the predictions.

Although this should be *the easiest possible labor*, it often ends up a disaster. Everything possible is done to get labor started. The woman is kept emotionally tense for the "any minute now" occurrence.

How sad. This has to be the easiest possible way to dilate four and five centimeters and not even be aware of it. Most women have to work to dilate that far! When you force labor to start before it is ready, you are asking for a hard labor. Why turn this type of extra-easy first stage into an extra hard one?

Be patient. Don't look for labor to start any second. You'll reach a point where you will *feel* contractions and have to get to work. Then, and only then, will you know what day will be your baby's birthday. This is not at all uncommon.

When you do start, chances are very great that you will bypass the beginning signpost and get right to work! Although you generally tend to have a shorter first stage, there is no consistent effect on second stage. It too may zip along or it may just as easily take a couple of hours.

TO THE COACH

More people get to the hospital way too soon, rather than too late.

The surest way *not* to have a natural birth is to be psychologically beaten down and frustrated by a long stay in the hospital with all its routines and disturbances. Hospital personnel are accustomed to medicated mothers; they focus on complications, and these vibes come across with devastating effect on the laboring mother.

Coach, don't get a chip on your shoulder toward the hospital staff, though. They do not mean to hinder you. Certainly, they are not trying to make things difficult. You *must* develop good rapport with the staff. Never generate hostility because the laboring woman simply cannot relax in a hostile environment. There is no malice in hospital routines, but the fewer hours you are there the better your labor will go.

OUR BIRTH STORY: STEPHEN AND JAKAI YIP; FIRST BABY

Putterer

APRIL 9, Beginning Emotional Signpost
Steve spent the last four days in New Orleans at a sports medicine conference; I picked him up from the airport at 6:30 p.m. We had our last date night that evening. In the shower, my bloody show appeared. This was followed by my water bag leaking for the next hour. No contractions started, so we decided to go to bed.

APRIL 10, Serious Emotional Signpost
FIRST STAGE OF LABOR
Contractions began at 5 a.m., continuing throughout the morning until they were six minutes apart, lasting more than sixty seconds. I became more serious and needed coaching from Steve in bed.

Steve notified our midwife team and sent out a message to close friends and family for prayer. Our midwives advised us to check my temperature every four hours and continue drinking and eating throughout the day. By the afternoon, my contractions stalled to every twelve to fifteen minutes, lasting fewer than forty-five seconds. *We were back to somewhere between the beginning emotional signpost and the beginning of the serious emotional signpost.*

We began to worry and decided to contact Susan for some insight. She reassured us it was a nice break and I should get some rest before contractions took off again. One of our midwives came by that evening to give me a gentle massage and support.

APRIL 11, Self-Doubt Signpost

My contractions started to progress to eight minutes apart, and around 2 a.m., I woke Steve up for more coaching. We were back at a solid *SERIOUS EMOTIONAL SIGN-POST*. My contractions progressed to five minutes apart, lasting more than forty-five seconds. The midwife returned around 7 a.m. to check on our progress. I was now showing the *SELF-DOUBT SIGNPOST*, such as not wanting to stay in bed and saying things like "This is too much" and "Help me, Jesus." The thought of giving in and needing an epidural crossed my mind during a few contractions as well, although I never vocalized this.

I had to get out of bed, due to a feeling of intense rectal pressure, so I alternated between pelvic rocking and sitting on the toilet during each contraction. I got into the shower and let hot water run down my back as Steve massaged me, then the urge to push began.

Contractions progressed to three minutes apart, lasting about two minutes. We decided to attempt pushing on the bed with the next two contractions. It felt relieving. At that point, our midwife advised us to meet her at the birthing center, as I was going into the pushing stage.

Before leaving the apartment, I had a contraction that felt much different, as if I felt my son's head emerge through my pelvis. I immediately felt a sense of panic and knew we needed to make our way to the birthing center as soon as possible. It was difficult to walk due to his position, and it was even more difficult not pushing with contractions in the car.

SECOND STAGE OF LABOR

Once we arrived at the birth center, our midwife asked us if she could perform a vaginal exam. We were hesitant at first because we knew we were complete due to observing all three emotional signposts; however, our midwife was not sure. She wanted to check my cervix because she could not tell how far along I was by how I appeared. She confirmed I was fully dilated and at a +1 station. They filled the birthing tub for me and I started pushing in the tub. I pushed in the pelvic-rock position a few times, and then switched to the squatting position. I felt the most awareness in this position and had a sense of how much pressure I needed with each contraction to move my baby's head farther down and out.

The midwife checked the baby's heart tones every third contraction. Steve continued coaching, and we felt

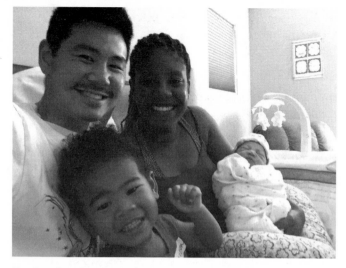

Dr. Stephen Yip and Jakai Yip, PA-C/MPH

the baby's head after each contraction. I felt intense burning in my vagina near full crowning. I also felt intense pressure and then numbness in my perineum with the last few pushes. His head fully emerged and Steve witnessed him perform the Heimlich maneuver. [Susan's note: The baby's chest is compressed by the vaginal barrel and this helps squeeze the amniotic fluid out of the baby's lungs. It's like a built-in natural Heimlich maneuver.] With one more contraction, his body came out and Steve caught him in the water. We did skin-to-skin immediately, and I was able to put our baby to my breast.

THIRD STAGE OF LABOR

The placenta came out after ten minutes with one last push. Steven then cut the cord after it stopped pulsating. We rejoiced over having a great birth and spent the next two days at the birth center getting to know and love our new baby.

OUR BIRTH STORY: STEPHEN AND JAKAI YIP; SECOND BABY

Putterer Again

JULY 12

I felt mild contractions in the early morning (5–8 a.m.) about every twenty to thirty minutes, but they never progressed.

JULY 13

The same contractions lasted throughout the entire day; they were manageable and felt more like menstrual cramps.

JULY 14

My contractions picked up and I needed coaching by 2 a.m. I was in active labor for almost eight hours, and then my water broke. Happiness!

After that, Steve says I definitely had the *self-doubt emotional signpost*, because I was confused about whether

I should push and if I would make it through this time around. Steve was great and focused on keeping me relaxed, but I got to a point where I was pushing involuntarily, lying on my side! So I got off the bed in an attempt to get to the bathtub, but with contractions every three minutes, lasting ninety seconds, the midwives though I might push the baby out on the floor.

Somehow I made it to the tub and pushed for about twenty-five minutes.

Once I was in the water, pushing felt good to do. But I remember feeling weary at the end of the pushing stage because I crowned through two contractions and kept thinking, "When is his head coming out!?" But thankfully I waited it out because he was *way* bigger than I expected him to be, almost two pounds larger than Jackson. I had no tears, just skid marks again. When he was born he did have the cord wrapped twice around his neck, but the midwives unwrapped him fast and he was fine.

I nursed him and tried to sit upright for the placenta to come out efficiently. There was no blood and after about forty minutes the midwife checked me and felt my placenta just sitting in my vagina and she lifted it out easily. They were impressed at how little blood I had lost. Sian Timothy Yip weighed 8 pounds, 12 ounces.

A TEXTBOOK RUN-THROUGH: THE FIRST STAGE

Now that we've covered all the various ways your labor might begin, let's erase all that and start at the beginning of a *textbook labor* for our rehearsal so you will have an opportunity to think about and try out everything.

The pieces of the puzzle for first stage all fall together for you now. It is important that the two of you find a time when you can go through this entire section from beginning to end like a drill.

You are ready for this rehearsal if you have carefully studied and put thought into the *six needs* of the laboring mother. You must know how to coach relaxation, breathing, and the "bag of muscles" technique. If needed, reread some of the coaching exercises before starting the rehearsal.

Do not skip over anything in this rehearsal, thinking you know it well enough already. If you do this rehearsal carefully and thoroughly, you'll have a good feel for labor. *Do it now*—tomorrow may be too late to practice!

Final Rehearsal of the First Stage—Textbook Labor

Your first contraction

You're standing at the sink doing dishes and you have your first contraction. Very minor really, only 30 seconds long. You just sag your tummy extremely and breathe with a steady, slow rhythm way down low in your abdomen. *Right now, at the beginning, think of relaxing your tummy extremely to avoid a crampy sensation.* Try it now in a sitting or standing position. Your coach can time a pretend contraction.

Your contraction at this point: 30 to 35 seconds long

Six to 7 minutes have passed, and you have another contraction. Again, you simply sag your tummy extremely and breathe with a steady rhythm way down low.

Contraction begins: 35 to 40 seconds long

Anything from 2 to 3 hours to several hours have gone by now. You say, "I'm getting uncomfortable trying to stand or sit up with these. I really need to lie down with them." *Don't lie down until you have to.* Nothing is more boring than lying down concentrating for more hours than necessary. This is the beginning of the serious emotional signpost.

CURVEBALL: Okay, here's a curveball. You go through the beginning emotional signpost of elation, excitement. You get to the serious emotional signpost, well, actually, you're just barely there, perhaps 40- to 45-second-long contractions (or whenever you feel a need for more than the relaxed, deep belly breathing) and you decide to lie down. You want some coaching and maybe a back rub. Now picture this: You are just at the *cusp* of the serious emotional signpost, just **starting** the working part of labor; so they're beginning to get stronger and you jump up!

(Recall, there's **starting serious, more serious,** and **most serious**—all part of the continuum of the serious emotional signpost as labor progresses, and after that there's the self-doubt signpost.)

If, when you were lying down, they were longer and stronger, say 40 to 45 seconds, but now standing up they are shorter, backing off to 30 and 35 seconds long, you want to ask yourself: WHY are you getting up? Are you trying to get away from the longer, stronger contractions? But that's the kind that puts your work behind you—long, strong flexes of the uterus! You want those, really.

But instead here you are standing up, making the contractions back off, perhaps back to 30 to 35 seconds. But they're coming closer, so you think standing is making things go faster, but remember, it is the long, strong contractions that get your work done and open that cervix. If lying down brings on longer, stronger contractions and you're getting up to get away from them, then you may be defeating yourself. Standing up may trigger *closer* contractions but frequently makes for *shorter* contractions. Less work is getting done **and** less rest time in between. Instead of 5 and 6 minutes' rest, perhaps they change to 4 minutes apart when standing up.

Recall the purpose of the side-lying position. The side-lying position is **physiologically best**, the position where the uterus is more fully perfused with blood and oxygen, and, being fully perfused, waste products made by working muscles can be carried away more efficiently. The uterine muscles can work better, while your baby is benefiting also. So again, WHY are you getting up—is it to get away from the contractions because they're shorter now and you like that better? It may not be the best thing to do.

For some women, **THIS IS THE COMMITMENT POINT OF LABOR.** Now, most Bradley moms have already made that commitment and don't go through this at all. But if *you* do, there's no shame in it. You undoubtedly *thought* you did make that commitment to want to work with your labor, but then you've never felt a working contraction in your life, and it takes your breath away; it takes you by surprise and scares you a bit. That's okay, but the sooner you make that commitment to want to work *with* your body and try lying down and going for it with the deepest relaxation you can achieve, the better it is.

COACH: If you have a mom who bumps into this commitment point, just coax her to lie down, to give it a dozen contractions, reassuring her you'll help her to get into the deep relaxation.

This can look like a self-doubt signpost, but it isn't. How can you know this? You know it because she's only *just started* the serious signpost; the contractions are not and have not been 2 and 3 minutes apart, nor were they lasting 60, 65, or 70 seconds. Remember, we look at all three things to know where she is, and two of them don't match up here. That's how you differentiate the woman who is trying to get away from contractions from the woman who is in the self-doubt signpost. Do not even think about scolding her or telling her she is trying to get away from them or that she is "fighting it." You never criticize a woman in labor. She needs some time to adjust. She needs total acceptance of her feelings and some time to come to terms with it and make that commitment now. She'll get there.

A CURIOUSLY ODD AND INTERESTING THING TO KNOW:

Once she has made that commitment, she will be handling much harder contractions later on and doing it beautifully!

Contraction begins: 45 seconds long, 5 minutes apart

COACH: Coach her from head to toe in relaxation and in quiet, relaxed abdominal breathing. Coach her in mental imagery ("bag of muscles" technique), keeping in mind the purpose of each technique.

Breathing=Control
Relaxation=Comfort
"Bag of muscles" technique aids in perception

Rub her back if there is any backache at all. You should be serious and alert. Don't let tension build up. Be ahead of things, Coach.

You see she is *MORE* SERIOUS NOW.

Another contraction: 50 to 55 seconds

COACH: Repeat the sequence above. Remind her not to hold herself still, imitating relaxing, but to really let go!

In between contractions

COACH: Offer her a wet washrag; wipe off her brow and the back of her neck, if she lets you. It can be nice, too, to have sweaty palms wiped. Continue to rub her shoulders in between contractions. Talk to her about relaxing. Do not let tension build up anywhere. The hours are going by.

You see she is *MOST SERIOUS NOW.*

Another 1-minute contraction

COACH: Coach her in everything. Don't forget key phrases: slack open mouth, loose limp hands.

In between contractions

COACH: About every hour and a half, remind her to go to the bathroom, and encourage her to turn over onto her other side.

(A contraction is not your enemy. It is just your own big bag of muscles flexing for you, to get the door open. As you feel the flex, think of opening and opening.)

Another contraction begins

Oops, no, it dwindled away before it got started.

Contraction begins: 60 seconds long, 5 minutes apart

Practice through it with your coach. Do not skip any practice contractions.

Contraction begins: 60 seconds long, 4 minutes apart

On this practice contraction, we are going to do a little play-acting and pretend that a contraction is starting to get away from you. You don't think you can relax, you tighten up a bit, maybe clench your hand, open your eyes, contract your tummy muscles slightly, and breathe rapidly. Respond to your coach *only* after he has coached you firmly!

COACH: Firm coaching does not mean harsh coaching, and, of course, you never criticize the laboring mother. Never tell her, "No, you're doing it all wrong!" If you say something like that, her whole body will immediately go "twang" with tension. This is not helpful. Instead, look for tension, listen for frantic breathing. Give her *specific coaching in whatever she needs help with*, and continue to give it in an absolutely confident, warm, strong voice.

Many women never get off the track with a single contraction. Others lose one or two. If they do, it's not a big deal. It helps for both of you to remember what happens if she tightens up on a contraction. She just makes it last longer, and it's very painful for her to work against.

Breathing is the key to control: calm, normal breathing. The coach should jump on the breathing first, because it's the simplest way to get her back on the track. It calms her immediately to slow her breathing down and get rhythmical once again, and encourages her that she indeed is able to respond and to help herself. But breathing is not enough. *Breathing is the key to control, but not to comfort!*

Relaxation is the key to comfort! Immediately after getting the breathing rhythm established (which occurs quickly simply by listening to slow it down), go right on to firm relaxation coaching.

Contraction begins: 60 to 65 seconds long, 3 to 4 minutes apart

Wait. Rewind a bit. Go back to just before the start of this contraction.

These are hot and heavy contractions. They are close. She almost snoozes off in between them; so the contractions can sneak up on her. It's under way before she really registers it, and now she is tightening up against it because it got ahead of her.

You both know that total relaxation is the key here; that bag of muscles works better and she feels better when she stays out of its way with a totally limp body.

So, Coach, how can you adapt your coaching?

Well, you've been timing contractions and you know that most of them are now coming about 2 or 3 minutes apart. You coach her to know when to expect another one.

Start coaching before it begins, about the time you think another one is due, so she isn't caught unaware.

Coaching before it begins sounds like this:

"The next time you *barely* begin to feel that bag of muscles starting to flex, you want to *greet* it with a limp, yielding body, releasing everywhere all at once, *welcome* it; let it come on strong as you let go. At the barest hint of another flex beginning, *embrace* it by melting down into the bed."

Coach, what are you accomplishing here? You are speaking softly and gently with this pre-contraction coaching and giving her a heads-up that another flex is expected soon. And she needs that heads-up because of the almost snooze state that so many women exhibit in the last few hours of first-stage labor. The most important words here are *greet, welcome, embrace.* And here's a word about words. Words are not magical, but words are powerful. They contribute to attitude and perception.

Now, let me mention how NOT to give her a heads-up. Don't say things like "Another one is coming any second now" (tense); "A contraction is going to hit you soon" (duck); "Get ready for one" (suggesting activity); and the worst one I've heard, "Brace yourself"! All tension promoting. Take great care with the words you use.

ON TO THE HOSPITAL OR BIRTHING CENTER

Women who go to the hospital too early in labor have more complications, and that may be due to physician interventions. Researchers find that women arriving fewer than four centimeters dilated have more infections (chorioamnionitis), more arrested labor, and, consequently, more Pitocin is used to get the uterus back to work or to make the uterus work faster.[1,2]

I see the best results with doctors who encourage first-time mothers to come in with one-minute-long contractions that are three minutes apart. Second-time mothers are encouraged to come in when contractions are one minute long and four minutes apart.

But **second-time moms** can have very scattered patterns. So if you feel you are having stop-the-world contractions, sixty seconds long or longer, you may need to go sooner.

Call the hospital before you leave and let them know you are coming and politely ask to have a nurse who is supportive of natural childbirth.

Note this interruption when you practice Master Exercise II and read the sequence that follows so that you are both familiar with the disturbance and routine of getting to the hospital, and the need to get settled and back on track with the contraction series.

Getting to the hospital. When you decide it's time to go, it usually is a good idea to call the hospital and ask them to "pull your charts," so there will be no delay when you arrive. The coach should put everything in the car except the pillows. Run back and coach her through one more contraction, and then go to the car with your pillows.

What if she has a contraction on the way to the car? (This may happen during a walk to the bathroom, too.) The most comfortable thing is for the woman to put her arms around her coach's neck and simply slump against his body. If his hands are free he can even rub her back this way as he talks her through a contraction that will often be a short or light one. Then, on to the waiting car.

Get her as comfortable as possible in the car. We suggest she sit up with a pillow on her lap supporting her arms. What if she has a contraction? Usually this is no problem. Most women get "anxious" going to a hospital and start pumping adrenaline. This negates the hormone

contracting the uterus, sufficiently impeding it so that the contractions are greatly reduced in strength or may stop altogether until she is in the hospital and settled down

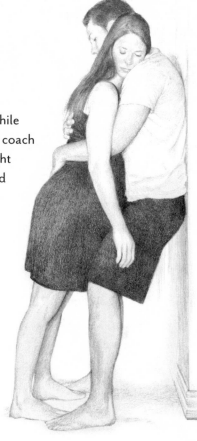

37. Contraction while standing. Let your coach support your weight while you relax and breathe normally.

ERICK INGRAHAM

again. (If she is such a relaxed lady that her contractions continue in strength, then we're not going to worry about her at all.)

The coach should coach as he drives, keeping eyes on the road and hands on the wheel. The most helpful thing the coach can do is to drive slowly and carefully, no sudden stops, jerky starts, or rough corners. You don't want to arrive at the hospital with an irritated teammate. Many of my students call me just as they get into the car and ask me to coach over the cell phone, just until they get to the hospital. It is definitely one of the "perks" of my job.

When you arrive at the hospital. You should have filled out all forms ahead of time so that you can just walk right in, sign your name, and get settled. This is very important to handle in advance. The red tape can easily take an hour otherwise.

When you first arrive at the hospital you may be examined before being admitted to determine if you are really in labor. If your coach has done his job, however, there shouldn't be much doubt about that.

Usually your blood pressure is checked, the baby's heartbeat is checked, and your pulse is taken. You may be asked to give a urine specimen.

Wear your own gown if it is short. A mother who has done this usually feels much better about it. Somehow she feels she's retaining her own identity this way, rather than becoming another cog on an assembly line. Her attitude toward the hospital in general seems to improve too.

A guy's T-shirt, large size, can be quite comfy.

Coach, get your wife back in stride with labor. *You alone are responsible for providing a warm, loving atmosphere for your wife to labor in. It is your very own specialty. Surround her with love and coach her diligently.*

Now, be sure to get her back into the proper side position or, if she prefers, a sitting position.

If you have been working away for hours at home and you arrive at the hospital to find that you are even three centimeters dilated, that's terrific. That's almost halfway to seven, and dilation usually goes slowly only up to seven. Once you get to seven or eight centimeters, you very often go the rest of the way in a half hour to two hours.

A couple of hours go by, and you are now five centimeters dilated. Another hour goes by. You are again examined and told you are still five centimeters. You should never get discouraged if you SEEM to be stuck somewhere. When progress doesn't show up in centimeters, then you are making progress in another way if you are still having contractions requiring diligent work. Maybe the baby has dropped lower or his head is molding or your pelvis is molding, or his head is turning. It isn't all about dilating, or you will jump a couple of centimeters all at once, very soon. If you were not being examined you would simply picture yourself making steady progress as your contractions get closer together and stronger, but if you are being examined, it can be discouraging not to make progress in steady increments.

TO THE COACH: THE PRACTICAL SIDE

A well-meaning nurse walks in while you are coaching in the middle of a contraction, with a cheery "Hello." Your wife is the one having the baby and is the most important person during that contraction. Keep coaching. The nurse will realize that you take your work seriously and will respect your intentions. After the contraction, be sure you show appreciation for her sensitivity and thank her for waiting for the contraction to end. It is up to you to create good communication and goodwill with the staff.

A couple of hours have gone by and she is now six or seven centimeters dilated. You are now seeing the third emotional signpost—*self-doubt*. She is really not sure she can do this. Remember *Praise, Encouragement, Progress.*

Step up your coaching now. Coach firmly in relaxation. Start using the floating technique or whole-body relaxation instead of or in addition to simple head-to-toe muscle-grouping.

You are nearing the end of the first stage. Soon you will start pushing.

SPEEDSTER REHEARSAL

Occasionally in class I hear a woman say, "Oh, I hope I have a fast labor." Be careful what you wish for. A fast labor with a first-time mother is very hard work. You take all the work that a textbook mom might do over 12 to 17 hours and cram it into 5 or 6. Whew!

I like to act out a speedster labor for my classes. Seeing what a speedster labor might look like prepares you better than just talking about it. So here we go, let's ink this picture into your store of birth knowledge.

I stand there, eyes closed, and say, "There's one," and I start moaning. The class is surprised, first because I'm standing and second because I'm moaning. They've learned about textbook labors and putterer labors, but this speedster labor looks and sounds different! I crack open an eye between moans and say, "Wow, I sure hope someone is going to jump up and help me." They freeze!

I continue moaning, picking up steam, and say, "Oh my gosh, somebody better help me!" Then one brave soul gets it together and runs over to me and starts coaching. He remembers or the class calls out to him: breathing is for control. (Fast, ragged breathing is a reflection of fear and a little panic and not good for the mother or the baby.) So he coaches breathing first and foremost, because mine is clearly too fast. But I make him work for it, and moan a little longer, so he has to simply repeat the coaching in a strong coaxing voice; he stays with it and finally I listen to him (because he simply hangs in there coaching, not scolding), and I slow down my breathing and then relax my shoulders, etc., and I handle the harder part of that contraction much better. Well, that's the speedster.

Don't let a little noise scare you! Step up—step in, be there for her, first by helping her calm and slow her breathing, by guiding her to simply *listen* to the sound of her breathing and let it slow down. If she doesn't respond immediately, breathe with her (make your own breathing loud, but calm and deliberate; ask her to follow your breath with hers). As soon as she slows her breathing, *acknowledge her immediately*: "You've got it, you're doing it, I heard you slow that breathing." She knows, in fact, she did, and your acknowledgment of *her* abilities encourages her further and adds to her confidence that she can handle it.

Move on now to the most obvious places that hold tension. Remind her to release her hands. (Did you *look* at her hands to see if they are clenched?) Say: "Relax your face, open mouth, relax jaw, *drop* your shoulders."

At this point there is usually applause from the class for the teamwork they just witnessed.

All right, let's back up and really look at this labor. There is no slow buildup. There are no short contractions

for her to have a chance to get good at this deep relaxation response and then ease her way into better, stronger contractions. No, she will probably not achieve the degree of relaxation that a textbook or putterer can achieve, but she will be able to relax enough to make a difference.

Most speedsters say that the breathing is the most important technique for them; in a hierarchy of what helped most, mindful breathing is at the top for a fast-laboring mom, since she doesn't really have a chance to get into deep relaxation before the strongest contractions come on.

Sometimes a speedster just cannot lie down. Remember, she's starting off in a different place than other mothers. She's skipped the beginning signpost and may have even skipped the beginning serious signpost. She plunges right in with the serious signpost and then on to self-doubt. This happens because she already has long, strong contractions, close together, which is exactly why she is a speedster.

Well, when this lady lies down, her contractions, which are already long and strong right out of the gate, can turn into seventy- and eighty-second contractions, and this for the mother who has had no chance to build up to stronger longer contractions with hours of using the relaxation techniques! So she jumps up and contractions back off to sixty to sixty-five seconds. We're not concerned with her making contractions shorter, since even standing and making them back off a bit the speedster is *still* having long, strong, cervix-opening contractions.

In case you're wondering, this is clearly not a woman who is just easing into the serious signpost with her first forty- to forty-five-second contractions after some hours of labor and jumping up because she needs to make that mental commitment. The speedster starts way past that. Don't worry about her standing if she needs to. She might like the pelvic-rock position, also.

She actually does better in the stronger part of the contraction than she will be doing at the beginning, where it just takes her breath away. The coach just has to be steadfast, stay with her. The woman is usually thinking something like, "Oh no, this one's too strong, I can't catch up." And then she turns to the sound of your voice, because the only way out of a contraction is through it, and the best way through it is to relax as much as possible, breathe with a calm, steady rhythm, and picture that bag of muscles working for you as you relax and let it happen.

SPEEDSTER LABOR STORY; FIRST BABY

Tillett Birth Announcement!

MONDAY, JANUARY 25, 2016, 12:01 PM

Hey Susan,

This is Todd Tillett, Nicole's husband, and we just wanted to share the good news with you: Nicole gave birth on Wednesday to a healthy baby boy. Jack Joseph Tillett was seven pounds, fifteen ounces, and 19.25 inches long.

Of all the types of labor we went over in class, I never thought that Nicole would be a speedster, but she was! Contractions started at 5:18 a.m. on Wednesday and Jack arrived at 12:38 p.m. that afternoon.

We spent the morning at home, timing contractions. I was coaching and Nicole's mother was on back duty, which came in handy as Nicole had some serious back labor pains. The tennis balls were a godsend, both for Nicole's back and for Pattie's (her mom) thumbs and wrists.

At 6:00 a.m., Nicole had hit the serious signpost.

At 7:20 a.m., we had Nicole's midwife on the phone, giving her the update; contractions were about 40 seconds long and about 4 minutes apart.

About 8:00 a.m., Nicole hit the self-doubt signpost, asking me if she was going to be able to do this. I did all that I could to reassure her that she could, and that I was there for her, no matter what she needed.

At 9:40 a.m., another call to Nicole's midwife, saying contractions were almost a minute long and 3:30 apart. They were going to send one of the midwives from Nicole's team out to our house to check on her. She showed up around 11:15 a.m. We decided a vaginal exam was the best thing to do to see the progress that had been made up to that point.

She was 8 centimeters dilated. Our midwife said we needed to get going to the birth center immediately. I ran around the house making sure the bags made it to the car, the cats were fed for a few days, and checking traffic on my phone to determine the best/quickest route to the center.

As I was doing all this, Nicole was being helped by her mother and her midwife, Joni. Nicole's water broke as she was walking out the door.

We got her into the car, and I drove to the birth center, arriving around 12:15 p.m. We got her into the room and onto the bed, and she began to push. Jack arrived just about 20 minutes later.

Total labor time: 7 hours, 20 minutes.

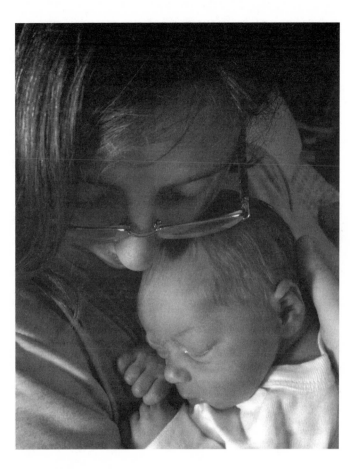

Nicole Tillett
Speedster; First Baby

It was quite an experience! Momma and baby are happy and healthy.

I know Nicole was looking forward to trying different positions we had gone over in class and wanted to try the tub, but there wasn't enough time. During contractions, Nicole was on all fours mostly, while trying to lie down and be comfortable in between. I would coach her from her side or front, while her mother was standing over her pressing the tennis balls as hard as she could into Nicole's lower back.

Thank you so much for getting me prepared for day of the birth. I believe that the lessons learned in your class helped me remain calm, steady, and there for Nicole during this time.

Thanks, Susan!

—Todd Tillett

P.S. I just wanted to add that Todd did an amazing job coaching me through such a hard and fast labor. It was much more difficult to remember to breathe normally than I thought it would be, but Todd was there to get me to calm my breathing and let my bag of muscles do its work! Thank you again for the tools we needed to give birth naturally.

—Nicole

[Susan's note: Go back and find the point where it was time to leave for the birth center.

Todd called it just right and phoned the midwives when the contractions were three minutes apart and one minute long, and Nicole was in the self-doubt signpost. He pegged it perfectly.

Can you see that if the midwives had concurred with Todd instead of telling them to stay home and wait for a midwife to arrive and check, they would have been at the birth center two-and-a-half hours before the birth instead of twenty minutes before the birth?

Trust yourself. Trust what you know. If you think it is time to go, you are looking at all these signs—*go*.]

PART III

THE SECOND STAGE
OF BIRTH

CHAPTER SEVENTEEN

Pushing: The Second Stage of Labor

Y OU'RE ALL THE WAY dilated, 10 centimeters or complete, as in completely dilated! You're there at last! The door is open!

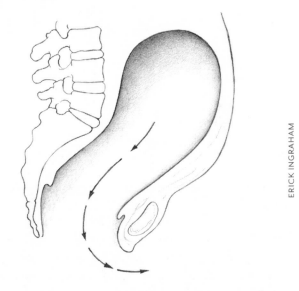

You no longer have two separate compartments; you have just one flowing canal.

ERICK INGRAHAM

And, as you would expect when a door opens, somebody is going to step through. Step through? In a way, that is what your baby will be doing. Babies born without drugs in their system will make stepping motions with their feet. In fact, when you lift your just-born baby up onto your abdomen, after he catches his breath, those stepping motions push him toward your breast! (See Dr. Lennart Righard's film *Delivery Self-Attachment* for more on that incredible phenomenon.)

Your baby makes the same stepping motion in your uterus before he is born. He can also push back with both feet simultaneously. In the pushing stage, the top of your uterus comes down *more* forcefully on your baby and you get an *action-reaction* as baby pushes back. Students watch a wonderful video in my classes (Alexander Tsiaras's *Conception to Birth*), where they see a baby toward the end of second stage use his foot to kick off against mom's sacrum and out he comes.

There's a lot to learn about the pushing stage. So here's how we'll do this. We'll build a bare hatrack of information by looking first at only a textbook pushing stage, with a woman who has an urge to push and has a baby in an A-1, Get Ready, Get Set, Go position.

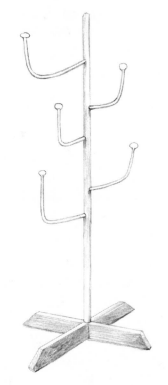

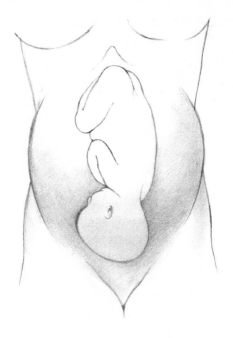

ERICK INGRAHAM

A-1, GET READY, GET SET, GO POSITION

(Baby's face looking somewhat toward mom's right or left shoulder)

Note: When I refer to the A-1 position, that doesn't mean that all other positions are wrong. Other positions are just different but may involve more work than this "get ready, get set, go" position.

ERICK INGRAHAM

When we are finished looking at the second stage in a textbook labor, then we'll add hats on this hatrack of information: We'll look at speedster second stages and putterer second stages, and babies in a common position that isn't Get Ready, Get Set, Go but is still perfectly normal (posterior babies). We'll also look at the laboring woman who has no urge to push, the woman who has an early urge to push, and the woman who has a complete time-out between first and second stage. Finally, we'll cover additional patterns seen with second-time moms. But right now, let's begin with that first-time mom having a textbook pushing stage.

WHAT'S HAPPENING: WHAT IS THE MOTHER DOING?

Remember, as you finished first stage, the last hour or so of it, your contractions were close, perhaps two minutes apart? Well, now, in our textbook pushing stage, your contractions have backed off somewhat. Perhaps you notice they've stretched out to five or eight minutes apart instead of two! (Lots of variation here, but certainly not two minutes apart anymore.)

Actually, Coach, you're the one who notices this first. Initially, you're confused. What's going on? Then you re-member. Could it be? Don't say anything. Let her get this extra rest and just wait. She's sliding into the pushing stage textbook style. At some point she might say: "I think I have to push." Think? Just think? Just wait. Let this urge develop. Let the picture of what is happening come into a sharp focus.

When the urge is just beginning, it often comes and goes, with a contraction here and there, before it really gets established, and that's why you're waiting. Wait for it. In a while she may say something more like: "I *have* to push!" Her hands may have a tendency to curl and her shoulders hunch down. Some women don't actually verbalize starting to feel the need to push; however, you will see a change as relaxation, during these contractions, definitely goes out the window. Relaxation does not work as it did in first stage; it's not supposed to; her body is telling her that she needs to *do* something and that something is push!

WHEN TO PUSH DURING A PUSHING CONTRACTION

You are still having contractions and, just like in the first stage, with each contraction, that bag of muscles starts to flex a little bit and then works a little more and builds to a crescendo or peak of work, after which it dwindles away.

So when do you begin pushing? At the very beginning, when it's barely starting to flex? No, you would wear yourself out when the uterus itself isn't working hard yet. You want to let the contraction get under way, to let it build a bit until the muscles are really flexing strongly for you, and you put your best effort behind your uterus's best effort. You want to synchronize your effort with that of your uterus.

Would you pull out a stopwatch and count off ten or twenty or thirty seconds? No, it just isn't that complicated. When you feel a contraction begin, simply pace yourself: Inhale and exhale once, inhale and exhale a second time (slowly, there's no hurry; be like a swimmer filling up her lungs, getting ready to hold her breath underwater for a short time).

Inhale a third time and by now, with your third inhale, that contraction will be under way, so hold your breath and push, but, oops, that *one* push won't get you all the way through, so exhale when you need to, then take another breath and give a second push.

Sometimes seeing it in a list, like 1, 2, 3, 4 helps you get the pattern down.

1. BREATHE IN DEEPLY—RELEASE BREATH CALMLY.

2. BREATHE IN SLOWLY—RELEASE BREATH COMPLETELY.

3. BREATHE IN, HOLD, AND PUSH. (Exhale when you need to.)

4. BREATHE IN, HOLD, AND PUSH AGAIN.

So twice you are just breathing in and out and twice you are holding and pushing.

Try it now (without pushing, you never push when *practicing*, you just hold your breath) and then we'll get more sophisticated, tweaking it a little by tuning in to your body.

You did try it, right? You're not just plunging on with the reading?

Okay, here's the best part. While you are taking the first two in-and-out breaths, you want to tune in to your body, sense how the flex is building. Is it strong as you move into the third breath you're planning to hold? Yes? Then do as planned, hold and push, and then push one more time.

What if the answer is no? No, it is not really strong yet? Then go ahead and take an *extra* "inhale-exhale" and *stay tuned in.*

What's that? As you took the time to take an extra inhale-exhale, you noticed the contraction was dwindling away, so it never took off? It was just a bump in the road? Aren't you glad you tuned in to your body and paid attention to the cues your body gave you instead of *blindly* following a pattern? Otherwise, you would have been working hard pushing when your uterus wasn't! The pattern is there to help you, not for you to follow blindly.

Why is a pattern helpful? Why not just wait and tune in? What about just relying on instinct? The hospital birth I attended the other night was like many others. Once the mother was pushing, eight people appeared, crowding into the room, bustling about, each one doing a different job: one getting out gloves; another, equipment; another starting up a baby-warming table. The message conveyed to the mother with all this hustle and bustle and too many people is not reassuring. It looks like everyone is getting ready for an emergency, not a birth. This is disturbing and distracting to many women. If there were such a thing as instinct, it would certainly be suppressed in this environment. Also, perhaps much of what we think of as instinct is actually learned behavior. Most women in our culture have not seen many, if any, other women give birth. This is why a pattern is helpful, and especially when you couple it with tuning in to your body!

What do women do when they don't have any pattern to guide them? They tend to do one of two things: Grab a breath and push immediately and frequently like a guppy (short, ineffective pushes), running out of steam just as the contraction is really beginning to work, or they wait until the contraction is just steamrolling over them and then they can't quite catch up and get a breath to stay on top of it and push; instead, they are moaning and groaning their way through.

Sometimes there are too many cooks in the kitchen, even in a home birth, with contradictory ideas of *how* to push; one says push now, quick, it's started; another says just do what your body tells you; another says, don't push at all—just breathe the baby down; another says get four or five little pushes with each contraction. Like a small boat in a storm, you are tossed this way and that with suggestions that don't match what you prepared to do and are ready to do. Ask everyone to have respect for you and to respect your choices. You chose a method that resonated with you, you practiced, you would like them to support what you chose. In the US, obstetricians do not learn about birthing normally (that is, without drugs). In fact, if you look up natural childbirth in the 2014 *Williams Obstetrics*, natural childbirth isn't even in the index! I always let my students know that their doctors or midwives or doulas are most welcome to join them through a series of classes. Why not invite your birth attendant?

TO THE COACH:

Remember that your role is to help her to help herself, and you can only do that well if you have learned everything she is planning to use. Your gentle, constant **verbal** coaching helps her to follow through with her plan and blocks out noise and distractions. What does that sound like?

She tells you there's one *now*, or maybe she is beyond talking and just grunts to alert you. Begin coaching. It sounds something like this:

1. "Take your first calm breath in."

(Don't say, "Inhale, exhale." You don't know when she is ready).

Observe her taking her first breath, so you can stay a beat ahead of her by saying:

2. "Take your second deep breath whenever *you're* ready."

You *see* her taking that second breath, so you stay a beat ahead of her, and as she is taking it you remind her what's coming up next, by saying:

3. "When you take your third breath, *if* the contraction is strong, hold that breath and push." (Emphasize that word *IF*.)

You continue to observe her and you *see* her taking the third breath, nodding her head to let you know it is strong, and she begins pushing. You stay a beat ahead of her and while she is pushing you say:

4. "Whenever you need to, let the air out completely, take one more breath, and get in a second push."

The two of you should stop and try that out now, and then we'll tweak it a bit.

Wait! Are you reading straight on *without trying that out?* Then you're not really comprehending how intense second stage can be. In first stage, you had a number of hours at home to become contraction pros, but second stage, if textbook, is an hour or two for a first-timer and anywhere from a mere three pushes to a half hour for a second-time mom. You won't have that quiet time alone to get smooth and comfortable with what you are doing. If you read without practicing, then you really won't be well prepared. Stop now and practice, until both of you put it together smoothly.

Now, we'll tweak that a bit. Run through that sequence one more time, but this time, on #3, where the coach says IF the contraction is strong, Mom should just shake her head no.

COACH: You are always watching out for her, you see her response, that shake of the head indicating no, it isn't strong yet and you immediately adapt your coaching to:

"Just take another calm breath and stay tuned in to what your body is telling you, just push when it's strong."

I'll wait for you while you try that out!

WHY PUSH AT ALL? WHY NOT JUST LET THE UTERUS PUSH THE BABY OUT?

1. Pushing is pain relief. If your body is clearly sending you signals to push and you don't push, it hurts. Which would you prefer?
2. If you don't push in the pushing stage, especially with a first baby, you *prolong the pushing stage*. We know this without a doubt. Paraplegic mothers, whose uteruses work just fine, but who cannot use their voluntary pushing muscles, have much longer second stages.[1] Prolonging the pushing stage can walk you right into interventions, such as a drug that forces your uterus to work harder, or an unnecessary "times-up" cesarean surgery, or a forceps or vacuum-extractor delivery. Really, doesn't it sound like a better idea to push?

PUSHING POSITIONS

Let's start with the pushing position you *don't want to use*. Lying flat on your back in a labor bed or on a delivery table is the worst possible position. You are literally pushing your baby uphill, increasing pressure directly against your perineum, which increases the likelihood of a tear, and I know you don't want that.

And don't forget, you have very large blood vessels running behind the uterus. When you are on your back, the baby is like a bowling ball compressing those blood vessels, impeding the flow of blood to the uterus. When you impede the flow of blood to the uterus, you impede the flow of oxygen to the baby. Since those very large blood vessels are sort of pinched when you are on your back, there is less *oxygenated* blood getting to the baby, which can lead to fetal distress.[2]

THE STARTING POSITION

Let's look at an easy *starting* position for pushing. This pushing position is actually a full squat, except that you are tipped back on your bottom to make it a sitting squat. This sitting squat was emphasized in previous editions of this book, as it was about the most a woman was *allowed* to do in a hospital setting. Today, that's changing. Women have more freedom to move around and to choose positions that work best for them. This change is not happening everywhere and not all at once, but more options are becoming available to women who seek them out.

Today, I teach women to use the sitting squat for no more than the first three contractions. It is just an *easy* way to get used to coordinating the breathing, the coaching, going into a position, and, at the same time, sensing where to put your best effort. After that there are many better positions.

Start by cranking the back of the hospital bed up at a 45-degree angle.

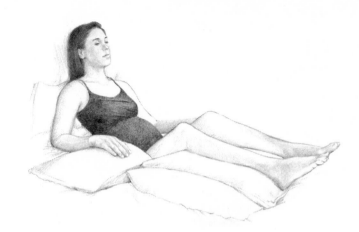

This woman is at the correct 45-degree angle.

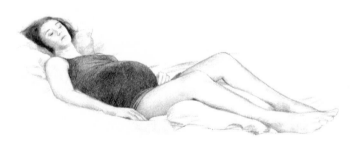

This woman's bed may be rolled up to a 45-degree angle but the woman's back is not. After pushing for a while, you will want to check for this common error.

ERICK INGRAHAM

So when do you lift your legs back—with the first breath? No.

With the second breath? No. Lift your legs back, as you take your third breath, and hold and push. Stay in this position when you need to exhale and take a fourth breath and push.

Then relax out and rest deeply in between contractions. If you remembered to plant your heels close to your bottom, it really should be as simple as lifting your legs and dropping them over your arms. You want to avoid lunging forward to grab your legs.

So now it looks like this:

1. BREATHE IN DEEPLY—RELEASE BREATH CALMLY.

   (No, don't lift your legs back yet.)

2. BREATHE IN SLOWLY—RELEASE BREATH COMPLETELY.

   (No, don't lift your legs back yet.)

3. AS YOU BREATHE IN CALMLY (this is the third time), SIMULTANEOUSLY LIFT YOUR LEGS GENTLY AND DROP THEM OVER YOUR ARMS, AND HOLD THIS BREATH AND PUSH. Exhale when you need to, but REMAIN IN POSITION as you exhale.

4. BREATHE IN DEEPLY, HOLD IT, PUSH AGAIN.

ERICK INGRAHAM

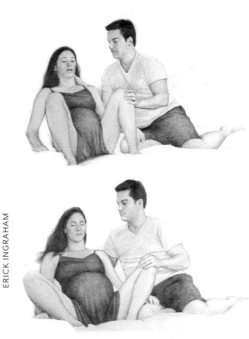

Take your first deep breath calmly and let it all out.

Take your second breath whenever you're ready, relaxing completely as you exhale.

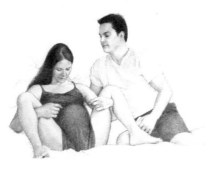

As you take your third breath, gently lift your legs back to you, chin toward the chest. This breath you hold and begin to push as long as you comfortably can.

When you feel the
need to breathe, lift
your chin, exhaling
completely, and take
just one more calm
breath.

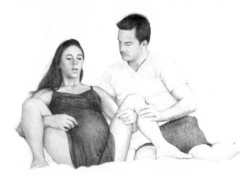

That's all there is to it. You finished that contraction.
Now, hang in there. You know what I'm going to say. Stop
now and try out that final instruction. This time you put
the breathing pattern, the pushing position, and the verbal
coaching all together.

Here's something for the coach to double-check:

Chin once again
toward the chest.
Push downward and
outward as you relax
your legs and your
bottom. Relax your
face and shoulders as
you let all the energy
go downward.

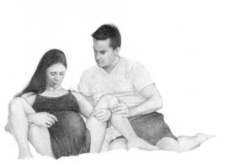

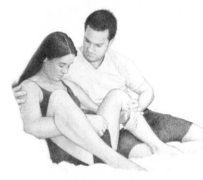

This picture is
correct. The mother
brings her legs back
to her. This is just
like being in a full
squat, but she is
tipped back in a
sitting position.

Relax completely out
of the position and get
the rest you deserve.

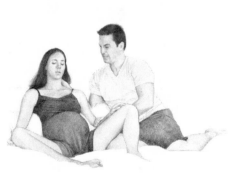

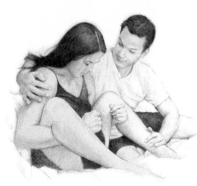

This picture is
wrong. Do not
push her down to
her legs. It is too
compressed.

WHY MOVE ON TO OTHER POSITIONS?

Why not just continue with the sitting squat? It has a serious disadvantage, which you can demonstrate for yourself right now. Remember how you shaped your hand like your sacrum and placed it at the bottom of your spine when you learned the squatting exercise? *Do that now; keep your hand in place and sit down and lean back, as you would in the sitting-squat position.* Now press the heel of your hand more firmly against your spine while trying to move your fingers back away from your spine. Can't do it? But that is exactly what your sacrum and your coccyx bone are designed to do in order to make plenty of room for your baby to come out.

The sitting squat and lying flat on a delivery table (or labor bed) defeat nature's plan. Both positions interfere with the normal, amazing expansion movements of your well-engineered pelvis. That's why you want to do no more than the first three pushes in the sitting squat. It's just an easy, no-commotion way to get the hang of things, but then it's time to move on to other positions.

I've also shown you the sitting squat for another reason. Many natural-birth moms are hustled into this position just as they are about to give birth. It is more convenient for your birth attendant, even though it interferes with normal birthing physiology. I hope you will have a discussion with your birth attendant so that you retain freedom of choice in the positions you want to use; if not, then this is the best you will be able to do.

INTRODUCING THE BIRTH BALL

The birth ball is a great new addition to the pushing stage. You can find them in sports stores. (Not a beach ball, a *sports* ball.) You can use the pelvic-rock position you've learned previously, but instead of holding yourself up, arms getting tired, you can let the birth ball hold you up. Be sure to have a towel to drape over the ball; otherwise, your face is in contact with that rubber and that's not too pleasant.

How to push from this position? Simple. Do you remember which breath is the one where you go into a pushing position? Right, the third breath. When you have a pushing contraction, stay resting on the ball as you take your first deep breath.

ERICK INGRAHAM

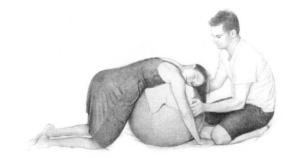

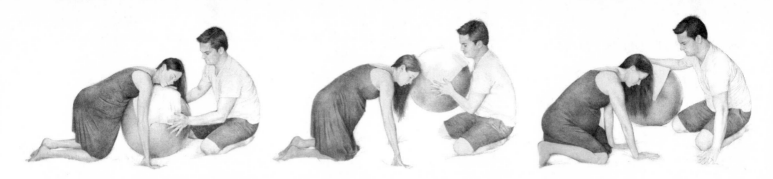

Stay resting on the ball as you take your second deep breath. On the third deep breath, your coach removes the ball; you walk back with your hands into the full squat position.

You can do this while you are taking that third breath, and arriving in position. You hold that very breath and push, and then one more breath and push.

Relax out of the full squat by walking forward with your hands, and your coach is replacing the ball for you to rest upon. Do not stay in the full squat; you *need* to relax and rest.

COACH: When you gently pull the ball forward and away from her, park it on the side, on something that prevents it from rolling away (like a large beach towel rolled lengthwise and then shaped into a circle, with a couple of the hospital's sterile pads [chux] under it), and then move forward immediately to support her with your

hands on her shoulders or by grasping each other's wrists; if you're holding wrists, both of you keep your arms out straight, not bent at the elbows, and lean slightly away from each other. This will provide the most stable support. If you acquire a birth ball, come back here and practice with it. If you already have a birth ball, then practice once or twice right now.

I like the twenty-six-inch diameter ball. The height is perfect, allowing for a correct pelvic-rock position. A bigger ball and I'm reaching up and over it with an upward slant to my back. If you are a tall lady, you might need a bigger ball. Finally, go to a garden center and get three spongy kneeling pads, one for each of her knees, and, Coach, you need one for yourself. Each time she rests out of the squat, by coming back to the pelvic-rock position, you will need to slide those pads under her knees.

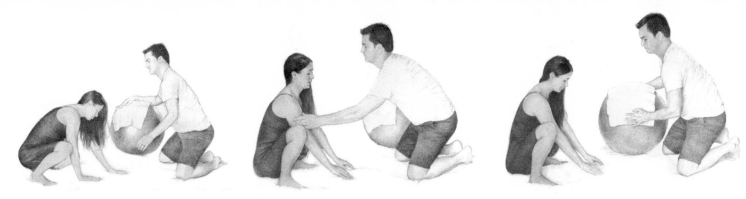

WHERE ARE YOU SQUATTING?

What's wrong with squatting in a bed? Your heels sink back into the mattress and your feet end up at an unnatural angle with the potential to cause damage. And don't assume the bed is a sterile place to birth. Many times I have seen a mother in labor jump out of bed and run to the bathroom, too absorbed in her labor to bother with the slippers by the bed. Those feet of hers, the very ones that just traipsed across the floor, go right back to the bed with her.

COACH: The woman in advanced labor just doesn't care about all these things; she's too absorbed with her labor, so the job falls to you to be mindful and be prepared to grab those slippers and get them on her feet. Hospitals harbor some of the worst bacteria; after all, except for birthing mothers, nearly everyone else in a hospital is sick.

Some women enlist their doctor's help or their nurse's help to make a safe, dedicated space on the floor for squatting. I watched as a mother asked her doctor to help her do this. She told him she brought a quilted pad and a fresh sheet. He helped her spread the fresh sheet out, and on top of that my students put down a quilted pad, like the kind you find for diaper tables in baby stores. Others have used a quilted pad for a twin bed. (Get it washed ahead of the due date and baked dry in a hot dryer; pick a flat one, not one with corners.) Over that, the nurses put down a few chux pads, which you can find in most drugstores. Hospitals have them, but take some of your own so you have them readily available the minute you want them.

Set up near a wall, in case you want to sit for a moment and have some back support. A rolled-up towel provides a comfy as well as a slightly raised place for you to sit when the head emerges. That makes it easier for the baby's head to drop down a bit and the shoulder to emerge.

Another mother, wanting to use the full squat in a different hospital, enlisted the nurse's help. This brilliant nurse came up with an innovative idea! This mom did not want a water birth, but the nurse encouraged her to use the *empty* water-birth tub for squatting and pushing. This obviated the need to set up a sterile place on the floor.

Remember, here's something I said when we started talking about positions, but it bears repeating: Women should have more freedom to move around and to choose positions that work best for them. This change is not happening everywhere, and not all at once, but more options are becoming available for women who seek them out.

When you are in a full squat (not the sitting squat), your weight is a force. When I taught physics classes, I always made my students rewrite any physics math problems that included weight, so that it stated weight-force in the problem, not just the word *weight*. Then they never forgot that weight was a force and needed to be converted to Newtons and calculated into the problem. Will you remember that when you squat, your own weight-force helps open your pelvic outlet optimally? Your weight-force is not in play when you use a *sitting* squat. It is in full play when you do a full squat. Here's what we know:

The abducted femora and flexed knees act as levers to force the outlet open.[3]

The femora refers to your two femurs. A femur is your upper leg bone between your knee and hip. It is the lever. It's the longest and strongest bone in your body. And a force is a push or a pull. In this case a pull, and it comes most optimally from your **weight-force**. You're applying that force when you do a full upright squat and you open the bony pelvic outlet a lot.

ANOTHER WAY TO GO INTO A FULL SQUAT

Take your first two breaths while still standing. As you take your third breath, slowly lower yourself into a squat and push, and then another breath and push. Once again, you need to relax out of the squat. Will you stand up now or go to the pelvic rock with the birth ball?

SIDE POSITION FOR PUSHING

If you are very tired and just want to lie down for three or four contractions, you can certainly do that! That's the benefit of the side position for pushing. Simply tuck your arm under your upper leg and draw your leg back and apart as you take your pushing breath. The drawback is that it puts extra stress on one side of the vaginal barrel, and Dr. Kegel noted that women were more likely to have a tear on that side, so don't stay in this position for more than three or four contractions and avoid it if you are already seeing the baby's head.

STAY STANDING AND PUSH STANDING

Put the birth ball on the bed. Now you can stand beside the bed and huddle over the birth ball, letting it support you. When you have a contraction you may want to stay just like that, huddled over the ball, and push. This is particularly good when the baby is high and if you are a first-time mother. Check with your birth attendant. If your baby is low or you are a second-time mom, she will either direct you to choose another position for pushing, or she will stay right there in attendance, ready to catch the baby for you.

ERICK INGRAHAM

STAY IN THE PELVIC-ROCK POSITION AND PUSH

Go back to the pelvic-rock position with the birth ball supporting you. On your third breath you just stay right as you are and push, take another breath, and push again.

Before we look at the grand finale to the second act (the second stage of labor), before your new family member puts in his/her appearance, let's sum up what's been going on so far.

As a first-time mom, in a textbook pushing stage, it can take an hour or two or more to move your baby down and out. You don't see any progress; you don't feel any progress. (You don't, until the moment your baby's head appears.) About every four pushes, you change and try another pushing position. Why? Because every time you change positions, you change the dimensions of your pelvis and that helps your baby wiggle down. Your baby is actually moving his head from side to side, like the clapper in a bell, but *ever so slowly*. (It's called "asynclitic" when he rocks his head to one side, and "synclitic" as he rocks back to the midpoint, and asynclitic again as he rocks to the other side.) This successive shifting of his head, to one side or the other, aids descent.[4]

Finally, at the peak of a push, your coach says he can see a dime's worth of the baby's head! Then your uterus stops to rest and you stop to rest and it disappears. Remember, it's a sort of two steps down, one step back process.

Next push he sees a nickel's worth of head; it too disappears after the contraction. And then a quarter's worth of head appears and disappears. Soon, it's fifty cent's worth of head when you push, and now, when it slides back it doesn't completely disappear anymore; instead, you have maybe a nickel's worth of head to see. You make a little more progress with each push.

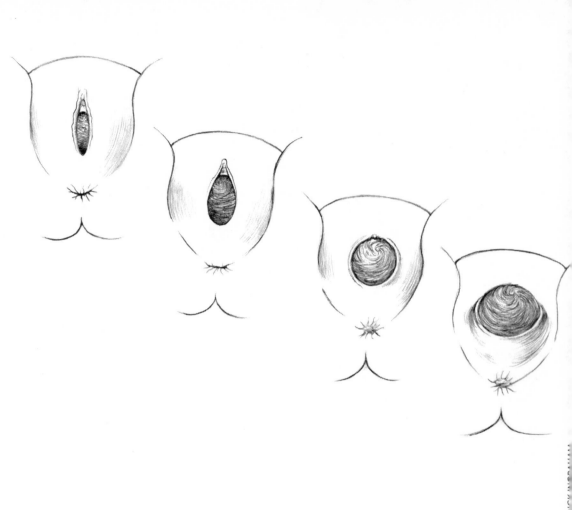

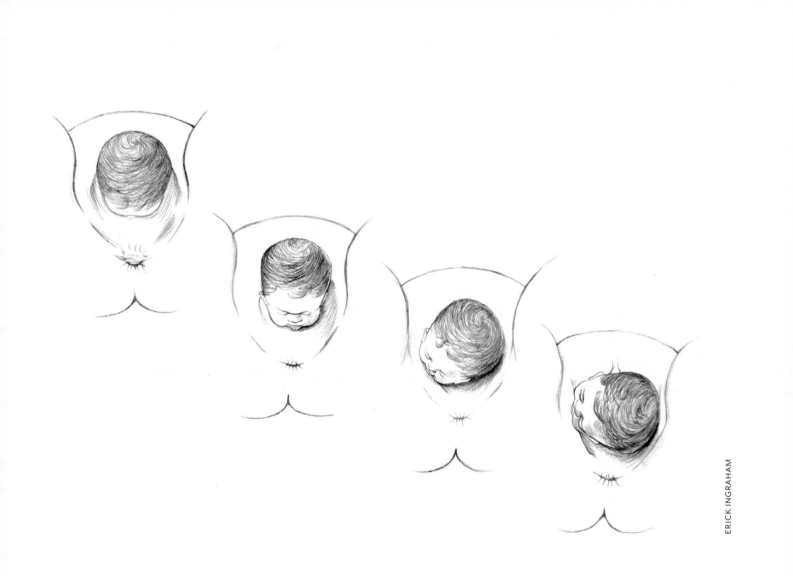

ERICK INGRAHAM

Note that the artist begins the illustration when enough of the baby's head is showing to make an *oval*-shaped appearance at the vaginal outlet. With subsequent pushes you get to the third picture in the series, where the vaginal outlet is a *circle* around the baby's head.

In the fourth picture, there are two important things to look at. The first is to notice that the circle is surrounding the widest diameter of the baby's head. It looks like a crown around his head, and this is called **crowning**.

The second thing to notice is the **vulvo-vaginal ring**. The vagina is beginning to extend, somewhat tubelike. If you turned this mother up into a full squat, the baby would not be coming out toward the floor but rather straightforward. I was surprised once at a birth where the doctor, unfamiliar with squatting birth but willing to accommodate the mother, wondered out loud: "Am I supposed to get underneath her to catch the baby?" I didn't need to respond, as the baby came straight out toward him, into his waiting hands, in the next moment.

What does crowning feel like? Startling! In fact, I call it the **startle reaction.** The mother sucks in a startled breath, which is a great natural response actually, because *you want to stop pushing right now*, and it's impossible to push effectively when you are breathing in. If the baby crowns slowly, then the circulation in your bottom is impeded, causing the perineum to feel numb, tingly, a little

weird, like sitting on your leg too long—same thing, interfering with circulation. Some women describe it as burning, stinging.

Either way, I see women let fear crowd in sometimes, a little bit of panic, of "Oh, my God, I'll just push hard and get it out quick!" You don't want to do that. Don't let fear and a minute or two of that crowning sensation, cause you to shove the baby out in a hurry, tearing the perineum and resulting in weeks of pain, instead of a few minutes of a burning sensation! So here's how to *stop pushing: just keep breathing*. Oh, and slow it down; you don't want to pant. Some women like to think of opening up like the petals of a flower. Get ready to reach for your baby; you're almost there.

We're usually talking just a few minutes here, so there's not a lot of time for you to remember not to panic and what to do. So you and your coach need to have this down, with lots of practice.

COACH: If you don't have this down, like an automatic response, it will be all over before you get it together to help her to help herself.

You only need to say, 1. Don't push; 2. Just breathe; 3. Slow down your breathing (you don't want her to hyperventilate with rapid breathing). It's also nice if you remind her to open her eyes, Kegel release, and that the baby is almost here, but the first three items are the most important, so here's a little coaching quiz to help you to show up on cue.

Because this often occurs quickly, a first-time coach can drop the ball. Since it is so important for the woman's comfort in the next few weeks after birth, let's write that down again. I'm serious, Coach. You need it on the tip of your tongue. It needs to be an automatic response: See crowning—say stop pushing, just breathe, slow breaths. It wouldn't hurt for *you* to write it out ten times or say it out loud ten times, but it might hurt *her* if you don't.

Your doctor or midwife may tell you when to stop pushing. Coach, you should just assume that the mom didn't register that, no matter how loud it was announced. You relay that information right away. She would not be the first mom so tuned in to your voice that she just didn't register another voice at this particular moment of intense sensation.

CURVEBALL: Yes, I'm going to throw you a curveball here. Once in a while a mom just has to keep on pushing; there is no stop-pushing time for her. When might

that happen? Well, sometimes a baby has his hand beside his head. You might even see little fingers waggling at you as the head appears at the outlet. When that happens, your added pushing will probably be needed until the head is all the way out. Your birth attendant should guide you through that.

We're almost done with the textbook pushing stage. Well, here's a surprise! Remember the First Stage Emotional Signposts? In a textbook pushing stage, the emotional signposts *reset* all over again.

When you started pushing, your contractions were a little further apart than they were at the end of the First Act (first-stage labor). If that happens, then your emotional signposts reset. You might become chatty again, as in the beginning emotional signpost. (You have more time between the contractions. I've watched moms take telephone calls from friends in between these early pushing contractions. See the first or second edition of this book to view a photograph of a first-time mom doing just that.) Don't forget to take a picture of that emotional signpost.

Soon, contractions are already getting a little closer and stronger, once again, and as your uterus gets serious again, you get serious (serious emotional signpost), not so chatty and getting much more focused. Take a picture!

COACH: If you were hoping to have a moment to go pee or eat a sandwich, you needed to seize the opportunity back when she reset with the beginning emotional signpost—too late now!

When you have been pushing for a longer period of time, you get to the self-doubt emotional signpost, not sure this is working, not sure you can do this. Is this baby ever coming? Are you really getting anywhere? You snooze off heavily in between contractions, without even being aware of the rest you get in between, so that when a contraction comes, you might actually think there was no break at all!

COACH: Remember one of the reasons you take pictures of the signposts? You can use them to visually show her that she has progressed past the previous signposts and that encourages her; it's a useful coaching tool.

This snoozing off between contractions is normal toward the end of the second stage. It gives a woman an *appearance* of being wiped out—utterly exhausted! But this is not really the case; this is not clinical exhaustion. (Real clinical exhaustion has specific changes in health parameters and can be easily differentiated by your birth attendant.) She's fine. Don't read too much into this. You'll be surprised when you see this same woman, who looked like she didn't have enough oomph left to raise a finger, light up with supercharged electric energy the moment the baby is out. It is a stunning day-and-night change!

SPEEDSTER SECOND STAGE

Let's push on to the Speedster Second Stage. It doesn't take as much time to explain it, just as it doesn't take as much time for you to push your baby out. When a first-time mom is in second stage for just thirty or forty minutes, that's what I call a speedster.

You won't see that brief spacing out of contractions, where the textbook mom was sliding into second stage. Instead you steam right on from those close, long, strong contractions you were having at the very end of first stage to a *continuation* of fairly close, long, strong contractions as you enter the second stage. Of course, that is exactly why you produce your baby faster than the mom having a textbook pushing stage.

Your emotional signposts reset, but just like the woman who is a speedster in first stage, you skip the Beginning Emotional Signpost. You are serious, very serious, probably, in fact, overwhelmed as these pushing contractions just seem to take over. Whoa, Nellie! You feel like your uterus is running away with you. You don't have as much of a slow buildup with each wave; it's more like a steep takeoff. You find it hard to catch a breath and get on top of them, and there you are, moaning through them, and not liking this all that much. (Well, of course, remember, pushing is pain relief, and here you are finding it hard to get that breath in order to push.)

Recall what you learned about the pushing pattern? It's there to help you, not to follow blindly. You modify it when you need to. In this speedster pushing stage, you just need to get a breath, any breath, and push to the point that gives you the relief you seek.

COACH: At all times, you take your cues from the woman. By observing, you figure out what might be happening. Okay, so you don't figure it out with the first four contractions, but now the picture has come into sharp focus, and you adapt your coaching accordingly. Just help her to get a breath at the very beginning and if it is indeed strong, remind her to go ahead and push. Recall that waiting for the third breath was about waiting for the contraction to get under way, but you're watching a woman whose contractions are clearly under way almost immediately. In other words, a steep takeoff. So who needs to wait? Remember the mantra here: She gets her cues from the uterus; you get your cues from her by careful observation and listening to her.

And heads-up, Coach. Think ahead. You will most certainly want to be prepared for that moment, later, when she is crowning. It may be harder for your speedster to stop pushing.

SECOND-TIME MOTHERS

(First-timers: cover your eyes so you don't get confused.) Assuming your baby is in the Get Ready, Get Set, Go position, you second-timers may find your baby coming down fast. It's not the same as a speedster first-time mom. You've done this before. It's like this: The first time you blow up a balloon, it takes more work. You let the air out and the balloon returns pretty much to its former shape. The second time you blow up the balloon, it's easier, it expands faster.

When you try that first push or two, do it *tentatively*, lightly, and see what happens. Are you already looking at some of the baby's head? (My own second baby crowned with three pushes.)

You are the one who might benefit by backing *off* the pushing. You could push just little grunty pushes (puff pushes) and see how it goes.

You want your vaginal tissues to have a chance to expand and the perineum to spread nicely. Here's how this worked for Andrea and Josh:

The doctor and I stood quietly by the side of the bed as Josh murmured soothing words of encouragement to Andrea and rubbed her back in precisely the spot she had indicated. Andrea had that appearance of sleep; she was relaxing so well during contractions. This was the doctor's first natural birth and he was more than interested; he wanted to stay right there and observe this couple using the Bradley techniques. First-stage labor continued.

Andrea was lying on her side when she suddenly sucked in her breath, her eyes flying open, a soft "Oh" escaping her lips, and she locked eyes with me; I smiled. (I'm sure you recognized the STARTLE REACTION, just as I did, at that moment.) I said, "Don't push; I'll just take a look, if that's okay with you." Andrea nodded and with a quick glance, I could see a nickel's worth of the baby's head. The doctor was standing beside me, but didn't have the same view I had, as he was closer to the mother's shoulders. He said, "Oh no, she's not that far along yet." (Remember this was his first natural birth and he was not used to seeing a mother so calm and relaxed without drugs.)

Looking at me, Andrea said, "Should I turn over and get into the sitting-squat?" I said, "You look pretty comfortable as you are; your baby's coming down easily and fast, and your perineum is spreading open nicely; why don't you just stay as you are." She was happy to do so and had another contraction. Josh was a very tuned-in coach and asked, "No pushing then or light puffy pushes, right?" I nodded. Andrea didn't feel a need for pain relief by pushing, and with the baby coming quickly and easily, she chose not to push at all. The doctor moved to take a look with this contraction and, surprised, he nodded his head encouragingly. Two contractions later the baby's head was out and then the body slid out abruptly without a push.

Andrea had birthed in the labor bed (which the doctor had kindly left as a bed instead of breaking it down like an exam table), and she and Josh scooped up their baby girl and held her close and laughed and cried. There were no tears, and about twenty minutes later, the placenta detached. Andrea handed off the baby to Josh while she gave a push or two for the placenta, and out it came.

But remember, second-timer, there is no guarantee your baby is in the ready-set-go position. For example, my third baby was not, and it was a longer pushing stage. It was more like the work the first-time mom does. In any case, you may have a pushing stage much like a first-time mother, so you need to be flexible, ready to go either way as the picture unfolds.

You're finished learning about a textbook pushing stage and the speedster pushing stage. You've acquired a good hatrack of information. Unless you're due tomorrow or next week, I suggest you stop here and give yourself a few days to digest all this information; let it jell. Then come back and read the next chapter, where we'll add more hats to the rack, until you have the whole story!

CHAPTER EIGHTEEN

Completing the Pushing Stage

WELL, HERE YOU ARE, back again, ready to finish learning about second-stage labor. This is where you will put all the hats on that hat rack of information you built in the previous chapter.

POSTERIOR BIRTHS

So far we have only prepared you for pushing when the baby is in the most common position. But your knowledge of pushing is not complete until you have learned all about the posterior position. This occurs about 20 percent of the time, so it is certainly not rare. The physical sensations are going to be different, and the coaching requires some special tips, too.

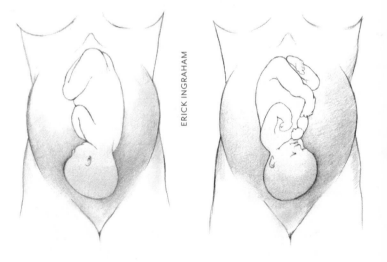

The "Ready-Get Set-Go" Position   Posterior

Notice the difference in the pictures on page 179. In the anterior position, the baby starts off facing somewhat to the mother's side and then turns to face her spine as she is pushing the baby out. You can see that the *baby in the posterior position faces more toward the mother's front*, either slightly to the left or right. Most of these babies will also turn, like a key fitting into a lock, until they are facing their mother's spine as she is pushing the baby out. *The posterior baby just has more of a turn to make.* If your baby is posterior, you will turn him with your pushing, and you will tend to do a lot more of it than the mother with an anterior baby. In a natural birth this is seldom a problem because the mother is quite capable of pushing well on her own, but in a medicated delivery this normal variation often turns into a complicated procedure.

That's because epidurals are known to interfere with the rotation of the baby's head, that turning of the head to the spine.[1] Remember learning about the top part of the bony pelvis (the inlet), the middle part of the bony pelvis, and the bottom part of the bony pelvis (the outlet)? When your baby reaches the **midpoint of the pelvis**, his head needs to find the roomiest part in order to fit through, and he finds the best way through when his head turns to the spine, lining up his head with the roomiest part of the pelvic shape at that midpoint. When he turns his face to your spine, now his head fits that shape best, just like that

toy kids play with: the plastic ball with different shapes that they must turn this way and that until the fit is just right.

Epidurals cause the encircling muscle support (think Kegel muscle) to go slack, flaccid, toneless. The muscles now offer no resistance to the baby's head, but that resistance is essential;[2] it is the very thing that gets the baby wiggling his head, trying to find a way through, and he finds it when his head turns to the spine, lining his head up with roomiest part of the pelvic shape at that midpoint.

The epidural can delay or prevent rotation even when a baby is in a ready-set-go position for labor! A posterior position, however, is not a ready-set-go position for the baby to be in. It is a normal variation, as I said, but it will take more work; it is more of a turn, and it is not just the baby's head that needs to turn when the baby is posterior.

With a posterior baby, his body and his head need to rotate all the way to the mother's side, and then rotate some more, as if the baby is looking in the direction of the mother's shoulder. At last, he has reached the position that the anterior baby—the ready-get set-go baby—started in. Now it is only his head that needs to rotate to the spine, just like all those anterior babies.

You can see that there is more work to do here, but it is just more of the same kind of work that you already know how to do. You're just going to have more contractions to do it. Yes, it usually takes longer; of course it does, he has more turning to do, so naturally the pushing stage usually takes more time.

For a posterior baby with a greater turn to make, having an epidural is far too often a one-way ticket to a vacuum extraction, forceps delivery, or cesarean. I find that when mothers know why second stage is taking longer, when they know ahead of time what can help and what can hinder them in this work, and when they have birth attendants who encourage them and do not hurry them, they handle these labors well.

If someone offers you an epidural, before you consent they are supposed to inform you of the risks, not just the benefits. That's why it's called *informed* consent. Ask to be informed of the risks. But people get busy and people forget, so just in case this well-known risk isn't mentioned, well, we've covered it here.

Oh, and one more thing. Infrequently, some posteriors don't do this turn to the spine and, instead, turn to face completely forward, toward the mother's front, and yes, they can come out this way, too.

The first stage of a posterior birth is the same as a regular birth, except that it may take longer to go from seven to ten centimeters because the uterus may already be trying to do some of the work of turning the baby. And the woman with a posterior baby does not want just any old back rub in the first stage, but really strong pressure. "I couldn't believe how hard she wanted me to rub," one coach told me. "She kept telling me to push harder and I kept thinking that if I rubbed any harder I would push her right off the bed."

Now, instead of the backache disappearing as this woman switches over to pushing, the backache gets harder with each push, at least until the baby turns for her. So this woman may look quite distressed and uncomfortable during the pushing stage when she is well into it. My first and third children were posterior. The first one turned early on in the pushing stage and I had a pretty comfortable second stage that was just a lot of work. The third one took her sweet time turning, and with each push I experienced what I would call a damned uncomfortable backache.

How do you help yourself with a posterior birth? *Push and think of moving the backache down and out.* The better you push, the farther down you move it. Sort out the difference between the contractions and the backache. I found myself thinking, "Well, the contractions are okay, that's about the same as I have been doing all along. It is just the backache that is different, and I can work with that."

COACH: It is important that you help her recognize that the contraction itself is something she has already been working with and handling well. Help her acknowledge the backache sensation and separate it from the contraction. This laboring woman needs a lot more direction to stay "on top" of the push. Your coaching, remember, should always match the intensity of the work as you take your cues from her. Although she still sets the pace, she may be quite distracted by the backache, and you must give her firm direction so she can just tune into your voice and follow. Remember, progress is often slow with a posterior birth, so don't stumble over the self-doubt signpost.

REHEARSING THE SECOND STAGE

There are ten ways that labor might begin, but there are really only four ways to start the pushing stage. We will look at those.

Scene #1: ALL THE WAY DILATED; AN URGE TO PUSH

You feel an urge to push, and it is impossible to continue to relax. Your coach asks the birth attendant (or, he asks one of the nurses) to check you. You are told you are completely dilated and ready to start pushing, so go ahead. Great!

Scene #2: HOQUET REFLEX; ALL THE WAY DILATED (WITH OR WITHOUT URGE TO PUSH)

You were seven centimeters or more in the last exam an hour ago. Your contractions have been close and strong. You feel relaxed and calm, and your coach is telling you that you are beautiful to watch. But now your fingers half close during a contraction, your shoulders seem to move downward, and *your smooth breathing catches like a hiccup toward the peak of the contraction.* You suddenly feel that you *cannot* relax. You are experiencing the *Hoquet* (ho-kay) breathing reflex, and you are actually entering the pushing stage. Your uterus is moving down powerfully to push the baby out, and the diaphragm actually bows downward as if to brace the uterus and force you to suck in air to push. Of course you cannot relax. In the second stage, relaxation does not work; *pushing* does. Women are often dismayed by this experience, thinking they have lost control when in fact they have not. They have simply slipped into another part of labor. It can be confusing for three or four contractions until someone figures out where you are in labor. Your birth attendant will now probably examine you and tell you to go ahead and push.

Scene #3: ALL THE WAY DILATED; NO URGE TO PUSH

You are examined and discovered to be completely dilated. Although you do not feel an urge to push, you will probably be instructed to start. If your doctor has a two- to three-hour time limit, it makes sense to try pushing even without the urge as long as you are having contractions. Better this than to let the time run out (in the doctor's head) and have him wanting to intervene. Thankfully, it is finally acknowledged in *Williams Obstetrics* that six-plus hours of the pushing stage is still within the range of normal.[3,4]

I have seen some doctors, nurses, and nurse-midwives instruct the laboring woman to wait and see if she got an urge to push in a while, *as long as she was comfortable* with the contractions. In two or three hours the urge to push often establishes itself, and the woman begins to push. In this case she gets a nice rest between the first and second stage. These were birth attendants tuned in to the woman's body, not just to the clock. And they were not afraid to let some relaxed time go by to allow the picture of her labor to come into focus.

What if the time goes by and there is still no urge to push? Finally, the birth attendant will say, "Well, you got a nice rest anyway, now let's start pushing as long as you are having contractions."

But if you are going to begin pushing without a strong urge, you must start in a different position than you have learned so far, a position with legs extended. The most common reason a woman does not have the urge to push, even when fully dilated, is that the baby has not yet dropped low enough to press on the muscles that give her the feeling of having to bear down. This happens more often when the baby is in the posterior position.

In the first stage of labor, you recall, progress in dilation is measured in centimeters from one to ten. In the pushing stage, progress is measured in stations. Look at picture 38 on page 184 to see where those stations are. Your birth attendant can determine the baby's station during an examination. When the attendant's fingers bump into the baby's head and find it even with two bony points known as the ischial spines that protrude from the pelvis, the baby is said to be at zero station. Before that, the baby is at a minus station. Generally, when a woman has an undeniable urge to push, the baby will be at a zero or lower—that is, plus—station.

So, if you have no urge to push but have been told to begin by your birth attendant (especially one who sets a time limit on the pushing stage), it would be a good time for your coach to ask what station the baby is at. If the

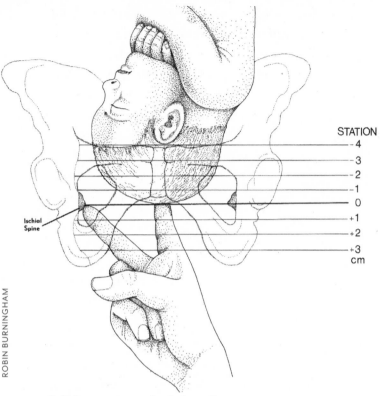

STATION
— 4
— 3
— 2
— 1
 0
+1
+2
+3
cm

Ischial
Spine

38. What station is this baby at?

answer is *a minus station, you do not want to start right away in the full or sitting squat.* Why? As you know, squatting opens up the bottom part of the pelvis at the outlet by making it up to one-and-a-half centimeters wider. But to gain that room at the bottom, it is lost at the top or inlet to the pelvis. If the baby is high, then by squatting the woman is decreasing the space at the top of the pelvis and slowing down or stopping the work of the pushing stage.

If the baby is at a minus station and the birth attendant is telling you to push but you do not have an urge to, you should not push with your legs flexed back as they are in a squat. You can push lying on your side with legs extended, or you can push standing up and leaning on your coach or bent over the bed for support. This leaves the upper part of the pelvis open to its maximum and allows you to begin effective pushing. *As soon as you either get an actual strong urge to push or are told the baby has dropped into a zero or plus station,* you can move into the sitting- or full-squat position and begin to really move along with the work of pushing your baby out. It would be great if all birth attendants knew to start women who do not have an urge to push in the legs-extended position (and even better if no birth attendant had a short, arbitrary time limit on a normal pushing stage). But this is not the case. You may want to talk over in advance how your birth attendant would handle this situation. But it will still probably be *up to the coach to remember—if the woman has been told to push but has no strong urge—to ask what station the baby is at and to recommend a pushing position accordingly.*

Scene #4: NOT ALL THE WAY DILATED; A STRONG URGE TO PUSH

You have a very strong urge to push. You can't wait to get started. You are examined and told you are eight or nine centimeters dilated and you should not start pushing yet. The rationale here is that you may tear the cervix. You should be prepared for a short but difficult time now. It is quite impossible to relax with genuine pushing contractions. The uterus is pushing anyway, cervix complete or not, and of course this is what gives you the pushing urge as the baby drops lower.

To deny the mother the comfort she gets from pushing when she has a strong urge is very hard on her. Fortunately, some doctors feel that if the cervix is very soft—that is, thin and pliable—it is all right to push anyway. The result is almost always a completely dilated cervix in a short time, usually four or five pushes. I have seen this happen many times, and the doctors reported no damage to the cervix. In my experience, doctors who do this get the best results and women are happiest for it. The criteria are that the cervix should be soft, thin, and pliable and that the urge to push should be undeniably strong. It should be very difficult for the woman not to push. This definitely does *not* describe the woman who says, "Oh, I *think* I have to push," or one who has a slight urge to push in the middle of the contraction only.

The final test is that when the mother does give a good, strong, fearless push, it feels right. It should not hurt. The birth attendant waits to hear this. This applies, of course, *only to a labor proceeding without obstetrical intervention*. It does not apply to an induced labor, one started by stripping the membranes or by an IV drip with Pitocin, or any other unnaturally started labor. It also does not apply when the bag of waters is artificially ruptured during labor. Any form of intervention can create real problems. When labor proceeds naturally without any obstetrical interference, you can pretty well count on your body to give you the right cues.

The other side of the coin is the doctor who will not allow the mother to push until she is "complete," in spite of her overwhelming desire to bear down. The woman is told she will cause the cervix to swell if she pushes. What often happens here is that after two or three hours of the mother's fighting a tremendous urge to push (and having a most difficult time), her uterus just sort of quits, as if it has done the work necessary to expel the baby and is now too tired to continue. This seems a much rougher course of action (or inaction) than simply allowing her to try several good pushes.

I have also seen women eight or nine centimeters dilated (or having so little cervix left that it is referred to as a "lip" or "rim") who were told to hold off on the strong urge to push, again resulting in great discomfort. Twenty minutes to an hour or so later, these women were *crowning*. Obviously, the uterus was pushing away, and the mother was being denied the comfort of pushing with it. This is most dissatisfying. In such a situation, we can only hope you have a *flexible* birth attendant. You should talk this over with your attendant (and, of course, your coach) and decide ahead of time how you would want each of these situations handled. You will not be able to make decisions at the time, in the midst of it. Go to Dr. Rachel Reed's website, *Midwife Thinking*. Look on the sidebar for "How to ruin a perfectly good birth." She writes about the "anterior lip."

THE ANTERIOR LIP

OUR BIRTH STORY:
JENNIFER SUNG AND RYAN MEHAN

Labor went really well! We decided not to induce but went into labor naturally late on Tuesday the 16th about 11:30 p.m., about six days before our due date. We labored at home for several hours. The contractions started at about a minute long and ten to eleven minutes apart, and steadily got closer together. My water broke at about 3:30 a.m. We labored at home for a while longer and then called the hospital to let them know my water broke. They asked us to come in, so we slowly got ready and went to the hospital. The contractions were about three to four minutes apart at that time.

Ryan's coaching and the relaxation techniques worked well throughout stage one. Ryan also used some acupressure that our friend taught us, which was also very helpful in decreasing pain/making it easier to stay relaxed.

Eventually I started feeling stronger contractions that extended to my backside, and my body was shuddering with each contraction. [Susan's note: Jennifer is going into the pushing stage right here—first stage is over.] I went into the tub for a while, which helped relieve some of the pain and helped me to stay relaxed through the contraction. Ryan continued to be a great coach and support pillar. He kept me hydrated and fed and as comfortable as possible and supported me during every contraction. After a while, I realized that the shuddering felt better when I gave in to it and that I felt like pushing. [Susan's note: This misinstruction denies what her body is telling her to do and denies the mother the pain relief of pushing.] The midwife said I should not push until I felt like pushing in between contractions, not just during. That went on for a while and eventually the midwife suggested doing a cervical exam to see if I was ready to push. We agreed and when she checked she asked with a note of surprise if I wanted to feel the baby's head! I reached down and felt our baby. She said that I was basically fully dilated and just had an anterior lip, and that I could start pushing. However, they did not want me to do full-on pushing, but I was allowed to give in to the feeling of pushing during the contraction. I continued that way for a while, but my contractions were far apart. The midwife expressed some concern because the contractions were so far apart and suggested that we consider Pitocin.

I refused the Pit, as I thought there was no rush and I was okay if the pushing stage took a while. At some point I was given the green light to really push and the baby's head was visible during the contractions but then went back when the contraction ended. I think that went on for some time.

Eventually, the nurse said she thought that the baby would be coming out soon and called the midwife to come back. I pushed as hard as I could for several contractions and next thing I knew they said our baby's head was out and she was completely out and being placed on my chest.

Someone asked if the baby was a boy or girl and at first Ryan couldn't tell because the umbilical cord was in the way. He was also convinced baby would be a boy, so I think it took a while for him to realize she was a girl! She was very alert. We were tired but ecstatic. We delivered at 5:34 p.m., so labor took a total of about eighteen hours from the time the contractions started on Tuesday evening to delivery. I had a small tear but felt fine (just exhausted).

I don't think I ever had a real self-doubt stage, mostly because I was aware that if it did come that it would be just a phase, so I kind of chose not to have one. The closest I came to feeling self-doubt was when the midwife suggested I take Pitocin—and I became worried about the fact that my pushing contractions were so far apart. But ultimately her concern just made me more determined to push as hard as I could when the contractions did come, and in the end that was enough!

Ryan fed me a lot of chocolate throughout labor and that was the only "drug" we needed—the nurse was very amused about our chocolate-fueled delivery. Both she and the midwife commented repeatedly on what a fantastic partner Ryan was and said that I was very lucky because "most men don't do all that." The midwife even suggested to Ryan that he consider becoming a professional doula!

It was pretty clear from the nurse's comments that we were unusual in sticking with our natural childbirth plan. We know that we were able to do that because we were so well prepared from taking your class—knowing what to expect, understanding the different possibilities that were all within the range of "normal," feeling informed enough to say "no" to interventions, and having a variety of tools to help stay relaxed but focused through the contractions all made our natural childbirth a reality.

Thank you so much for all your support.

You have learned the four ways that the pushing stage begins, so we will go on with a rehearsal of the textbook pushing stage, with a baby in the ready-set-go position and you have an urge to push.

Do you have all your props? Let's do this right. Pull together anything you are planning to use in second stage:

Birth ball

Garden kneeling pads (3)

A towel rolled up for her to sit on when the baby is emerging; use it in this rehearsal

Water bottle

2 tennis balls stuffed in a sock, then tie off the opening to the sock

Washcloth

Chux

Camera or cell phone for pictures

Quilted pad for squatting on

MASTER EXERCISE III

Final Rehearsal of the Second Stage (do not push when practicing)

You are in the hospital or, better yet, a birthing center. You are ten centimeters dilated, and you have an urge to push.

COACH: Did you find out how to work the bed controls when you first arrived? Great! Then you won't be folding her up in it when you're excited and in a hurry to set things up. Get the back of the bed up at that 45-degree angle.

Put pillows under her arms to support them when she is resting in between contractions, and a pillow under her knees. Let her hear your confident, gentle anticipation.

Pushing contraction begins: one-and-a-half minutes

Use the starting position, remove the pillow under her knees, and help her plant her heels back toward her body. If you need to, go back to the pushing chapter and review this. Put the breathing, breath holding, position, and coaching together. We'll just do this position once in the rehearsal, but three times is better when it's the birth day.

In between contractions

Since we're mocking up a textbook labor, you're likely back again in the beginning signpost with perhaps 7 or 8 minutes' rest. Take a picture of her smile right now in the rehearsal. Give her sips of water or ice chips. See if she would like her shoulders massaged.

Pushing contraction begins: one-and-a-half minutes

Now choose a better pushing position. Coach: Remind her to tune in to her body and sense where the contraction is building. If it's strong on the third breath, stay with the pattern. If it's building faster or slower, modify where to begin pushing.

You should know in advance what her first-choice position is and her second choice, etc., so you can help her follow through with *her* preferences. You should ask her, after the rehearsal, to list them in the order she thinks she would like best. But right now, do a pushing contraction.

In between contractions

COACH: Keep the atmosphere cheerful and light if she is still chatty. If she feels that she is not doing this right, remind her that she's just starting; she's never done this before in her life, and it often takes several contractions before she feels she has the hang of it. Sips of water again; shoulder rub, anyone? If she's hot and sweaty, she might like that damp washrag.

Pushing contraction begins: one-and-a-half minutes

We'll pretend you used the previous position three or four times, so pick another one for this contraction. Use that verbal coaching, and let's pretend she has backache. If she has a backache, try the tennis balls, rolling back and forth in the exact spot where she aches. (Easiest to do if she is using a standing or pelvic-rock pushing position.)

In between contractions

You noticed the rest time is getting shorter, perhaps five or six minutes, and she is beginning to show a more serious demeanor. Take a picture of the serious emotional signpost. Be quiet when *she* is quiet. When she really gets into it, she may not be able to ask you for what she needs, so just offer the water bottle or begin rubbing her shoulders. Just do it. If you ask *her* you are likely to get, "I don't know" (so just do what you think would be helpful. Interestingly, she'll have no trouble telling you what she *doesn't* want).

Pushing contraction begins

We'll pretend you used the previous position three or four times, so pick yet another pushing position. Start the contraction (take two breaths) and now she says, "Oops, no, it dwindled off."

Pushing contraction begins: two minutes

Go ahead and do this contraction.
COACH: You notice the rest time is even shorter and the contractions are more work, and she is looking so tired. You're wondering if she can do this? No, no, Coach, you don't get to have a self-doubt signpost! She does, though, and that's where she is right now. She doesn't think anything is happening; she's discouraged.

You remember what PEP stands for, right? Praise, Encouragement, Progress. She needs to hear that now, during and after the practice contraction.

Note: If you are using a birthing tub, you can use the pelvic-rock position, the squat, and the standing position.

In between contractions

Wow! Did you just see a dime's worth of the baby's head right at the peak of that last contraction? I sincerely hope you are birthing in a place where things remain quiet, calm, and relaxed, perhaps a freestanding birthing center with a midwife. But it's more likely you are somewhere else, where you now have three or more people in the room.

Did you want to birth in the labor bed? Was that on your birth plan? Did you discuss it in advance with your birth attendant? If so, remind everyone that you do not want the bed to be broken down into a delivery table, where the bottom part disappears, just like an exam table, because then you're not birthing in a bed; you're birthing on a mock delivery table. Stirrups may be attached. You're encouraged to bring your bottom to the edge of the now shortened bed. Side railings may be raised; you've just been caged. You've just lost mobility.

You might be one of those first-time mothers who sometimes need to give two or three extra-hard pushes to bring the baby down under the pubic bone. If so, you'll want the benefit of the extra room the full-squat position gives you. You'll find that option difficult to exercise once a bed is converted to delivery-table mode. Prevention is easier than trying to get something undone.

Well, lucky for you, in our rehearsal, we'll just rewind and assume that you had this on your birth plan, discussed it in advance with birth attendants and your bed is left as is, which allows you the mobility to change positions as you wish or as you need to change.

Contraction begins

Pretending you did three or four in the previously chosen position, change position again, and do this contraction.

In between contractions

With each push you see more of the head. Does your baby have hair or is he fairly bald? When your baby's head is bald, the scalp can look rumpled like a walnut. That's due to the vaginal lips compressing the scalp. It's fine.

Contraction begins

CROWNING!! STARTLE REACTION.

COACH: I know you have this on the tip of your tongue, right?

Stop pushing, just keep breathing, and slow it down. Try to analyze what it feels like, rather than just reacting emotionally to a startling sensation. Relax your Kegel muscle; you're almost done.

Are you in a full squat? If so, Coach: Tuck that rolled-up towel under her for sitting when the head is out. It should raise her up a bit. Or she could decide to move forward to a pelvic-rock position.

Your baby's head emerges facedown, quickly turning to face your leg. The body usually follows very quickly.

You will have a surge of oxytocin. Oxytocin has been called the love hormone. Ride that surge by keeping your attention on your baby and your partner. As you pick up your baby and hold him in your arms, he is searching for you; he's not a blank slate.

A newborn's brain expects faces: Even when they are less than ten minutes old, babies will turn toward face-like patterns, but not to scrambled versions of the same pattern.[5]

Where will you be looking when he is staring at you? There are so many people in the room at the moment of birth. I see mothers overcome with this surge of love hormone, dispensing the effects to the crowd rather than to her newborn, gushing, "Oh, thank you, I couldn't have done it without you;" she looks at the nurse attending a baby-warming crib, "Oh, thank you so much," and she looks at the doctor, "Thank you, thank you," and she looks at the nurse whose job is to document everything, "You're all wonderful!" Meanwhile, her baby's eyes are staring widely seeking hers, which are looking at everyone else. I tell you this so you will be aware of the effects of your natural hormone surge and use it to your benefit and your baby's benefit. You'll have plenty of time to thank the doctor, nurses, or midwives later.

The other distraction is the cell phone. It's tempting to call special people within five or ten minutes of the birth, but really, you and your baby deserve more time to focus on each other. Please try to give it an hour. When you call people right away, Dad, they want to talk to the new mom. I have seen moms chatting away happily on the cell phone while the baby is screaming. There is no other time in your life that you have as great a hormone surge as you have at birth. Enjoy the time.

THIRD STAGE: NURSING AND EXPULSION OF THE PLACENTA

This is pure anticlimax. Skin-to-skin contact and nursing the baby at once will help cause the uterus to contract efficiently and loosen the placenta in one piece from the uterine wall. Coach, ask the birth attendant if you can clamp and cut the umbilical cord yourself, and then stall a bit to make sure the baby gets all its cord blood. You will know this has happened when the cord turns white and stops pulsating completely. If you notice the doctor tugging on the cord to see if the placenta is loose, say something like, "Is it time to push the placenta out, Doctor?" This reminds him the mother wants to push the placenta out herself and would rather not have it pulled out or her tummy mashed. Usually a few pushes will expel the placenta. It normally takes from five to ten minutes, but can take up to forty-five minutes. Sometimes it helps to get into the full squat to expel the afterbirth, which you can do if you are birthing at home or in a labor bed.

An artificial hormone may be injected at this time to contract the uterus and expel the placenta. But sometimes the effects of this hormone shot can actually trap the placenta inside the uterus. The mother then has to be put under sedation while the doctor goes in after the placenta and scrapes it out of her. Second-time mothers can have unnecessarily violent postpartum contractions with this hormone that are often reported as more uncomfortable than labor. How much simpler if everyone would just wait a few minutes and let labor take its course!

Be sure the mother is again at a forty-five-degree angle for nursing. It is nearly impossible to do so lying flat on your back. If the baby is not interested in nursing right away, the mother should squeeze the nipple gently to express a little milk. Often the smell of dinner is enough to get the baby started. Nursing immediately after birth is beneficial to the baby as well as the mother. At that time the milk has colostrum, which is high in immunity factors that are important to the baby—especially if he is going into a central nursery to be exposed to unfriendly forms of bacteria. It also has a laxative effect on the baby and helps get that system working quickly. While the mother is putting the baby to the breast, if any stitches are needed the doctor will inject Novocaine into her bottom, but now that drug no longer matters, since the baby has been born. The new mother should have the baby for *at least* two hours at this time, even if it is to go to the nursery, since it takes a while to establish nursing. Surely weighing the baby and the like can wait a bit. It is far better for the two of you to have the baby with you completely for the first few hours so the three of you can get acquainted as a family.

Next the nurse will want to put drops in the baby's eyes, a legal requirement in most states to prevent blindness from venereal disease. See what is available where you live. As for a warming crib, which may be suggested at this time, the medicated baby's metabolism is not functioning normally at all, so the newborn may have a definite need to be in a warming crib. The normal, natural-birth baby, on the other hand, does not need one and may possibly find it detrimental to normal responses at birth. An initial cold stimulus may play an important role in the onset of breathing. And studies have also shown that heat loss in the mother's arms is insignificant.

Many Bradley Method® couples are able to walk out of the birth room together holding the baby. This is only possible if they have had a normal and totally unmedicated labor and birth. If you would like to leave together, and the mother feels up to it, be sure that she nurses the baby immediately after birth and that she drinks a glass of orange juice to restore her depleted blood sugar. The new mother will find that she feels fantastic after a totally unmedicated labor and birth. (The coach is probably showing more fatigue than she is.) Many Bradley mothers go home within a few hours after the birth. If you are planning to go home at once, you should talk this over with your pediatrician during your pregnancy. Make it clear that if the baby checks out fine, following a normal, unmedicated birth, you may like to go home within a few hours. Some doctors are more accustomed to this than others, and your pediatrician's attitude is important.

When you go home early, you should be prepared for the baby's first bowel movements. They are black or blackish-green. This is just the meconium, which plugs up the bowel tract when the baby is in the uterus. He clears this out first. Then the stools quickly turn a liquidy yellow. This is a typical breast-fed baby's stool and not diarrhea. Beyond this you will have to depend on other books for the care of your baby. Two of the best for getting started are *Nursing Your Baby* by Karen Pryor and *The Womanly Art of Breastfeeding*, published by La Leche League, which has groups meeting in almost every community in the country that are extremely helpful to new parents.

HAVING THE BABY ON THE WAY

So, Coach, after all this you're worried about having the baby in the car? (It's in the back of every coach's mind.)

It happened to Marty and Judy. Judy was a second-timer who had had a very bad, medicated, forceps delivery the first time. She was going to the hospital on a medical plan, which made it difficult to get agreements with the doctors about the upcoming birth. So, as Judy told me later, she decided she was going to wait until the last second to go to the hospital. Did she ever!

As Marty was driving her to the hospital in their van, Judy said, "Marty, I feel like pushing."

"Okay," he said. He stopped the van, flagged down a passing motorist to take the wheel, and got in back with Judy.

She was definitely pushing! A little head showed at the vaginal outlet. Marty put his arm around her and said, "Okay, honey, you are doing great. I think you're supposed to stop pushing now. Just breathe."

But with the next contraction the baby's head did not come forward, so he told her to go ahead and push a little more. Now he could see a lot more of the baby's head and, wondering if this was enough to call crowning, told her again to stop pushing.

She did, and the baby's head was born gently. With the next contraction and another push the entire body slipped out with a gush of amniotic fluid. (The bag of water was already broken; this was the water remaining in the bag behind the baby's shoulders.)

As Marty told the class later, "He breathed and then he let out a small cry. I cried a lot and Judy laughed and said she couldn't believe it!"

They put the baby to breast, and at first they were worried he wasn't going to nurse. Then he latched on and really went for it.

When they arrived at the hospital, Marty helped unbutton and rebutton Judy's bathrobe so the cord could protrude between the buttons. (The placenta was still attached.) Judy and Marty got out of the van and headed for the front door.

Just as they got there, they heard a great racket. They turned around to see the total stranger who had driven them to the hospital, jumping up and down and hollering, "HOORAY!"

The placenta came out about fifteen minutes later.

Another of my couples, Jan and Don, had their baby in the car, too. They had left for the hospital with contractions at three minutes apart, sixty seconds long, and a definitely serious signpost, after many hours of labor at home. They had called me to compare notes, and I agreed it certainly sounded like time to go. When Jan arrived at the hospital, she was examined (after waiting for about a half hour) and told she was only one centimeter dilated and probably in false labor. She was never admitted because no one believed she was in labor. (Relaxation techniques can sometimes cause attendants to underestimate how much work you are doing.)

But as they drove back home, the contractions got to be about two minutes apart and seventy to eighty seconds long. Jan told Don, "If this is false labor, I'm never going to be able to do this!"

Don said, "You are not supposed to have a third emotional signpost in false labor." Then he heard her grunt as she felt an overwhelming urge to push. They looked at each other, and Don turned the car around to head back to the hospital. They birthed as they pulled into the parking lot.

Neither one of these was a "blitz" labor. One couple stayed home past all the signs they knew to look for because that was the way they wanted to do it. The other couple went to the hospital at the perfect time after a number of hours of labor at home, but the staff looked only at how far dilated she was, rather than how much work she was doing or how close and how long the contractions were.

Neither of these couples was in an emergency situation. Simply having a baby outside the hospital does not constitute an emergency. This is just birthing. So here is what to do with the unexpected birth outside the hospital.

Do

Have the baby. Don't try to hold it back if it's ready to be born. Don't keep your legs closed. Don't pant.

When you can feel yourself stretching open and the baby's head is quite definitely right there at the outlet (you have that numb, tingly, burning, stretching feeling), stop pushing! Just breathe and let the head be born gently. This is important to avoid an unnecessary tear; it usually only takes two or three contractions.

If the cord permits, put the baby to breast. If not, perhaps if the mother tries a tailor-sitting position the cord will be able to reach without any pulling so the baby can nurse.

Do Not

Do not pull on the baby's head.

Do not get in a big hurry. The baby is still connected to the placenta and getting oxygen via the cord. And normally there is a pause now with the head out and the body still in. With the next contraction, push the body out.

Do not pull on the cord. This can pull the placenta off the uterine wall before it is ready and cause bleeding. It can also invert the uterus.

You don't have to worry about cutting the cord. If the placenta is still attached and you go on to the hospital, then you may want to use Marty and Judy's trick of weaving the cord between buttons. If the placenta comes out, just wrap it up with the baby. After all, he's been floating around beside it for nine months; he won't mind a bit.

Go on to the hospital to have them check the mother and baby, but I think you will be happiest if you can get right out of the hospital again. Otherwise your "contaminated" baby (who has been in touch with the real world outside) may be isolated in the nursery and from you!

OUR BIRTH STORY:
SUSAN WILLIS, RN, AND AIDAN WILLIS;
FIRST BABY

According to our doctor, our baby was due on December 12. That day came and went without even a Braxton-Hicks contraction to tease us. I was scheduled to see my doctor again on December 17 to do a nonstress test, which was "highly encouraged" by my doctor if I went past my arbitrary "due date," but not medically necessary. However, the night of December 16, I (Susan) noticed a bloody show before going to bed. I was feeling a bit "unsettled," almost like a carsick sensation, so I told Aidan about the latest symptoms, and we went to bed crossing our fingers that maybe labor would start up sooner than later.

In the middle of the night, I woke up to feeling "tightening" sensations in my abdomen. After getting up to use the bathroom, I noticed that they didn't fade with walking. I laid down for a while, keeping an eye on my watch. The tightening appeared to come and go pretty regularly (every five to ten minutes, lasting thirty or so seconds at a time). At this point, I woke Aidan up. This was

around 2:30 a.m. I was feeling good, excited, and a bit apprehensive about what was to come. We discussed for a bit if this really was labor starting or not, and came to the conclusion that, either way, maybe we should try to go back to sleep.

I may have dozed off once or twice, but the tightening feelings continued, and I was too excited to really sleep. Around 4:00 a.m., both of us were feeling wide

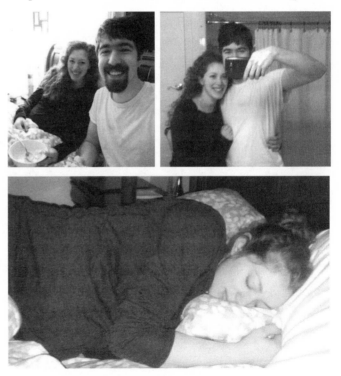

awake, so Aidan got up and made us some breakfast to eat in bed. The contractions didn't take much concentration at this point, but they were still regular (five to ten minutes apart, forty-five to sixty seconds long at rest, and thirty to forty seconds when I got up). Around 5:30 a.m., the contractions required some focus on my part, but, when I got up from bed, they were still less intense and shorter in length than they had been.

We got up around 7:30 a.m., showered, dressed, and tried to get on with our day until the contractions got more serious. I packed my hospital bag and tried to straighten up our room, but soon the contractions picked up again, and I needed to lie down (around 8:30/9 a.m.). Aidan coached me through them. He did an awesome job of making sure I got up to change positions or use the bathroom every thirty minutes or so.

By around noon, the contractions were taking a lot of concentration while I was lying down. I was having really strong back pains with each contraction, so I started thinking our baby might be in the posterior position. Consequently, it was getting harder to relax my body and not fight the contractions. Aidan coached me through each one, gave counterpressure to my back, and reminded me that my body was doing what it was supposed to do. At this time, while lying down, my contractions were three

to five minutes apart and were about forty-five to sixty seconds long. When I stood up, however, the spacing stayed the same, but contractions diminished to about twenty to forty-five seconds in length.

During a particularly painful series of contractions, lasting about one minute each, I got up in the middle of one to find relief. We wondered if it was time to start thinking about heading toward the hospital. We had seen progression, we had been at this for a while (in our minds), and we were approaching the contraction time markers that we had talked about in our Bradley class. However, since the contractions seemed to get easier and shorter when I changed positions or got up, we weren't sure it was *really* time to go yet, so we called our Bradley instructor, Susan McCutcheon.

Susan very kindly offered to time some contractions for us. The first set of contractions was similar to the shorter and easier contractions I had been having when I was up and moving. I was feeling a bit awkward and nervous about having someone other than Aidan timing my contractions, especially over the phone, which may have affected the contractions. However, as I relaxed and got used to the setup, the contractions picked back up and lasted for closer to a minute throughout the whole second set of contractions that Susan timed for us. Based on these observations, Susan assured us that we were *definitely* in labor, but it appeared that we might just be *starting* the second signpost. This was both reassuring and a bit discouraging news to hear, since it felt like we had been working hard for some time now. It did help to have a better idea of where we were in the process, though, so we were glad we called to ask.

For the next five hours we settled into our rhythm. Timing, coaching, changing positions, using the bathroom, and attempting to rest between. The contractions were still coming between three to five minutes apart, but they were gradually building in length and strength. Around 6:00 p.m. I (Aidan) convinced Susan that we should try to eat something. Nothing sounded good to her, but I made her a baked potato anyway. She was able to eat and felt more energized after eating.

Around 7:30 p.m. Susan's dad, a family medicine physician with experience delivering babies, came to check on us. He used his stethoscope to listen to the baby's heartbeat during a couple of contractions and reported that the heartbeat was reassuring and that we were doing great. Based on how "calm and relaxed" we seemed, he mentioned that he thought that maybe today's labor, up until now, had just been prodromal, and he predicted that the baby would maybe make her appearance by the next morning to after-noon. Although a bit discouraging to hear, this didn't square up with what we had been taught in our Bradley class about the "signposts." According to our class information, we were pretty sure that we were well into our serious signpost. We continued to labor as before.

Another contraction set completed, and Susan noticed a small amount of leaking when she got up to use the bathroom. Around 9:30 p.m. Susan's contractions were noticeably stronger. She was really having trouble lying still during them and was complaining of overwhelming back pain. After a particularly strong contraction, Susan asked for the trash can and threw up. At that point, there were slight "gushes" during contractions that soaked her pants, and she began insisting that we head to the hospital.

Our hospital was only seven minutes away, and Susan's dad offered to give us a ride, so it wasn't long before we were wheeled up to the Labor and Delivery floor, around 11 p.m. We told the staff that we believed that Susan's water had broken, but that we did not want to have vaginal exams unless they were medically necessary. The admitting nurse wanted to test to see if it was amniotic fluid and informed us that the swab wouldn't require a vaginal exam. We allowed this test, and it did confirm that Susan's water had indeed broken. We also allowed intermittent fetal monitoring (because the nurse insisted that it was necessary). The monitors were really aggravating for Susan, however, especially during contractions. As soon as Susan would have a contraction, the monitors would move out of place, which caused the nurse to keep adjusting them and insisting that Susan "lie still" on her back, which was the most uncomfortable position for her. Between monitor uses, Susan tried rolling on a ball during contractions and sitting in a bathtub, but these did little to relieve the back pain she was experiencing.

The doctor and nurse really wanted to examine Susan, but we were worried about the risk of infection due to her water being broken. We also didn't want to find out that we hadn't progressed as much as we had hoped.

Finally, around 1:15 a.m., Susan started asking for some sort of relief. She was doubting that she could continue without medication. In retrospect, we can see that this was the "self-doubt" signpost. The doctor again asked if he could do an exam, and we relented. As soon as he examined Susan, he incredulously reported that she was complete! The nurse didn't believe him, and proceeded to do her own check, which was followed by another gush of fluid. I (Susan) immediately felt relief and the contractions stopped for a few minutes.

Within about five to ten minutes, I felt a small urge to push with the next contraction. This was initially more pleasant than the previous labor stage. The

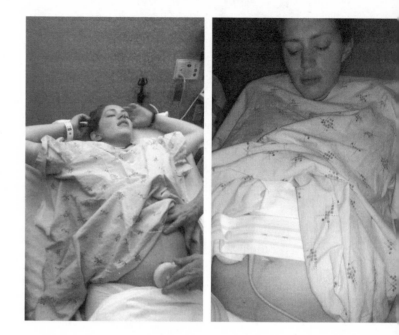

nurse wanted me to try sitting on the bed "tailor" style through a few pushes, which I felt was counterproductive, but we cooperated.

After a few pushes, we told the nurse that we would like to get out of bed and squat on the floor. She responded with, "Would you like me to get the squatting bar? Then you can squat while in bed!" We politely declined her offer and told her we would like to have our feet firmly planted on the ground. She looked at us quizzically, and then asked with a hint of disapproval if we meant to give birth to the baby on the floor. We showed her that we had brought a waterproof mat with us to lay on the floor so that the baby would be protected from direct contact with the floor. She then protested that the fetal monitor wouldn't stretch that far, so we assured her that we could move closer to her monitor, if that would help. Reluctantly, she agreed.

We proceeded to squat through a couple of urges to push, but soon, I felt the need to move to all fours, for stability. I stayed in this position for the remainder of the pushing, ultimately moving toward more of a "child's pose." Aidan coached me through the pushing, and the baby crowned soon after I assumed this position. We told the nurse, who (after verifying for herself) called the doctor into the room. He casually walked into the room as though he didn't quite believe that we had progressed this fast, and when he saw the top of the baby's head, he quickly moved to gown up. He next commented on our birthing position, but given the fact that our baby was confirmed to be posterior, he agreed that this position made sense to him. After another couple of pushes, the doctor told me to give one more good push to deliver the head and then to stop. [Susan's note: Oops! See crowning; stop pushing.] I gave one more good push like he told me to, and our baby's head AND body came out all at once! In a total of about forty minutes of pushing, our baby girl was delivered to my arms at 2:10 a.m. on December 18.

Susan and our sweet baby moved back to the bed and snuggled skin-to-skin on Susan's chest. We asked that they delay the cord clamping until the cord had at least stopped pulsing, and I (Aidan) got to cut the cord. Susan attempted to nurse the baby, and the baby latched right on! There was a second-degree tear due to the baby's fast departure during pushing, so Susan needed to get stitched up after the placenta was delivered, but overall, everything went smoothly and Mama and baby were healthy and strong during and after labor and delivery. The medical staff kept saying how they initially hadn't believed that we had labored at home for so long before coming to the hospital and that they were impressed with how prepared we were to have a natural birth—especially for the first baby!

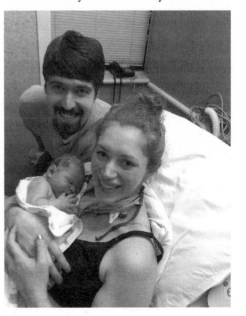

CHAPTER NINETEEN

Drugs During Labor

THE BRADLEY METHOD® IS an effective approach to natural, unmedicated childbirth. But why have an unmedicated birth? Because you want to do everything in your power to protect the well-being of your new baby. Actually, it is most often the medicated mother who talks about pain and being out of control during birth. And despite what you may be told, there are no drugs for labor that are without risks to your baby and to you.

For example, Nicentil, Stadol, and Fentanyl are commonly used drugs, especially for the first stage of labor. Drugs can cause depression of fetal breathing and decreased responsiveness in newborns. Babies are less alert and are less vigorous in nursing.[1] And frequently used drugs have been detected in infants *several weeks after birth*.[2]

But some people think that natural, unmedicated childbirth is just for the sake of babies. It is for the baby, of course, but with natural childbirth both the baby and the mother have a better experience. *Drugs affect mothers, too*. Choices disappear from the scene as soon as a woman is medicated. Drugs can affect the bearing-down reflex, and even though you want to push the baby out yourself, you end up with a forceps or vacuum-extraction delivery. [3,4]

Sometimes women are told that they are going to be given "just a local" and that it won't interfere with pushing or get through to the baby. This is not true. The so-called "local" anesthetics all cross the placenta rapidly. Some examples of these drugs are: Xylocaine, Carbocaine, Novocaine, and Pontocaine. They may depress the baby directly or indirectly by causing maternal hypotension if used for regional anesthesia, such as spinal or epidural anesthesia.[5]

Paracervical anesthesia (injections directly into the cervix) may interfere with the baby's blood supply by increasing the tension in the muscles of the uterus. A drop in fetal heart rate is not uncommon when the mother receives a paracervical block, and there is an increased incidence of a lower Apgar score for the infant. Dr. Avis Erickson warns, "Any drug which artificially changes the mother's blood chemistry or alters the intrauterine environment can jeopardize the fetus."[6]

Too often labor slows down or comes to a complete halt right after a woman gets "a shot of something." Then she has to wait for the drug to wear off to begin again where she left off. The work still has to be done, so the effect of giving her a shot is too frequently to prolong the labor. Sometimes, to counteract this common drug-caused slowdown, the mother will be given Pitocin, a drug that forces the uterus to contract. It is usually administered through an IV, an intravenous drip.

Epidurals increase the number of babies who need to be delivered by instruments, a number that increases regardless of fetal position or size.[7]

Drugs and medical technology can be enormously beneficial when used to take care of real complications, but too often they are abused when applied to women birthing normally. These women are thus subjected to unnecessary risks. The key to this problem is *informed consent*, an ideal too seldom realized. Informed consent means that no woman during pregnancy or labor should ever be deceived into thinking that any drug or procedure (Seconal, epidurals, paracervical block, etc.) is guaranteed safe. Not only are there no guaranteed safe drugs, but many of them have well-known, recognized side effects and potential side effects.

Informed consent should mean that no woman would ever hear such falsehoods as, "This is harmless," or "I only give it in such a small dose that it can't affect the baby," or "This is just a local and won't reach the baby." These falsehoods would not be possible if consumers demanded that informed consent be practiced properly. I have seen women given statements to sign and told only, "Sign here. This is just a standard form." These statements sometimes give permission to use drugs or perform procedures on the woman and her unborn baby, stating that she has given her "informed consent." This must be the grossest misuse of the term possible.

Sometimes informed consent means that the laboring woman and her coach are told all the possible benefits of a drug or procedure in glowing terms but none of the possible negative outcomes. For example, before giving permission to use a fetal monitor, a woman is often told how valuable it will be to be able to tell when a contraction is about to begin (as if she can't tell very easily herself what her body is doing). She gets a sales pitch about how safe the baby will be because they will be able to tell at once if the baby is in trouble, and if so do cesarean surgery immediately.

What she is almost never told in this so-called informed consent is that *the fetal monitor is known to*

increase the rate of infections and unnecessary cesarean sur-
geries, and, of course, there is a higher maternal mortality rate associated with major surgery. She is not told of a government-funded study indicating that electronic fetal monitoring is potentially dangerous and that effective-ness of such monitoring has not been proved scientifi-cally. She is not told that, in effect, she is consenting to unproved techniques and therefore allowing experimenta-tion on herself and her unborn child. (We will look at fetal monitoring and unneeded C-sections in detail in Chapter Twenty-Six.)

The point here is that informed consent is not really being practiced in most hospitals today, beyond the "sign here" on a paper that means you have gotten a sales pitch with little—or more often no—information about potential hazards. Yet informed consent is essential as a corner-stone for parents to formulate intelligent decisions about drugs, routine procedures, and birthing.

PART IV

CONTROVERSIES IN CHILDBIRTH

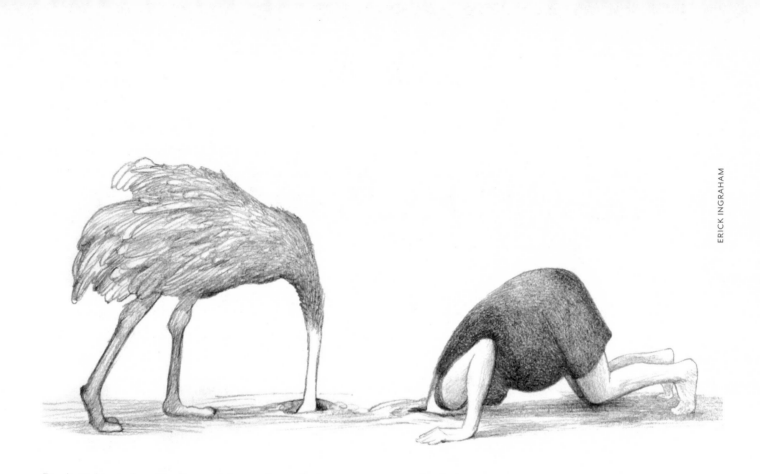

Don't stick your head in the sand. Learn about the important issues in birthing.

SOME PEOPLE FEEL THREATENED by the part of class where we cover the controversial issues in childbirth. They don't want to hear it. But there's no need to feel threatened. After all, *you* are the one who will decide whether or not to *apply* some, all, or none of the information that follows.

Other folks feel that they only want to hear positive, glowing, fluffy information, with the idea that this is going to help them achieve their goal of a natural birth. They believe firmly in the power of positive thinking. Well, so do I. But positive thinking does not mean *blinkered thinking*. Here's an example of blinkered thinking.

A young man gets a great new job with a wonderful salary. There's a six-month probationary period. He goes to work and he knows he is doing a good job and he is also well-liked by his boss and fellow employees. After a while he goes shopping for a house. Before the probationary period is up, he puts his hard-earned deposit down and takes on a mortgage that is quite reasonable with his current salary.

But at the end of the six months, they let him go, no job. He loses the house and his hard-earned thousands in the deposit. It turns out they hired two people at the same time with the idea that they would keep the one who worked out best. The other guy did an equally good job, was also well liked, but had more years of experience, so they kept him instead.

Our young man would have been better served by not ignoring the circumstances, and while waiting for the probationary period to come to an end, he could have used positive thinking to learn all about the housing market, the best neighborhoods, etc., and be prepared to move forward once the probationary period ended. So he was a blinkered thinker rather than a positive thinker.

I urge you not to stick your head in the sand and not hear about the issues because, ironically, by not knowing about them, you are more likely to experience them. Too often I hear mothers taking my class for the first time, but having a second baby, saying, If they had only known, with their first baby, they would not have allowed something to happen that they regret . . . if they had only known!

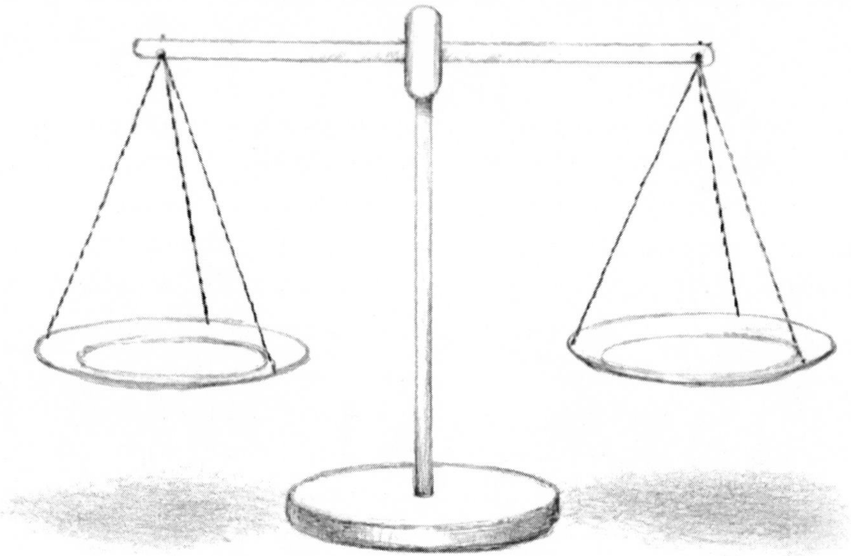

ERICK INGRAHAM

CHAPTER TWENTY

Evidence-Based Medicine versus Belief-Based Medicine

IF YOU LIKE CRITICAL thinking, you will enjoy this chapter. First, there are three concepts to define, and these will be your most important critical thinking tools. The application of these concepts can be enormously helpful whenever you have important decisions to make before and during labor.

First concept: Evidence-based medicine. The phrase is self-explanatory. It means medical practices that are backed up by evidence, by rigorous scientific research, preferably randomized controlled trials, that gold standard of the scientific method.

Evidenced-based medicine is a buzzword right now in the news media as well as medical circles. I recently walked into a hospital with signs in the hallways stating, "We practice evidence-based medicine—we wash our hands." Well, seriously, we all certainly hope so, because it has been determined that many life-threatening, hospital-acquired infections were due to medical personnel failing to wash

their hands, so studies were done to demonstrate the difference that hand washing could make. We're not talking about the days of Florence Nightingale; we're talking about contemporary times. Overreliance on gloves and antibiotics had created a false belief that rigorous hand washing was no longer so important.

Second concept: Belief-based medicine. It means a medical practice that is not supported by scientific evidence. (Like the idea that gloves and antibiotics make hand washing less important.) When a practice is based on belief, the habit of doing it over and over again reinforces that belief. Belief-based practitioners are fond of saying, "Based on my clinical experience this is the best way to do things." That should be a red flag! Clinical experience is an opinion, based on personal observations, not on rigorous scientific support, and those observations might be absolutely valid, but they might also be absolutely wrong. Clinical experience alone is just another term for *belief-based* (and that might be a belief held by one person or many people collectively), but it is not a substitute for evidence-based practice.

Third concept: The standard of practice, or the practicing norm, and recently renamed as "best practice." The practicing norm is what everyone in mainstream medical practice is doing. This is the standard of practice. A standard of practice might or might not be evidence-based. The only thing you know for sure about a standard of practice is that everybody believes in it and everybody is doing it.

Now you have the following concepts to keep in mind: 1. Evidence-based medical practices; 2. Belief-based medical practices; and 3. The practicing norm, also called the standard of practice or best practice. So here we go.

BELIEF-BASED MEDICINE VERSUS EVIDENCE-BASED MEDICINE

Even as he slashed open a vein so his very ill patient, George Washington, could bleed out into a bowl, the attending doctor believed, as did his fellow doctors, that as the patient's lifeblood drained out, so would all the bad things in George's blood that were making him sick. George Washington had pneumonia.

No doubt Washington's doctor thought of himself as a modern man of science, and he would come back the next day and the next to do some more bloodletting. If the patient got better, in spite of his doctor's **belief-based practice**, then this modern man of medicine (considered modern in his time) would point to the success of this medical treatment. If the patient died, it couldn't have been the doctor's treatment that caused or hastened George's death, because *everyone else in medicine was doing the same thing,* and most of his fellow doctors fervently *believed* in it.

If someone in the room questioned the practice, as the patient seemed weaker after each bloodletting, the doctor would say, "Do you really want to take a chance with his life by ignoring best medical practice?" And the relative or friend would be cowed into acquiescence.

This is an example of a **belief-based practice**, as there were no scientifically conducted studies to provide evidence to support bloodletting. But doctors believed it, and they acted on that belief, with the best of intentions; nevertheless, they caused a great deal of harm with this belief. This is how George Washington died. Perhaps he would have died anyway, from the pneumonia, but, certainly, bloodletting did not increase his chance of recovering, did not benefit him in any way.

Why do we study history? We study history with the idea that it helps enlighten us so that we do not repeat the same mistakes over and over again. And I have chosen to present you with a historical example because it is nonthreatening—nonthreatening in that none of you will ever have to say, "No, Doctor, I'm not submitting to this belief-based bloodletting procedure," because absolutely no doctor does this anymore.

So now, let's try jumping to the 1900s and move into obstetrics. When the X-ray machine was first developed for medical application, obstetricians were excited. Now they could take a picture of a pregnant woman and see the baby's head as well as the mother's pelvic bones. They thought, what a great idea! They would X-ray pregnant women and look at the picture to see if the baby's head would fit through the mother's pelvis. If not, they could just do a cesarean.

I can see how they could think that, and I'm sure you can, too. It sounds logical, doesn't it? The benefits seemed perfectly obvious to obstetricians, so why wait for studies to prove that it was safe or that it actually worked for that particular purpose? (Do you recall learning about squatting in the exercise chapter, and that the FDA published a booklet for obstetricians letting them know that X-rays didn't work for that purpose, since just changing a woman's position, like squatting, could change the dimensions of her pelvis?)

And babies were still born breathing and not deformed, so that was all the proof needed that it was safe. Why not use it on any woman who seemed to be having a slow labor; maybe it was because her pelvis was too small, and any petite woman, who surely must have too small a pelvis, and first-time mothers, because they had not yet proved they had an adequate pelvis by giving birth to a previous child. This meant that quite a lot of women were X-rayed during labor.

Along came Dr. Alice Stuart in the 1950s. Leukemia and other malignant tumors in young children had increased significantly (by 50 percent) and no one had a clue as to why this had happened. Dr. Stuart looked for anything that might be a common denominator and she found it! By a rate of 2 to 1, the children who died of leukemia had mothers who were X-rayed in labor.

Her data was reported in a respected British medical journal. And later, a study by Brian MacMahon published in a US journal reported the same problem. This led to the FDA special publication on the Pelvimetry Examination. Here's an excerpt:

> There is a considerable body of evidence that ionizing radiation exposure of humans involves potential for long-term biological injury. Exposure of the fetus is of special concern. For example, the data from the Oxford Survey of Childhood Cancers have suggested that radiation exposure in utero increases the cancer risk by 50 percent during the first 15 years of the child's life. A study by MacMahon in the United States also showed an increased risk of leukemia in children who were exposed in utero to diagnostic x-rays.[1]

But how did obstetricians respond? "This is too new to act on; more studies are needed before we can accept this as valid. Ten years later, "These studies are too old to be valid." In the meantime, it was business as usual.

X-raying pregnant women had passed into **the practicing norm,** the standard of practice; it was considered a "best practice" without any evidence of safety or any evidence that it even worked for what it was purported to do.

Now there was evidence of actual harm done, but it was not what obstetricians wanted to hear. This is a very human reaction, but not a scientific one. There were egos and reputations involved: the head of the obstetrics departments in each hospital that had insisted they needed a bigger budget for X-ray capabilities in obstetrics, the professors in medical schools who had taught thousands of doctors that X-raying was not only safe but a desirable practice for any good obstetrician. And, of course, there was this expensive machine and specialist to operate it, which had to be paid for by using it and billing the patient.

Isn't it ironic that no evidence was needed to adopt this practice *overnight* in hospitals everywhere, but now that there was evidence clearly delineating the harm done, it was pooh-poohed as being information that was too new, needed more studies, and then too old to be valid?

Here's the problem—and it's a huge problem: Once something passes into **the practicing norm** (everybody does it, everybody is in the habit of doing it, and everybody believes in it), it is incredibly hard to get rid of it! It was twenty-five years before obstetricians stopped this practice. In the meantime, "a child a week was dying."[2]

If we want medicine to be practiced like a science, then nothing should be allowed to pass into the practicing norm or the standard of practice or titled as a "best practice" until it is first subjected to rigorous testing in randomized controlled trials and proven to work and to be safe. This should come first, not the other way around. That's putting the cart before the horse. As a matter of fact, if it isn't evidenced based, then it is actually experimenting on pregnant women and their babies.

Every doctor who used X-rays on pregnant women would have said they thought it was safe and effective based on *their clinical experience* and they would have believed that. Certainly no physician intended harm. Physicians are good people; certainly none of them wanted to cause the tragedy of increasing the number of children with leukemia and other cancers. None of these physicians were acting out of mean-spiritedness and yet they did indeed cause harm by not practicing medicine as a *science*, by not waiting for evidence first of efficacy and safety!

When I first started teaching birth classes, women were still being X-rayed in labor, years after Alice Stuart's study (and MacMahon's). Every woman who took my classes heard about these studies. Some of the mothers I taught had the courage to say "no" to this belief-based practice and some did not. It takes a great deal of courage to say no to a doctor, even when the evidence (produced by scientists and medical researchers) is readily available and easily accessible.

Fortunately for you, obstetricians have finally abandoned this practice. But throughout this book, you will learn of several "standards of practice" that will require close examination, where you will be using your critical-thinking skills by applying the three concepts you learned at the start of this chapter.

CHAPTER TWENTY-ONE

Inductions (Early Inductions)

AN INDUCTION IS THE chemical management of labor, using synthetic chemicals (Pitocin or Syntocinon) to force your body into labor and to force your baby out now!

In contrast, spontaneous labor starts naturally, when your body and your baby are ready for labor. There are some good reasons to do an induction, and when used judiciously (which means rarely) mothers and babies benefit.

For example: A mother developing preeclampsia, with her blood pressure climbing, will be lucky that today she can be induced before this goes too far. While induction itself comes with risks, her preeclampsia is a *greater* risk. When used for essential situations it is a *lifesaving tool*.

But today, Pitocin is not being reserved for the rare life-threatening situation. Instead, it is used in 55 percent of labors.[1] In the US, about one million women per year are undergoing inductions and another million women per year are getting Pitocin to make their labors go faster. Pitocin is a "high alert" drug with major risks for mother and baby. When used unnecessarily it becomes a *life-threatening* tool.

Let's explore what is happening by dividing this into three parts.

FIRST: We'll look at what we know about early inductions.

SECOND: You'll get a description of what to expect in an induction.

THIRD: We'll look at late (going past your due date) inductions

THE EARLY INDUCTION

My phone rings. I pick it up. My friend is on the line. He works for a major health insurance company and in an incredulous voice he says, "Susan, you won't believe this!"

I'm all ears, waiting to hear something I won't believe.

He says: "The statistical analysts in our department figured out we've been *hemorrhaging* money, steadily and increasingly, over the past ten years or more. Neonatal Intensive Care Units (NICUs) are a primary cause. There's just this huge steady increase in very sick babies, which statistically stands out to the analysts. More babies are going to the NICU and more of them are spending longer periods of time in the NICU. So the analysts did what analysts do; they looked for common denominators and found one: a direct correlation with elective inductions!"

Sadly, I believed him. Childbirth educators across the country have been talking about this "induction epidemic" for the past ten to twenty years. We're not the only ones who are seeing this.

Here's what Dr. Regina Benjamin, US surgeon general, had to say in a public service announcement uploaded by the March of Dimes.

> Our country has one of the highest rates of preterm birth in the world. We must do better.
>
> Hospitals need to insure that babies are delivered early only when medically necessary. . . .
>
> Remember forty weeks is a full-term pregnancy, and every week of pregnancy counts.

The key line is, "Hospitals need to insure that babies are delivered early only when medically necessary."

Dr. Benjamin is not talking about the mom who goes into labor on her own at five, six, or seven months, producing a severely premature baby. Hospitals have little control over a woman walking in already in spontaneous premature labor. She is talking about women who are induced toward the last weeks or month of pregnancy. This is called a "*late*-preterm baby." She is talking about medically unnecessary induced labors causing us to have one of the highest preterm birth rates in the world.

One strong administrator answered the call, stepping right up to the plate. He stood up for women and their babies, and he accomplished meaningful changes with his actions. Dr. Brent James, chief quality officer at Intermountain Health Care, helped establish an intervention system. When women were sent in by their obstetricians to be induced inappropriately, they were sent home, and the obstetrician would receive a phone call letting him know that his patient did not meet the professional criteria for an induction and they'd need to meet with a department chair or high-risk pregnancy consultant.

Amazingly, the elective induction rate plunged to 3 percent and along with that they had a "massive drop in unplanned C-sections." You can see and hear him talk about this in a fascinating movie called *Money and*

Medicine. I'm most impressed when Dr. James says, "Our NICU turned into a ghost town, and that's a lovely thing." In the meantime, elsewhere in the country, our NICUs are crowded. (If you do get a copy of the movie, go to the menu and select #2, "Too Many Cesarean Sections." Do you get the connection? Elective inductions have a high failure rate and lead to cesareans. [2])

I feel compelled to pause and point out that it could not have been an easy task for Dr. James. It was probably done at personal cost to himself. Imagine obstetricians getting such a phone call; they were probably offended and angry and not used to being monitored. It couldn't have been easy for this administrator to make these changes. It is unlikely that it made him popular. But he had the character and the integrity to put mothers and babies before any concern for himself. We need more leaders like Dr. James!

Babies born early, even a few weeks early, have more breathing problems. They have more infections, jaundice, and feeding problems (and as a group they tend to spend more days in the hospital).

Dr. Betsy Lozoff, a professor of pediatrics at the University of Michigan, conducted a study recently to see what effect these early deliveries were having on brain development, as the brain changes dramatically in the last weeks of pregnancy. She discovered that with each decreasing week in the womb there was a concurrent decrease in mental development that was measurable at one year of age. [3]

She said, "To give some reference point, the differences observed in this study are as large as those observed with low-level lead exposure." The researchers suggested that it's best to wait forty or forty-one weeks, unless there's a real medical indication to do otherwise.

I recall opening the *New York Times* in 2011 to see this headline: A CAMPAIGN TO CARRY PREGNANCIES TO TERM BY JANE E. BRODY.

What a title! It now takes a *campaign* to allow mothers to let their babies complete their growth and development in the uterus!

The March of Dimes did actually open a campaign to rein in the ever-increasing number of early-induced labors. They launched a program to "reeducate" obstetricians. Their slogan is "Healthy babies are worth the wait!" Imagine having to "reeducate" (their word, not mine) obstetricians to the idea that babies are better off when they are allowed to finish growing in the uterus. Their focus is to get obstetricians to *voluntarily* stop doing elective inductions when there is no compelling medical reason for it.

The March of Dimes is drawing a line in the sand at thirty-nine weeks, pushing to have doctors let babies grow *at least* that long. That's a starting point, but a "line in the sand" doesn't mean it's a good idea to induce *at* thirty-nine weeks. It means the damage done is so glaringly obvious *before* thirty-nine weeks that it cannot be allowed to continue. They have given a special program at more than two hundred hospitals, but the March of Dimes does not actually wield any power over obstetricians. It's a call for obstetricians to *voluntarily* stop this harmful practice. If you're pregnant, you'll find out soon whether or not your doctor has complied.

Do we really have to rely on insurance companies and volunteer groups to watch out for pernicious practicing norms that hurt our babies? How is it that insurance companies and a volunteer group like the March of Dimes notices the harm done, the damage to these babies, but apparently many practicing obstetricians, perinatologists, and neonatologists hadn't noticed the harm caused by the induction epidemic?

Let's explore some of the answers:

One: We've become too compartmentalized. Once the obstetrician hands off the baby, she's done with the baby. A baby in trouble is passed off to another "expert." The obstetrician's job is over. Out of sight, out of mind.

Two: Everybody else is doing it, it's a practicing norm, so it must be a safe practice to force babies out early instead of waiting for spontaneous labor.

Three: We're currently inducing 25 percent of all births and accelerating another 25 percent. We didn't get here overnight. It's been a gradual, steady climb. At each step along the way, we became *habituated* to a new norm, a new level of babies in trouble, and habituation leads to unthinking acceptance of that new norm, *as if it is normal!* When something is common, that doesn't necessarily make it normal!

Four: Inducing women early is convenient. Babies who are allowed to finish their development in the uterus and come out when they are ready usually pick inconvenient times to do so—during office hours, requiring the doctor to rearrange or hand off appointments; during dinner; just as the doctor was planning to get to bed early tonight; on the weekend; or just when his vacation is about to begin. Hospital health plans with a constant staff don't really escape this "convenient scheduling" problem. Staffing is often lighter on weekends and holidays, and certain hours of the day or night.

THE EARLY INDUCTION MYTH

Well, if the baby is a few weeks' early, it's okay; she'll catch up, won't she? After all, they do keep growing after they are out of the uterus, so she'll make up the difference in growth eventually, right?

Not exactly. Let's take a baby who is born a few months early, as a way to emphasize what's wrong with this idea. Most of these babies will need glasses (the Coke bottle variety). They are *expected* to have impaired vision. Now this baby will keep growing once he's out of the uterus, but the eye development that was supposed to occur during his time in the uterus is now cut off. The baby's body is out of the uterus and the body moves into different kinds of growth and development (just as the teenage body turns on a different kind of growth and development at a specified point in his body's programming). So, yes, the baby keeps growing but the eye is done, out of the oven. The kind of development that is programmed to occur in the uterus is done once the baby is out. It's not just her eyes; her other organs are also affected.

THE LATE PRETERM BABY

Now let's look at the late-preterm baby, who is out a few weeks, rather than months, early. The brain is growing most of all in the final weeks of pregnancy. Neurons are still moving to get themselves into the right place in the brain. The brain looks more and more like a cauliflower as it develops what looks like deep crevices (which is associated with higher-level thinking). Babies born early have smoother brains.

"Although many women think that weight gain is all that happens to babies during the last few weeks of pregnancy," Dr. Eve Lackritz, chief of the maternal and infant health branch of the National Centers for Disease Control and Prevention in Atlanta, said, "vital organs like the brain, lungs, and liver are still developing. There are also fewer vision and hearing problems among babies born at full term."[4]

Dr. Uma M. Reddy of the National Institute of Child Health and Human Development said in an interview that the textbook definition of "term pregnancy" as one that lasts from thirty-seven to forty-one weeks "is arbitrary—it has no biological basis."[5]

ARE WOMEN DEMANDING INDUCTIONS?

Are women themselves causing the induction epidemic? I'm sure there are some women who ask to be induced, but for the most part that's not quite what happens.

Few women actually say to their doctors: "I'd like to have this baby next Tuesday. Would you schedule that for me, please?"

No, the conversation is usually initiated by the doctor. Here's an example of how that sounds. Jill's doctor started the ball rolling by recommending an induction as soon as she reached thirty-nine weeks. When she was alarmed at this recommendation, he reassured her that the baby was doing fine and so was she. Puzzled, she asked him why, then, did he recommend an induction. He told her there's *no benefit* to the baby to stay in the uterus after thirty-nine weeks, so why wait? If my student hadn't known better, she probably would have agreed. And that would have been documented in her record as, "Mother *requested* induction."

Some of my students have been told "It's safer for the baby, even when there is no compelling medical reason, to be induced early, so *if* you care about your baby, we can schedule an induction for you right now." So the woman agrees and that is written in the record as, "Mother *requested* elective induction."

Coming up in the next chapter we'll explore what happens when you are induced. What does it look like? Is an induced labor the same as a spontaneous labor? What are the risks and the benefits? Don't skip it, assuming that *you* won't be induced; 25 percent of labors, overall, are being induced (and it's more like 35 or 40 percent for first-time mothers in many hospitals).

And when that happens, your baby does not get to finish his/her development, and your body does not get to benefit from hormones and changes that naturally occur in the days before a normal, spontaneous labor.

CHAPTER TWENTY-TWO

What to Expect with an Induction

AN INDUCED LABOR IS nothing like a spontaneous labor. Women who have experienced both an induced labor and a spontaneous labor are quick to tell you that an induced contraction feels quite different and is quite painful.

Women usually can't tell quite where the peak is in an induced contraction. Your own hormone (the one your body makes) oxytocin causes the longitudinal muscles to flex *first* at the top of the uterus and then continue in a wavelike progression down toward the cervix. Pitocin (the synthetic version) causes the longitudinal muscles to flex at the top, middle, and bottom all at once and at the same time. It feels like one big crunch because it *is* one big crunch. There is no gradual buildup during the contraction.

If you are having an induced labor, you cannot count on the emotional signposts that you have learned for a spontaneous labor. (I'm always surprised when women forget this and they wonder what happened.) Perhaps you should read that sentence again. Women usually start right off with the self-doubt signpost and stay that way through the whole labor. Very few women manage to get through an induced labor without pain drugs. (The few who do absolutely amaze me.)

HERE'S HOW AN INDUCTION STARTS

An induction is not usually just one intervention. Most often it is a series of interventions.

During an office visit, your birth attendant decides to "strip the membranes." This has several different names: stripping the membranes, sweeping the membranes, stimulating the membranes, and the latest thing is to describe it as "massaging the cervix," which sounds most innocuous.

But what exactly is happening? A finger is pushed through the cervical canal, dislodging some or all of the mucous plug. That plug is there as a barrier to prevent infection. Now that finger is inserted farther up into the lower part of the uterus itself and swept around in a circle, separating the lower part of the amniotic sac from the wall of the uterus.

Stripping the membranes doesn't usually work (studies show that you would have to do this to eight women to avoid one regular induction—so it fails for seven out of eight women).[1] It's just the first step. But it can make a woman feel miserable for a few days with a constant naggy backache and constant tight, crampy feeling in the lower abdomen. That's when I get a phone call from a woman in tears, who hasn't been able to sleep and who's worn down. She isn't in labor yet. She's not having definable contractions.

Next: This might be repeated in three or four days, but in addition you may have a "ripening agent" (prostaglandin gel or Cervidil) inserted in the vagina to get the cervix to soften and thin. Your birth attendant should, of course, have gone over the risks of these drugs before this step is taken. Cervidil carries some of the same risks as Pitocin—mainly hyperstimulation of the uterus causing violent contractions that can last too long. But often this is downplayed and it is even suggested that this is just a "mini induction" since Pitocin isn't used at this point. (Read Kim West's experience at the end of this section.)

Next: You're soon sent to the hospital. If you are less than three centimeters dilated—and if you are a first-timer this is probably the case—a Foley balloon might be inserted into your cervix. The balloon is filled and expanded with sterile water. It is designed to mechanically force your cervix open. When you are dilated to three or four centimeters, it falls out. In addition to increasing the rate of infections, it can cause the body to turn into a breech position and result in a cesarean.[2,3]

Next: By now you are hooked up to an IV. The stage is finally set to further hook you up to a Pitocin or Syntocinon drip (synthetic oxytocin). Your bag of water will be broken so an internal fetal monitor can be screwed into your baby's scalp. In this instance, the fetal monitor is essential. This is not normal birthing, and it is not at all uncommon for these chemical inductions to cause serious fetal distress. How does this happen? If Pitocin causes you to have contractions that are way too long, then your baby is cut off from oxygen for too long a period of time. This is one of the well-known risks, and leads to brain damage or death.

Pitocin can also cause contractions that are so powerful that the uterus can rupture (tear itself apart). This is why you *must* be on the monitor, so they can know sooner rather than later if this is happening and stop the Pitocin. However, Pitocin has about a three-minute half-life, so things don't quite stop immediately. This is an emergency

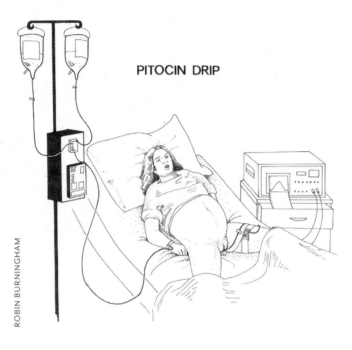

PITOCIN DRIP

when it occurs. What is most amazing is that when this emergency happens, women seldom connect this to the induction. They think they have been rescued from the process of birth rather than from the process of inducing labor. And there are many other known risks. For example, postpartum hemorrhaging is more common when labor is induced or accelerated. Hemorrhaging leads to an increase in the rate of emergency hysterectomies associated with elective induction.[4,5] This kind of intractable hemorrhage (resistant to stopping) is no small thing. All your organs are deprived of optimal blood and oxygen and organ damage can occur. Your brain is an organ.

Next: If you're a first-time mother, the failure rate is quite high with an induction, and then you have a cesarean—at least, that's how it used to go. Inductions used to be stopped if they didn't work after a number of hours, but in recognition that failed inductions are a major cause of our sky-high surgery rates, inductions are now run for up to three days in an attempt to avoid the cesarean.

Three days of an induced labor is the new horror story women share with one another, as if this represented childbirth rather than intervention-caused complications. And why this push to reduce the cesarean rate? Recent statistics show that *more* mothers are dying now that the cesarean surgery rate is so high (all surgery carries the risk of death, so it was inevitable that doing more and more cesareans would lead to this increase).

Recently, in a popular medical journal for obstetricians, I perused a column written by a lawyer who writes for doctors, helping them keep up with lawsuit information: who is sued for what and who wins and who loses. She analyzed for them a case involving an induction. She informed them that when a jury hears the risks associated with induction drugs, the jury members are left wondering why anyone would use such drugs.[6]

In such cases the risks are read to a jury directly from the drug company's literature, so there is no chance to minimize or downplay the risks. Imagine, juries get to hear those risks; don't you think mothers should get to hear those risks right from the company's literature? In fact, a mother is supposed to hear those risks so that her consent is informed, but since they are so often glossed over, if covered at all, we've covered them here, all but his last one, which you can keep in mind as you read Kim's story.

Partial separation of the placenta before the baby is born is called partial placenta abruption. It causes heavy bleeding and fetal distress and is an emergency. It is a known risk of induction.

Kim West shares her experience with her first baby.

At forty-two weeks, all tests showed that Kim and her baby were doing well. Yet she was told it was safer to induce than to wait. As you read her story, you might wonder if it *was* safer to induce than to wait.

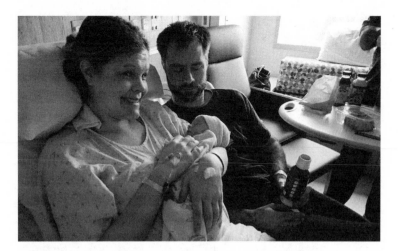

OUR BIRTH STORY:
KIM AND CHRIS WEST; FIRST BABY

I understood getting induced was not allowing my body to go into natural labor. That's where my regrets are. At thirty-nine weeks, my doctor brought up induction for the next week. I let her know I didn't want to be induced. At forty-one weeks, she said she wouldn't let me go past Thursday (two days later), and I would need to be induced at that time.

Since I was going to be at forty-two weeks, I felt like I didn't have a choice. When Thursday night came, I felt conflicted. When getting to the hospital, I regretted not pushing for more time and not asking questions of what this scheduled induction entailed. I think because we were able to get to almost forty-two weeks from the initial induction conversation at thirty-nine weeks, I felt like I couldn't say no. I do believe it went down the way it did because of the Cervidil.

We had the cervix softener, Cervidil, around 9 p.m., and I woke up to pretty intense contractions at 4 a.m. At 5 a.m. (just one hour later) I seemed to be losing a lot of blood and Chris called the nurse. The nurse said it was my mucous plug. Twenty minutes later, the blood kept coming, and I knew it wasn't "normal." Chris called the nurse again, and she called the doctor.

I remember the pain being so intense and thinking, "Am I going to be able to endure this?" Soon after the doctor arrived, they couldn't find the baby's heart rate and said we were going to the operating room (OR). They were concerned and needed to get this baby out. Chris was mainly doing the communication, as I was fully aware of these conversations but I wasn't participating in them; I was in my own zone getting through the pain.

When getting to the OR, the doctor said again we are in an emergency situation and we need the baby out. She said she would allow me to try to push with help of the vacuum extractor, or we needed to do a cesarean. I chose pushing with the vacuum; I hadn't had an epidural, fortunately, so I was able to push very well. With that final push our baby boy was born at 8:30 a.m. Four-and-a-half hours of labor.

CHAPTER TWENTY-THREE

Late Inductions

ALL THE APPLES ON a tree do not ripen and fall on the same day. Some ripen earlier than others, most fall around the same time, and some ripen later.

Plotted on a graph it would make a standard bell-shaped curve. You would see the *normal range* of ripening.

You could do the same thing with a large group of healthy, normal women, pregnant with their first babies, and if allowed to go into labor spontaneously, no inductions, then you would see a similar spread. Women don't all grow their babies the same number of days. Some

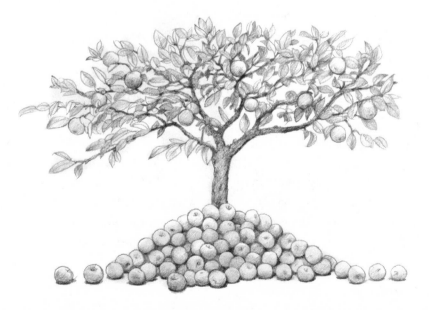

ERICK INGRAHAM

women grow their babies faster than most; most grow their babies approximately around the same number of days; and some take more days to grow their babies.

Some babies are indeed actually ready at thirty-nine weeks, on the early side of the bell-shaped curve, and when they are, the mother goes into labor *spontaneously*. Most babies, however, need more time to grow. For decades now, obstetricians thought forty weeks was average and based due dates on that average. *It turns out forty weeks is wrong. First babies average forty-one weeks and one day.* Is your birth attendant keeping up? Is your due date calculated on an evidenced-based average or the old, now discredited average? And babies fall on either side of that average, two weeks either way in the normal bell-shaped curve, yielding a range of thirty-nine to forty-three weeks.

We've already looked at the early induction scandal that has led to the United States having one of the highest preterm birth rates in the developed world.

GOING-PAST-YOUR-DUE-DATE INDUCTIONS

But there's another major component of the induction epidemic, and that's the so-called **prolonged pregnancy**, otherwise known as the going-past-your-due-date induction.

This is causing intense anxiety for many pregnant women. It's all they talk about when they first come to class. They are so anxious about going past the due date. Most don't want to be induced, so as their due date nears, they start going for acupuncture, trying castor oil, going jogging, drinking herbal teas that supposedly initiate labor, using nipple stimulation—anything and everything they can to self-induce. But an induction is an induction is an induction. Your body is not ready for labor and your baby is not ready for labor or you would be in labor spontaneously.

Dr. Bradley had this to say:

> In healthy, normal mothers with healthy, normal babies there is no such thing as overdue.

Let me be clear that we are not talking about a mother or baby in trouble, where medical intervention could be helpful; we're talking about nothing more than going past the estimated due date. Some doctors call it "post term," some call it "post mature." To avoid confusion, *Williams Obstetrics* calls it "prolonged pregnancy"; so that is the term we will use.

How long is a so-called prolonged pregnancy? One normal, healthy mother comes into my class and announces that she's been told thirty-nine weeks is it and then she must be induced because there are *so many* stillbirths after that. Another pipes up and says her doctor told her forty weeks, because there are *so many* stillbirths after that; another says her doctor told her it's forty-one weeks and then after that there are *so many* stillbirths; and yet another says she was told forty-two weeks is the cutoff, after which there are *so many* stillbirths, and that's when she has to be induced.

So this begs two questions:

First: Which is it: thirty-nine, forty, forty-one, or forty-two weeks?

Second: How many is *so many*?

So here's what you'll want to know. The international definition of **prolonged pregnancy** is forty-two *completed* weeks, and this is the definition endorsed by the American College of Obstetricians and Gynecologists.

The 2014 edition of *Williams Obstetrics* states:

It is important to emphasize the phrase "42 completed weeks." Pregnancies between 41 weeks 1 day and 41 weeks 6 days, although in the 42nd week, do not complete 42 weeks until the seventh day has elapsed.[1]

By definition, then, you are not even in a prolonged pregnancy until you have completed the very last day of the forty-second week!

Yet many normal, healthy women with normal, healthy babies are pushed into inductions before they have

even reached forty-two completed weeks. What happens *after* forty-two completed weeks?

To answer that, we need to look at the second question. Since women are told that "so many" babies die after forty-two weeks, then let's put a number on it and find out how many is "so many." You know where we look, of course—the Cochrane Review. If you look at 100 babies, all of whom are past forty-two weeks, how many babies do you think will be stillborn? None. Okay, so how many babies out of 200 going past forty-two weeks? Would you be surprised to know that the answer is still none? How about 300 babies past forty-two weeks? It's still zero. How about 400 babies going past forty-two weeks? The answer is 1 stillbirth in 410 babies past forty-two weeks, according to the Cochrane Review, June 13, 2012.[2]

To suggest to women that "so many" babies are stillborn after forty-two weeks, rather than giving them the actual facts, robs them of the opportunity to weigh risks and benefits. Such hyperbole almost guarantees that mothers will submit to induction before getting all the facts. There are risks to the induction itself, for both mother and baby, but those are never weighed properly on the scale, as they are glossed over. It's like someone puts a heavy thumb on the "induce now" side of the scale and puts nothing on the risks of induction side of the scale. Yet the Cochrane Review states it this way:

However, the absolute risk of perinatal death is small. Women should be appropriately counseled in order to make an informed choice between scheduled induction for a post-term pregnancy or monitoring without induction (or delayed induction).

It is interesting to note that the abstract of the same Cochrane Review states:

> Such deaths were rare with either policy.

But women aren't being told that such deaths are "rare" whether induced or whether they wait for labor to start on its own. They're being told that there are *so many* deaths if they wait, *and that effectively ends any discussion*!

What a difference between the wording used in the Cochrane Review as they refer to:

> Births after 42 weeks seem to carry a slightly increased risk for the baby. . . .

and the way this information is usually presented to women today.

If 410 mothers, all past forty-two completed weeks are induced, 409 of those mothers and babies will be subjected to the risks associated with induction with no benefit to them or to their babies.

It isn't *so many* babies, according to the Cochrane Summaries, it is *so few* babies, and women are not being counseled to make an informed choice when accurate information is withheld from them.

Here's yet another twist to the going-past-your-due-date-induction.

Many women are told that their placenta will get too old and stop working. It is usually referred to as placental insufficiency. This comes from a hypothesis proposed in 1954, although the person proposing it could find no evidence of placental degeneration when he looked for it histologically. In fact, *Williams Obstetrics* states:

> Still, the concept that post maturity is due to placental insufficiency has persisted despite an absence of morphological or significant quantitative findings (Larsen and co-workers, 1995; Rushton, 1991).[3]

In plain English, the 1954 theory is unsupported by evidence. When researchers looked for evidence in 1991 and again in 1995, they couldn't find it. What do you think? Is this evidence-based or belief-based?

There are women who are, understandably, afraid to participate in decisions concerning their bodies and their babies, and so leave all decisions to the birth attendant. That's a choice.

Other women find that our appalling world ranking in infant mortality, shocking at forty-one, compels them to participate in decisions and to insist on evidence-based care, and to check on the quality of the evidence, and engage in discussions with their birth attendants and, finally, to expect to be accurately and thoroughly informed before anyone should expect their informed consent.

"Being a critical thinker starts with resisting the urge to be a pleaser."

—Margaret Heffernan

"Everyone believes in informed consent, until a woman does not consent."

—Susan McCutcheon

CHAPTER TWENTY-FOUR

The Mother's Dilemma and the Doctor's Dilemma

NOTHING I'VE TOLD YOU so far will help you avoid an *unnecessary* induction. Everything we've covered up to this point merely alerts you to the induction epidemic, the process itself, and the inherent risks.

No one ever says to a woman, "And now, Mrs. Smith, we'll schedule your unnecessary induction." If that were the case, it would be easy. You might say, "No, I don't think I will accept the risks of an unnecessary induction."

So what can you do? You can be aware, in advance, of two big drivers of the induction epidemic: low amniotic fluid and small-for-date baby. Then you can apply the critical-thinking tools you have already learned. You know about the Cochrane Review and how highly respected they are. You know that RCTs are the heavyweights when it comes to evidence. You know the difference between evidence-based and belief-based medical tests, procedures, and practices. And you know you are supposed to be informed not just of benefits but also of risks for any tests you are asked to take, *and any proposed procedures that might follow due to taking a test;* it is part of the process of informed consent or dissent. You can know all of these things, but it will come down to this: Will you *apply* these tools?

Why wouldn't you? Sometimes it is easier to be "willfully blind." Margaret Heffernan states it succinctly in her fascinating and thought-provoking book *Willful Blindness*:

> When we are willfully blind, it is in the presence of information that we could know, and should know, but don't know because it makes us feel better not to know.[1]

Heffernan tells us the price we pay for willful blindness:

> We make ourselves powerless when we choose not to know.[2]

So you have a choice. You can default and leave all decisions to your birth attendant, or you can choose to use the tools you've learned, to acquire information, and to, *at the very least,* use the information to have a discussion with your birth attendant.

So let's put the top two drivers of the induction epidemic under the microscope.

You go in for an office visit and you are assured that your baby sounds fine and you are also doing fine. And now you're going to have an ultrasound exam. Notice the starting point here is that everybody is healthy and well.

But then the attendant frowns. The sonographer leaves the room and you wait awhile, and the doctor shows up, frowning, and says, "Well, you have very low amniotic fluid, called oligohydramnios, and we're concerned about your baby."

He talks about a chart where you are below "normal" with your fluid levels. You might hear the terms *AFI* or *single vertical pocket measurement.*

You are to go directly to the hospital and this evening or tomorrow morning you will be induced. You might tell him you would rather not be induced. Your doctor tells you your baby could die, so if you want a live baby (if?) then you need to be induced. "You don't want to take a chance with your baby's life, do you?" he says. This pretty much stops the conversation, as it is intended to. There is no discussion about how reliable the test may be or not be. There is no discussion of the evidence demonstrating whether or not an induction has benefited babies when mothers *are* induced for low amniotic fluid. There is no acknowledgment that a baby can die from induction itself.

I am enormously pleased to tell you that the American College of Obstetrics and Gynecology released a committee opinion, #664, that deals with this very situation. Obstetricians are urged not to use coercion or manipulation or refer to a woman's conscience to push her to comply with care that she does not want. It acknowledges that data and technology are not perfect and results are not always predictable. It acknowledges that coercion and failure to discuss risks of a proposed treatment has been a problem and needs to change. It is quite an enlightened paper and runs about seven pages. You can go online and read it. ACOG has stepped forward to address these issues and provide leadership in this important area of concern.

How could we modify the above-described experience?

If you know that this is one of the top reasons for pushing inductions, you should have already researched it. It's happening far too often for you to be a wishful thinker and believe it won't happen to you. Be informed. Give yourself a chance to look at the information in the Cochrane Review, and to look at RCTs ahead of time.

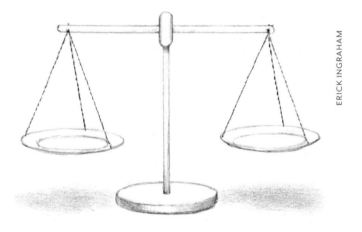

ERICK INGRAHAM

Let's do that now. Let's practice the application of the tools you've learned. You know what the starting point is:

THE BIOPHYSICAL PROFILE

FIRST STEP: How reliable is the test?

Using ultrasound to measure amniotic fluid is one of the components of the BioPhysical Profile, but there have been no definitive RCTs to support the BioPhysical Profile. In fact, *Williams Obstetrics* is careful to state that there are no RCTs supporting this testing and they clearly state this testing is based on *circumstantial* evidence only.[3]

You know where to go next, don't you? What about Cochrane?

Lalor and Associates performed a Cochrane Review and determined that there is insufficient evidence to support the use of the BioPhysical Profile as a fetal well-being test in high-risk pregnancies.[4]

Enkin and colleagues (2000) reviewed evidence in the Cochrane Library from controlled trials for antepartum fetal surveillance. They concluded that "despite their widespread use, most tests of fetal well-being should be considered of experimental value only rather than validated clinical tools."[5]

These late-pregnancy routine ultrasounds, when there is no compelling medical reason to be having one in the first place, are driving up the induction rate. Yet women are getting routine ultrasounds simply because they are thirty-six weeks' pregnant, and many are getting ultrasounds twice a week any time after thirty-nine weeks.

The American College of Obstetricians and Gynecologists states that sonography should be performed only when there is a valid medical reason.

As time passes, will this information still be valid? The tools that you just saw applied here will remain valid. You can use those tools to check and see if anything has changed, at any time in the future.

SECOND STEP: If you do submit to a late-pregnancy ultrasound, you'll want to know what happens if you are induced for low amniotic fluid. *Are babies better off? That's always the next question to ask.* What is the evidence that the proposed intervention actually makes a difference in outcomes for babies? Do they benefit by being pulled out early? You are now weighing benefits versus risks, thinking about that picture of a scale.

Williams Obstetrics reports that the only randomized trial today, Conway and colleagues (2000), showed that nonintervention and just waiting for spontaneous labor was as effective as induction in term pregnancies with amniotic fluid index values less than five centimeters. It makes no difference in outcome if you are induced or if you just wait for labor to start on its own?[6] Which would you prefer?

• • •

The next top driver of the induction epidemic is, again, having a routine sonogram in late pregnancy and being told that you have a small-for-date baby. This is also called IUGR (intrauterine growth retardation).

Sarah and George Economu were thirty-seven weeks pregnant. Sarah was told she was the picture of health and the baby sounded great. Then she had a "routine" ultrasound exam. Now they were told that the baby was too small for gestational age and it would be better off if the doctors got it out and put the baby in the NICU—where it would thrive, because the baby was failing to thrive in the uterus. An induction would be scheduled for the following Monday morning.

Sarah and George's first step was to take themselves off the hot seat. In the absence of an emergency situation, they let their birth attendant know that this was a lot to digest, and they were going to take some time to process the information before consenting to the induction. Taking themselves off the hot seat in the absence of an imminent emergency was a good idea. Too many parents have regretted making a hasty decision to just go along to get along, in the pressure of the moment, even though they experienced grave concerns about proceeding and felt they needed more information.

They went through the process, using the tools that we used above. They discovered that while we may be getting better at identifying small-for-date babies, intervention (inducing) did not improve outcomes.[7] The same number of babies died whether induced or not induced—no improvement in outcome. Sarah and George decided to decline the induction.

Five weeks later Sarah gave birth at forty-two weeks to a vibrant, healthy, six-pound baby. Her baby was alert and did not need to go to the NICU. The baby, who went home with Mom and Dad, would have been robbed of five weeks of growth! And what develops most in the final weeks? The brain.

Six pounds at forty-two weeks—what would she have been five weeks earlier, four pounds? She most certainly would have been a baby in trouble and would have needed the intensive care nursery. They had been told at thirty-seven weeks that the baby would lose only a few weeks, that thirty-nine weeks was a full-term baby. For this baby, forty-two weeks was a full-term baby!

George and Sarah came back and told their experience at the next series of birth classes, and here's what they said.

It was a hard decision and once we made it, the decision was hard to stick to, primarily because we got no

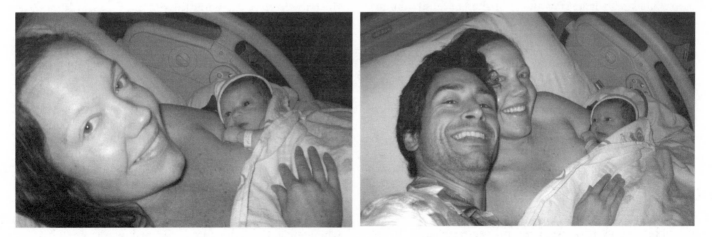

Sarah and George Economu; First baby

support for choosing the option of waiting. Our birth attendants made us feel like we were bad parents, as if we didn't care about our baby. As if waiting wasn't an option, but that just didn't line up with the evidence. Waiting was an option. We are enormously relieved we didn't choose the induction.

HOLD THEIR FEET TO THE FIRE

Here's something important you will want to know about "informed consent." When my copy of *Contemporary OB/ GYN News* comes in the mail, I read it from cover to cover. It is written by doctors for doctors. I'm a childbirth educator, but I read it to stay ahead of the curve, so I know what's coming up next in obstetrics. One of the most interesting sections is called "Legally Speaking."

A leading attorney analyzes lawsuit cases and looks at who wins, who loses, and why. Again and again I read about cases where a patient has suffered some terrible harm, but *the patient lost the case because the harm suffered was a known risk of the procedure, and she gave her informed consent.* So if you give your consent, be sure you have been informed of the risks. It's important! I call it "holding their feet to the fire."

Here's how it works. I recently acted as a doula for Stephanie at a local hospital. The doctor wanted to speed up labor with Pitocin. The mother knew to ask, "What are the risks?"

Her doctor replied, "Oh, there aren't any risks. It works just like your own hormone, oxytocin."

A doula is a patient advocate, among other duties. I looked at the doctor and mentioned quietly that I give all my students a copy of the Mayo Clinic list of risks. The doctor paused a moment and then amicably said, "Oh, where is it, we can go over it." I replied that Stephanie didn't have it with her, but she was aware of it and would like to review those risks at that time.

Following that, the doctor explained the risks of hyperstimulation of the uterus with the potential to cut off the baby from oxygen and the potential to tear the uterus and also the increased incidence of hemorrhaging after the birth, which, if uncontrolled, could lead to hysterectomy.

That's holding their feet to the fire, but it can be done without accusation or animosity. Why wouldn't the doctor have been forthcoming in the first place? Because most of her clients wouldn't want to know and would probably just ask her to decide for them. When that happens over and over, they just fall out of the habit. But natural-birth moms *do* want to know. There was no malintention in this young doctor. In fact, she was enormously pleased for Stephanie when she gave birth naturally a few hours later.

THE DOCTOR'S DILEMMA

When we get to talking about controversial issues like too many cesarean surgeries and too many inductions actually hurting mothers' and babies' health, rather than promoting health, some of my students wonder what's wrong with obstetricians. Why are they doing this and not "policing" themselves? How did we get to a million surgeries a year and climbing? How did obstetricians not notice the harm done to so many babies coming from early inductions?

Some students wonder if obstetricians are doing more harm than good when a normal bodily function, which works just fine when left alone the vast majority of the time, has now become the most common surgery performed, year after year! And usually, someone in the class will ask, "Is it about doing what's most convenient for the obstetrician, rather than what's best for mother and baby?" (Cesareans take a lot less time and inductions can be scheduled during hours that don't conflict with office appointments or weekend plans.) And someone else wants to know if this escalation of surgeries is driven by greed.

So I would like to show you the doctor's dilemma. Then, instead of seeing the doctor as the enemy, you will see him as just as human as the rest of us. This is important. It will help you communicate more amicably with your birth attendants, doctors, or midwives.

Use your imagination. Pretend you are a young obstetrician. You spent years going through medical school and it wasn't easy. While many of your friends were starting families, purchasing homes, and launching their lives, you had to delay all of these gratifications while you kept your focus on getting through the rigors of medical training. You racked up a tremendous amount of debt to do this. The debt is scary because there are no guarantees that you will actually get through medical school; you could become ill; you could be in an accident, or you just might not be able to handle the stress, the hours, the grueling demands of medical training. This huge debt will still be there, in any case, whether you get through or not.

Well, now you've made it. Whew! You finished all the requirements and now you have arrived; you are a practicing obstetrician. You happen to be the best of all doctors, and by that I mean you keep up with the literature about evidence-based practices, because you really want to be an excellent doctor.

Now I have to pause. What issue shall we pick to demonstrate the doctor's dilemma? Let's pick the electronic fetal monitor.

Some of your clients do not want to consent to electronic fetal monitoring and request monitoring by stethoscope only. You are puzzled. Why in the world would any woman reject this modern technological machinery? You research the literature and discover that while you were trained to use the electronic monitor in medical school and during your residency, that, actually, babies do not benefit when electronic monitoring is used. Babies do just as well when only the stethoscope is used. But mothers don't do as well when they are on electronic monitoring. They are greatly harmed by suffering a tripled rate of cesareans. Since the babies don't benefit by this monitoring, then this increase of surgery represents unnecessary surgery. You see that this fact has been demonstrated in RCT after RCT. Being the best of all doctors, you decide to stop using the electronic fetal monitor and have your clients monitored with the stethoscope.

And here's the dilemma. You know, as a doctor, that no doctor has a zero infant mortality rate. No doctor, no hospital, or country has a zero infant mortality rate. There are a certain number of babies who will die no matter what; even if they are in the best hospital in the country, attended by the best obstetrician in the country—no one has a zero infant mortality rate. There is always that inevitable baby that comes up for every doctor, everywhere. And what are you doing? Well, here you are going against the practicing norm, the standard of practice. First, you will be gossiped about in the hospital as a bad doctor because you are not doing what everyone else is doing. The staff at the hospital is just waiting to condemn you when you lose a baby, and you *will* lose a baby; you know it before you stop using the electronic monitor. You know it happened when you did use the monitor and you know it will happen when you stop using the monitor, because no one has a zero infant mortality rate. It is an inevitable number that will come up. When it does, your peers will point the finger at you for not using the electronic fetal monitor, no matter what all the evidence says.

If you end up in a lawsuit, you will lose. In the courtroom it might sound like this:

LAWYER: Doctor, is it true you did not have this mother on the electronic fetal monitor?
DOCTOR: Yes, but . . .
LAWYER: That's all, Doctor, a yes-or-no answer will do. Isn't it true, Doctor, that using the electronic fetal monitor is the practicing norm in your hospital, in fact it is the practicing norm all over the country—isn't that true, Doctor?
DOCTOR: Yes, but the evi—
LAWYER: A yes-or-no answer, Doctor.
DOCTOR: Yes.
LAWYER: Isn't it true that you failed to follow the recognized standard of practice, Doctor?

And a lawyer can always find an "expert" to testify that, most assuredly, if this mother had been on the electronic fetal monitor, it is most likely that this baby would be alive today. It doesn't matter what the studies show—the jury is watching a live "expert," television drama–style.

Now, how do you think the jury will vote?

The lawyer, by the way, may be quite aware of the research and quite aware that the doctor was acting in the best interests of mother and baby, but the lawyer's job is to win the case for his client and accusing the doctor of not doing what everybody else is doing is a courtroom winner.

When you lose a lawsuit, your insurance goes up. You know this situation will come up again, after a few hundred more births. If you lose three or four lawsuits over time, the insurance company might cut you off. If you cannot get insurance, then you will not be able to practice, as hospitals require that you be insured. If you cannot practice, you can't do any good for mothers, and you essentially lose your career. All the hard work, the years of study, for nothing. Rather than let that happen, you are beaten into conformity. Your ideals of doing what is best for mother and baby will take a backseat to self-interest. And the next time you have a client who wants evidence-based care, you'll look around and decide to wait until the other guys are doing it. You won't be going against the practicing norm, no matter what the evidence says. I do not say that scornfully; I say it with compassion and understanding.

Next you have the hospital's attorney. The hospital attorney's job is to protect the hospital from lawsuits and he keeps an eye on what kind of case the hospital can lose. He informs the hospital administrator that "We better be sure everyone is on an electronic fetal monitor or we could lose a case for not following the practicing norm." The hospital administrator is alarmed and tells the obstetrical head of department that every mother in labor must be on the electronic fetal monitor. The head of the obstetrical department tells the nurses working obstetrics that every laboring mom must be on the electronic fetal monitor; those are the rules. The nurses tell the mom who does not want to consent that she does not have a choice. Those are the rules.

Now you see the dilemma. You can see that many people along the way are unintentional colluders, promoting and protecting a system that does not put mothers' and babies' health first and foremost.

Doctors themselves are not able to make changes. So it comes down to parents insisting on changes. And it's hard. It takes being informed about tests. Are they reliable and necessary tests? If not, then it takes being able to say, no, thank you. It takes insisting on knowing the risks of any test you take. It takes insisting on knowing the risks and not just the benefits of any procedure offered. It takes understanding the process of informed consent or dissent and insisting that the process is followed. You, the parents, are the only real engine of change.

CHAPTER TWENTY-FIVE

The Episiotomy

GOING, GOING, NO, NOT QUITE GONE!

Margaret comes to class and tells everyone that her doctor said no one does episiotomies anymore.

But the 2014 edition of *Williams Obstetrics* calls the episiotomy "a common obstetrical procedure." [1]

So, if that is the starting point, that it is still a common procedure, then it is important that you do not skip this chapter, no matter what you've been told by your own birth attendant or your friends. And the fact that the episiotomy has *decreased* over the past thirty years is not exactly a credit to the obstetrical community. The cesarean surgery rate, a much bigger surgery than an episiotomy, has steadily *increased* over the past thirty years. By swapping a cesarean surgery for an episiotomy, of course, there has been a decline in episiotomies. You don't do an episiotomy *and* a cesarean surgery on the same woman.

We now have a 32 percent cesarean surgery rate, so you have at least 32 percent fewer episiotomies. It's inverse proportionality.

Doctors who do give episiotomies too often lack the skills to help women give birth without a tear. Older doctors and midwives who know how to do this are dying off. For the first time in fifty years of teaching, I am now seeing women having bad tears as they give birth with attendants who don't know how to prevent a tear.

Obstetricians only need to invite midwives, who have done this successfully for years, to come teach them these skills, but I don't see anyone doing this. This is why there is so much emphasis in this book on the "startle reaction," on the mother feeling the progress of the head at crowning and defeating her fear so she can stop pushing and how to stop pushing, and on the coach keeping an eye on the progress.

Pulling and tugging on the baby's head, without waiting a beat for the baby's shoulders to rotate so he can come out on his own steam, also causes tears. With a mother on an epidural, this is probably necessary, as her uterus isn't working as effectively and her baby is not actively helping by pushing back and wiggling to come out. The natural birth mother and baby, however, rarely need this kind of assistance, but it is usually done routinely.

I fear that the episiotomy will simply come back with a vengeance. Why? The new 2014 guidelines for obstetricians are all about bringing down the cesarean surgery rate, which is a good thing, since an increase in major surgery increases the maternal mortality rate. The 2014 guidelines are an attempt to reduce maternal mortality.

But instead of urging a return to more natural methods of dealing with labor, the guidelines urge a return to forceps and vacuum-extraction deliveries. When forceps or vacuum extractors are used, more pulling force is applied than the mother herself would use in pushing. Pulling and hurrying can cause bad tears and will probably convince doctors to return to episiotomies.

Does it never occur to anyone to try supporting natural birth methods, giving women encouragement to try learning the techniques, to see how it might work for them, and having doctors themselves required to take at least one series of natural childbirth classes as part of their training?

We'll see what the future holds. In any case, when the episiotomy does finally essentially disappear as a common procedure, I would still not delete this chapter. We study history so we don't repeat the same kinds of mistakes, and the episiotomy story, from start to finish, is the epitome of a belief-based practice, with no evidence to support it but slick-sounding reasons for doing them.

The reasons, as you will see, besides lacking evidence, were terrifying-sounding and caused women to acquiesce and submit to a procedure that defied common sense. And finally, the episiotomy story is the epitome of why it is so wrong to allow experimental procedures to become the practicing norm without randomized controlled trials being performed first. Thirty years after exposing episiotomies as harmful, we still haven't gotten rid of it. At the very end of the chapter, you will find out what the 2014 edition of *Williams Obstetrics* now says about episiotomies. Use the episiotomy chapter as the lens through which you examine today's obstetrical practicing norms.

You will be glad to hear that by 1995 the ACOG (American College of Obstetricians and Gynecologists) had publicly withdrawn support of the routine episiotomy. However, the episiotomy is still common.

SO HERE IS THE INTACT EPISIOTOMY CHAPTER AS IT ORIGINALLY APPEARED

How common is the episiotomy? *Very.* It is done in *at least* 90 percent of first-time births in hospitals and again in most second or later hospital births.

How often is it really needed? A Maternity Center Association record of home births shows that out of almost 5,000 home births, there were only twenty-two episiotomies (and only one third-degree tear). That's an episiotomy rate of about one out of every two hundred women, or half a percent![2] (It is also interesting to note that in most European countries, the episiotomy rate is only 12 to 15 percent of hospital births.)

What is an episiotomy? Typical birth books describe it as a "small incision" made at the time of birth through your perineum to "get the widest part of the baby's head through the opening of the vagina."

This incision, made with scissors inserted into your vagina as the baby's head is crowning, can be two to four inches long. What's that? You say that doesn't sound like a "small cut"? You don't think that you have two to four inches around your vaginal outlet to cut?

Well, you will at birth. When the baby's head crowns, the perineum fans out, the thick, springy muscles flattening and spreading as they are designed to. At that time you easily have two to four inches between your vaginal opening and rectum spreading out for the surgeon's scissors. But once the baby is out, your perineum is no longer fanned out. It will return immediately to its thick, muscular form, meaning that the cut you are left with is about two inches on the outside, with the rest going up into your vaginal barrel.

That is a pretty serious bit of "minor surgery." And it is so frequently performed (at least in the US) that you would expect a lot of research has been done on its usefulness, wouldn't you?

Quite the contrary. Drs. David Banta and Stephen B. Thacker's research into the medical literature about episiotomy found that "there were little scientific data to support the widespread use of episiotomy. Indeed, if one restricts the definition of scientific data to that which is obtained from a randomized, controlled, clinical trial, there were *no* data to support widespread use of episiotomy."[3]

Considering the significant risks associated with the episiotomy, these medical doctors say that the episiotomy rate in the US could easily be cut in half without causing harm to either mothers or babies. That is probably conservative.

These risks include *pain*—swelling, burning, and aching in the perineum that stays for weeks, months, or longer, often interfering with sexual relations—and they include infection, which can lead to more serious complications.

Why is the episiotomy rate so high with no evidence that it is needed or useful? Banta and Thacker say, "Many physicians feel that clinical experience provides an adequate basis for good practice . . ." In other words, doctors say that this is the way they were taught and this is the way they do it; it works for them and they don't know any other way—and, frankly, it doesn't hurt them a bit.

This may seem a harsh indictment of physicians. Yet as Drs. Banta and Thacker point out, "While many obstetricians perceive it to be a minor problem, many women regard post-episiotomy pain as quite a serious matter." That pain can be severe for as many as 60 percent of the women who undergo the procedure.

In my classes I have seen many women who have a deep and sincere dread of the episiotomy. It is, after all, a serious surgical procedure performed on the most intimate part of their bodies. They want to know if the episiotomy is necessary, and they want to know how they can avoid it.

Some mothers who return to the class after their birth to share their experiences echo and intensify this concern.

This is not a pleasant subject. This was probably the hardest chapter in this book to write. But let's look a little more closely at the episiotomy.

The history of this surgery goes hand in hand with the shift to hospital deliveries and the development of new methods to intervene in what should be a natural, normal process.

When anesthetics first appeared on the scene, women were really "put under" for birth, completely "zonked out." Obviously, it was impossible for mothers to push their babies out in this condition. The baby still had to come out, though. If the mother couldn't push, then the doctor had to get it out. This was the real beginning of the "routine" forceps delivery, and with it came the "routine" episiotomy.

"Speed" was the watchword whenever the mother was completely put under because the baby was in great danger. It was necessary to get the baby out quickly, or it would be exceedingly difficult to get him to breathe. You could get a baby out faster by cutting the mother's perineum open and extracting the infant with forceps. So it was speed and efficiency (made necessary because the mother was medicated) that made the episiotomy and the forceps delivery the norm rather than an unusual form of delivery. The routine episiotomy is a legacy women bear of the history of intervention in childbirth.

As you know, an episiotomy need not be painful at the moment it is given because the baby's head cuts off your circulation and makes your bottom numb. This is the so-called pressure episiotomy that we discussed earlier and that requires no anesthetic. After your baby is out, an anesthetic will be needed as the obstetrician stitches up your sexual organ. When this wears off, the pain begins.

Episiotomy can do permanent harm to your PC muscle and set you up for future health problems. It also creates scar tissue in the perineum and leaves a numb spot in this sexually responsive part of your body. Psychologically, this intense, unnecessary pain associated with birthing can make women feel bitter.

Many women who are left with lingering pain (which may last several months and even return occasionally in twinges years later) have difficulty piecing together their expectations of being a mother (and a woman) and the reality of the ache in the very core of their sexual organs.

I have seen women burst into tears over the physical pain and frustration of trying to care for their baby during the prolonged recovery that often goes with the unnecessary loss of blood and the pain.

I had a mediolateral episiotomy with my first baby and decided having babies was great but episiotomies were not! I went on to have two more babies with no episiotomy and no tear. I simply forbade my OB to do an episiotomy, and I was amazed that after the birth there was nothing to recover from but a lost night's sleep.

This is not nearly as uncommon as women think it is. I have seen many babies born without tears or episiotomies, including some nine- and ten-pound first babies!

THREE KINDS OF EPISIOTOMY

The original episiotomy was the bilateral, a cut made sideways out toward the leg. This episiotomy is now obsolete. It has been abandoned due to excessive scarring, poor healing, and extreme pain. But at one time, women were told it was perfectly safe.

The three most common episiotomy techniques used at this time are: the mediolateral; the median, or midline; and the relatively new "hockey stick." We will look at them one by one.

Mediolateral Episiotomy

This incision is a slanting cut to one side of the perineum. It cuts through nerves, muscle, and tissue. This may be the most painful episiotomy. The fact it is so painful should alert both the woman and the doctor that the perineum is a highly sensitive, sexually responsive area.

But—besides the perineum—Dr. Arnold Kegel (who as you'll recall, invented the PC muscle exercises you have been doing) made an entire film to document the permanent harm the mediolateral episiotomy can do to your PC muscle.[4] One of the main reasons doctors say they give every woman a routine episiotomy is to prevent "stretching" of that PC muscle. The doctor who gives you this reason believes stretching will cause your muscles to sag permanently and your inner organs to fall downward. He believes the episiotomy preserves the muscles in good condition and prevents this future problem. But Dr. Kegel's film clearly shows that the mediolateral episiotomy does *not* prevent this problem and, in fact, can be a major factor contributing to it.

The reason for this is that the PC muscle is wrapped around the vaginal barrel. This muscle extends down toward the perineum as the baby moves through the vaginal barrel. When the cut is made in your perineum, the PC muscle, which can't be seen, may be included. It is usually not completely severed, but it frequently may be partly cut. Since it can't be seen, it is not sewn up as the perineum is after the cut. This results in permanent damage to your supportive muscle that was caused, not prevented, by the episiotomy.

Women who have had mediolateral episiotomies and suffered this damage can feel for it and find it if they know what to look for. Simply insert two fingers into the vagina and press firmly right at the outlet, around in a circle. You will feel the damage. Where you were not cut, the perineal muscles feel thick and springy against your fingers. Where a cut was made, your fingers will not feel that counterpressure, but instead will feel no support. It will feel as if this part is a thin, not a thick, muscle.

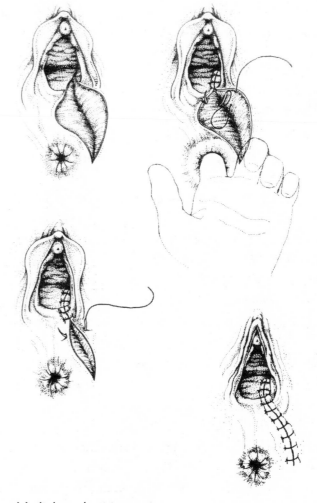

ROBIN BURNINGHAM

39. Mediolateral episiotomy

You can also use a mirror, and you may notice that the tissues surrounding your outlet are slightly bulgier on one side than on the other. This is the musculature trying to compensate by overdeveloping on the unharmed side.

The Median or Midline Episiotomy

So what if your doctor says not to worry, he hardly ever does a mediolateral episiotomy. Instead he uses a median or midline episiotomy.

The median goes through connective tissue, rather than nerves, straight down the middle of your bottom toward the rectum. It is less painful than the mediolateral and does not include the PC muscle, but this one has many other problems.

The biggest and rather frequent problem is that it tends to tear right on through the rectum. The perineum is stretched thin like a piece of cloth at the moment of birth. Cutting the perineum now is like cutting a piece of cloth and adding pressure. Anyone who sews knows what happens. It tears straight on through.

When this happens, of course, you are right back to facing a long, painful recovery; and in addition, your sphincter muscle has been severed and permanently weakened.

This happens much more often than any doctor I've ever known cares to admit. After having my student cou-

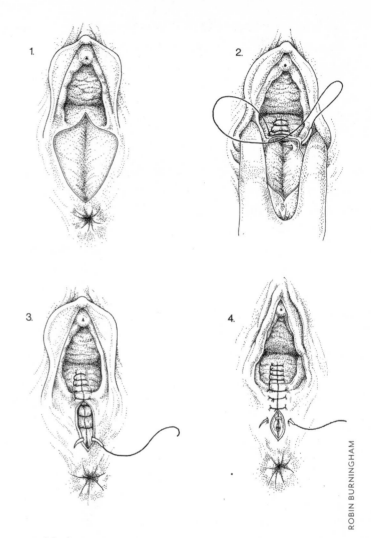

40. Median episiotomy

ROBIN BURNINGHAM

ples go to a hundred or more different doctors through the years, it has become apparent to me that the doctor's skill as a surgeon does not prevent this from happening.

The Hockey Stick

This episiotomy goes straight back toward the rectum like a median and then veers off at the end like a mediolateral. The fact that this one was invented makes it quite clear that doctors are aware of the dangers of both of the other kinds of episiotomy.

So somehow this technique is at one and the same time an admission of the hazards of both median and mediolateral episiotomies and a compounding of the problems of both.

I have seen women given this "compromise" technique and then tear in both directions, through the rectum *and* off to the side. Where you cut into the thin-stretched perineum, you are risking an extension into a longer tear. The hockey stick solves nothing and risks the dangers of both episiotomies in one.

TEARS

I have never seen a tear happen when no incision was made that was as bad as an episiotomy. I have seen some bad tears *with* episiotomies. But when no cut is made, most tears (if they occur at all) consist of the following: (1) a little split in the *surface* of the skin inside the vaginal barrel; (2) a small tear in the perineum, usually less than a quarter of an inch long. (Much less than an episiotomy.)

The word *tear* strikes fear into the hearts of most women, but when you take a close look at what a tear usually consists of, and what an episiotomy consists of, it is the episiotomy that should make women more apprehensive.

An episiotomy is a complete severing of all the layers of tissue, muscle, and nerves *and is no guarantee of not tearing.* In fact, it can contribute to a much more serious extension. Again, to quote Drs. Banta and Thacker, who reviewed all the available medical literature, "These studies give no clear indication that episiotomy prevents third-degree lacerations. It is also evident from these data that episiotomies sometimes tear further and can extend into the rectum."[5]

I have seen doctors very nonchalant about this complete surgical severing and yet very upset about a surface split in the skin or a quarter-inch tear.

Why? Because among a doctor's colleagues episiotomy is acceptable. It is considered proper obstetrical technique; but a tear is considered careless. Imagine the pressure this puts on the young doctor, new and anxious for his peers' approval. Even when he wants to help women out with this, there are strong forces pressuring him to conform to "prevailing standards of practice."

It is sometimes said that it is better to cut the perineum than to risk the possibility of a tear up by the clitoris. This hardly ever happens, but even when it does, I challenge the idea that the clitoris is more important than the perineum. This is a male concept.

The perineum itself is a highly sexually responsive area, and it is certainly difficult to enjoy intercourse with the penis directly rubbing a cut, stitched, and scarred area in the very organ that holds it during intercourse.

OTHER REASONS GIVEN FOR EPISIOTOMY

When women question doctors about episiotomies, they are often told about tearing, but this is not the rationale that most physicians are themselves sold on. It is just the one women accept the most readily. It pushes all the fear buttons and ends the questioning.

The reasons given in obstetrical texts, however, include:

1. To shorten the second stage.

Yes, it does shorten second stage by all of *several to sometimes a dozen contractions* (say, fifteen minutes). This is a kind of cruel joke from the woman's point of view, since she has just experienced perhaps a couple of hundred contractions.

2. To prevent the baby's head from pounding on the perineum.

Pounding on the perineum? This is really reaching to support the "routine" episiotomy. The perineum is hardly a brick wall. Any baby who just came through the cervix, which took ten to fourteen hours to dilate with much more work, is not going to have any difficulty with the vagina and perineum.

3. To prevent overstretching of the muscles that support the inner organs, preventing uterine prolapse (uterus dropping down into or even out of the vagina), and incontinence (leaking of urine).

We already know what Dr. Kegel had to say about this, so suffice it to say that scar tissue does not make for strong muscles. Exercise does that.

4. To make repair easier. A clean cut is said to be easier to repair than a jagged tear.

But somehow doctors manage to repair the many tears caused by midline episiotomies without much hassle about it. There would be far fewer tears and less serious tears to repair in the first place if we gave up episiotomies.

ARE WOMEN ABLE TO GIVE BIRTH WITHOUT EPISIOTOMY?

There are physicians sensitive to the trauma of surgery performed on a sexual organ. I have the highest regard for them. My own faith in the normality and simplicity of birth is reaffirmed each time I accompany a mother to see her give birth with no episiotomy and no tear.

At a teacher-training workshop in the Bradley Method®, Dr. Victor Berman, who practices obstetrics in Los Angeles County, reported on a mother who gave birth to a thirteen-pound baby with no tear and no episiotomy. (He humbly spoke of catching the baby rather than delivering it.) Why do we expect it to be otherwise? Birth is a normal bodily function and women are designed for it. Most women *can* give birth without an episiotomy or a tear if they are allowed to assume a proper position for pushing, given adequate training to help them prepare the muscles involved in actually giving birth, and, most important, told when to stop pushing.

A woman must also have a doctor who is not in a hurry, who does not use his fingers to stretch her apart and grasp the baby's head to hasten its birth. All this hurry-up technique does not allow your tissues a chance to stretch gradually, as they should.

To Avoid an Episiotomy

Be sure you have selected your doctor carefully. Get one who *seldom* does episiotomies.

Prepare yourself by doing lots of squatting. Remember that a muscle in good tone has a much greater stretch ratio. You squat to make the perineum more flexible and to get into good tone.

Prepare yourself by doing your PC contractions. Again, you increase the stretch ratio of this muscle, too. You also get to know what it feels like to consciously relax and let go with this muscle.

Do not have a pudendal block or any "local" anesthetics. You can't tell when you are letting go or contracting the muscle.

Avoid anesthetics! Epidurals, caudal, and paracervical anesthesia interfere with pushing and can lead to an episiotomy to hasten the end of the anesthetic-slowed pushing stage.

If you don't want to do anything that would increase

the likelihood of a tear or an episiotomy, then don't take drugs that interfere with the way your body works.

And finally, you absolutely cannot be flat on your back to give birth. This position puts too much pressure on the perineum when the head is emerging, and at the same time makes it difficult to relax the perineum. A flat-on-the-back position *creates* the need for an episiotomy.

The physician who sees bad tears invariably also has the mothers in this position or is *hurrying the birth with manipulation.* Perhaps the reason I have never seen a bad tear when no episiotomy is performed is because I have attended births with physicians who do not require the woman to be flat, who do not hurry, and who do not use anesthetics that interfere with the perineal reflex.

The episiotomy is one of those unpleasant, unnecessary things that happens to a woman at birth that is being questioned more and more by those concerned about women's health issues. We may not be able to revolutionize the practice of obstetrics in this country during the nine months of your pregnancy, but you can take steps to avoid having this initiation ritual of motherhood performed on you.

In the next chapters we will look at some of the other risks that you face when going to the hospital to have your baby.

WHAT DOES *WILLIAMS OBSTETRICS* NOW SAY ABOUT EPISIOTOMIES?

Williams Obstetrics states that episiotomy never protected a woman from incontinence, never helped preserve the integrity of the pelvic-floor muscles, and when compared with spontaneous lacerations, episiotomy is worse than a spontaneous tear, as it increases the risk of tearing through the rectum, increases the risk of a second-degree tear fivefold, and actually triples the risk of fecal incontinence.[6]

We also know that doing episiotomies does not protect a baby from brain damage, by lowering the rate of cerebral palsy, as the incidence of cerebral palsy does not decrease.

We knew as early as 1982 that there was no evidence to support doing episiotomies and that they actually caused harm.[7] And yet, obstetrical textbooks didn't start reporting this in such a definitive way until 2010, and in 2014 textbooks we are told it is still a common procedure.

If nothing else, these stories should help women realize that it is essential that they get involved in their care, that they insist on evidence-based care, and somehow we need to insist that our discussions with birth attendants be more factual and free from emotionally terrifying overstatement of risks that push toward a practicing norm, even if and when there are no randomized controlled trials to support whatever the proposed intervention might be.

Consider: Why did women consent to episiotomies even after telling their doctors they really would rather not have one? What would you have said if you were told, "Your baby can end up brain damaged with his head pounding needlessly on the perineum? You don't want to overstretch your perineal muscles and then have trouble with incontinence." Some even indicated you wouldn't have a very good sexual response if you didn't have an episiotomy. What woman wouldn't be terrorized into consenting to an episiotomy by these unfounded statements?

When obstetricians make these statements they believed what they said. They are not evil people with intention to do harm. They are true believers. They are naive about checking for evidence themselves, and practice as they were taught, and they fail to ask questions about inherited practicing norms. But they do think it is acceptable to conduct discussions in a manner that scare women into consenting. Hopefully the recent ACOG committee opinion on informed consent will facilitate factual, honest discussions about all *current* interventions.

WHAT HAPPENS WHEN A BRADLEY-TRAINED COUPLE ENCOUNTERS A COMPLICATION

Emily Sparks, RN, and Paul Simon learned that they had a placenta previa: that the placenta was at the bottom of the uterus rather than in the upper two-thirds, which means it would separate first, before the baby could come out, and lead to life-threatening bleeding.

It occurs only in one out of every four to five hundred births. I suggested that Paul and Emily go out to dinner and celebrate that they could have a cesarean and that if they had to have a placenta previa, they lived in the best of times.

Read how Emily and Paul used their Bradley training to get the best results. It helped a great deal that they had selected an excellent doctor.

OUR BIRTH STORY: EMILY SPARKS, RN, AND PAUL SIMON

We heard from a friend of ours, a mother of three, about the Bradley Method® and were instantly intrigued. It just so happened that there was a class being held that coincided with my expected delivery date. After signing up but before even the first class, however, we discovered I had

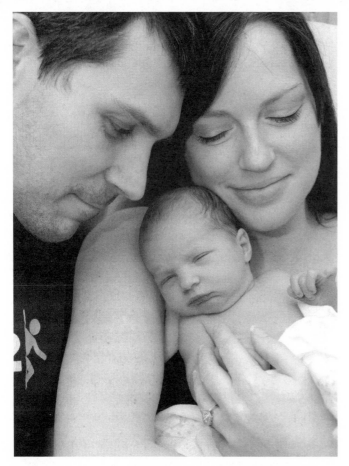

Emily is a cardiac nurse at Providence Portland Medical Center and Paul is a former accountant, now a stay-at-home husband and dad.

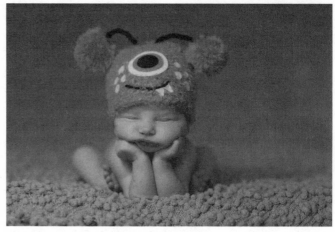

placenta previa. This meant that unless things changed drastically, I had to have a cesarean section, which neither of us were thrilled about. Regardless, we decided to stay in the class to learn as much about the birthing process as possible. It ended up being a great decision.

Although nothing changed and we did need to go through with the cesarean, what we learned in class changed the entire process. In regards to placenta previa, for the safety of the mother and child, the surgery is recommended to take place earlier rather than later. Typically, it is performed around thirty-six weeks. However, thanks to the research website we learned about in class, we discovered two recent research articles that stated it is considered safe to wait up to thirty-eight weeks with asymptomatic placenta previa (if there has been no bleeding). And a full two weeks of letting our baby continue to develop was very important.

Our surgeon had not read the same research we had, though, and still wanted to operate at thirty-six weeks. It was something we had anxiously expected. Armed with the techniques we learned in our Bradley Method® class, we presented our case to the surgeon amicably. Though she was not immediately convinced, we told her where we got our information and she looked it up on her phone on the spot. She was pleasantly surprised (and impressed, actually) that we had done our research and that it was now considered safe to wait on the cesarean until week thirty-eight. We did agree, however, that if any complications arose that we would be willing to come in early.

Ultimately, we were able to push back the birth of our child to the latest possible date while still remaining safe for both myself and our child. This wouldn't have been possible without the Bradley Method® class. We are both very grateful and recommend the class to everyone we talk to. If nothing else, knowing that doctors are not infallible and that doing our own research can lead to what's actually best for our family.

On a side note, I did not have any risk factors for placenta previa. Audrey was born December 28 at 5:49 p.m., six pounds, six ounces. Right after she was born they suctioned the fluid out of her lungs and then handed her right to me. After they were done they wheeled me to the recovery room and insisted on an hour of skin-to-skin. They refused to let anyone else in the room except for Paul so we could all bond together.

CHAPTER TWENTY-SIX

Cesarean Surgery

Nearly 25% of all U.S. births in recent years have been accomplished by Caesarean section, up from just 4.5% in 1965.

WALL STREET JOURNAL, JANUARY 20, 1993

Almost one million of the four million births annually in the U.S. involve Caesarean sections, according to a study to be released today by the Centers for Disease Control and Prevention.

WALL STREET JOURNAL, APRIL 23, 1993

About half the Caesarean section operations done each year in the United States are unnecessary.

WASHINGTON POST, MAY 19, 1994

Doctors performed 349,000 unnecessary Caesareans in this country in 1991 at a cost to the nation of more than $1 billion, the Centers for Disease Control and Prevention said today.

NEW YORK TIMES, APRIL 23, 1993

ANYONE WHO DOUBTS THAT there are many unnecessary cesarean surgeries is not paying attention to the World Health Organization. They have stated clearly that the outside number of women needing surgeries could not possibly exceed 10 to 15 percent at most. They have also clearly stated that anything over that is causing harm without a benefit of any kind to the mother or baby.

Think what that means. We currently have about a 32 percent cesarean surgery rate. That means that at least *every other* cesarean is an unnecessary major surgery with all the attendant risks of surgery and anesthesia.

Yet no one ever says to a mother, "And now, Mrs. Smith, we will do your unnecessary cesarean surgery." Put that way, any mother would simply say, "Oh no, you won't!" Every mother who gets a cesarean surgery is told she needs one, so every mother who gets a cesarean will tell you that hers was necessary to save her or her baby's life.

She's often told that the physician doing it has the lowest surgery rate in the hospital, maybe even in the whole state! Well, really, can you imagine a woman being told, "And by the way, your doctor has the highest cesarean rate in the hospital"?

At each revision of this book the cesarean section rate has climbed higher and higher. First, it tripled to about 15 or 16 percent, and there was talk of getting it back down to 10 percent. Instead it jumped to 20 percent, and then in light of media focus, there was talk of getting it back down to 15 percent. Then it jumped to 25 percent, and talk of getting it back down to 20 percent. Now, in the third edition of this book we are at 32 percent, and it's headline news if it wavers downward to 31 percent.

Women are actually being told this is because they are sicker, fatter, and older. Yet when you look at so-called low-risk mothers only (low risk because they do not have any chronic poor health conditions, aren't overweight, and aren't older), they are also getting cesarean surgery at high rates.[1] Notice that the victim is blamed in this scenario.

As you read this chapter, you'll find updates on the fetal monitor and the common "too big baby" cesarean.

• • •

When I started teaching, your odds of having cesarean surgery were thirty to one. Today, your odds are four to one. The cesarean section rate is now so high that even Congress has investigated it.

You don't really need to know what your hospital's C-section rate is, but you certainly *do* need to know your individual doctor's rate, because that will be the risk you personally run of having your birth turned into major surgery. Your independent Bradley teacher—not a hospital's or doctor's childbirth instructor—is your best source of information when you are seeking to reduce this risk.

I have actually had the experience of working for one group of doctors with a 3 percent surgery rate while working at the same time for another group with a 40 percent rate. As I worked for the two groups of doctors, I clearly saw the impact of a high group-practice surgery rate on the health of mothers and babies. I had taught for years with so few problems that at first I thought perhaps statistics were catching up with me, as four out of ten women from one doctors' group had their babies via major surgery. The difference was incredible, not just in rates of cesareans but in the condition of the mothers and babies. I had never seen so many washed-out, pale women with dark rings under their eyes. Many of them had to be rehospitalized to treat infected uteruses (rather common after cesarean surgery) and had to leave their nursing babies at home. Some of them came back to the class to tell their stories without their babies, since the babies were still hospitalized to recover from breathing difficulties and other problems common to cesarean delivery. And, of course, all of these mothers had to deal with more than their share of pain and frustration. Meanwhile, women who went to the doctors whose cesarean surgery rate was only 3 percent rarely had infections, experienced fewer days of hospitalization, and were far more successful at breast-feeding. Those mothers were simply happier and healthier—and so were their babies.

Almost half of all cesarean patients in a survey of 4,000 who had this surgery from 1959 to 1976 had one or more operative complications, "including a respectable number of severe complications which compromise future childbearing or are potentially lethal," according to L. T. Hibbard, writing in the *American Journal of Obstetrics and Gynecology*.[2]

What are these complications? Infection is fairly common: Intrauterine infection occurs in 35 to 65 percent of cases if the mother had internal electronic fetal monitoring and in 20 to 40 percent of cases without monitoring. Other categories of infection include cystitis, peritonitis, abscess, gangrene, and generalized sepsis.[3]

The list goes on and on. In a declining order of frequency it includes things like hemorrhage; accidental reopening of the wound; subsequent uterine rupture; injuries to adjacent parts of the body, like the bladder or bowels; complications with blood transfusions including hepatitis, aspiration pneumonia, anesthesia accidents; and even cardiac arrest. Death occurs for the baby more often with a cesarean and that is true even when there is no medical reason for the cesarean, according to the CDC.[4] This is about ten times more often than in vaginal births.

It stretches credibility beyond reason to really believe that 20 or 30 percent of all women need major abdominal surgery in order to have a healthy baby. In this cesarean-section chapter, unlike the class taught in the hospital, we won't prepare you for your highly likely cesarean surgery with no questions asked, but will teach you to know how to carefully pick your doctor to make a C-section highly *un*likely and also help you get information before you give your informed consent to anything.

First of all, your doctor's rate of C-sections should be no more than 3 to 5 percent—not 15, not 20, not 30 percent! But how do you know which C-sections make up the unnecessary increase and which fall into the necessary 3 percent category? We will take a look at some necessary C-sections, but first let's move in for close scrutiny of the reasons most commonly given for many of those unnecessary C-sections, and how you can avoid them.

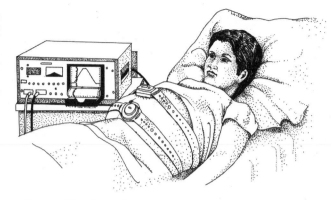

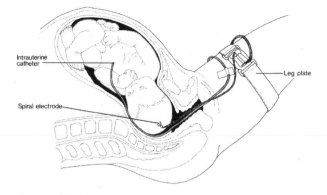

41. External fetal monitor

42. Internal fetal monitor

In figure 42: Intrauterine catheter, Spiral electrode, Leg plate

The three main categories into which the dramatic increase of unnecessary C-sections falls are:

1. *THE FETAL MONITOR C-SECTION.* Alias: Fetal distress, or inefficient or nonproductive uterine contractions.
2. *THE PUTTERER C-SECTION.* Alias: Failure to progress, or prolonged labor, or uterine inertia (lazy uterus); or it may even be called CPD (cephalopelvic disproportion).
3. *THE "YOUR TIME'S UP" C-SECTION.* Alias: Failure to progress, or CPD. Differs from the putterer C-section in that it occurs in the pushing stage.

THE FETAL MONITOR CESAREAN SECTION

We need to start with a little vocabulary. **EFM** means "electronic fetal monitoring." Let's take a look at the electronic fetal monitor and at the evidence stacked up against it as hazardous to the health of the mother.

With the external fetal monitor, two belts with sensors are strapped around your waist. One directs sound waves (ultrasound) at your baby, and as the sound waves are bounced back your baby's heart rate is recorded. The other belt with sensor records your uterus contracting. Already two hazards have been added. Lying on your back for this monitoring increases risk to the baby, and ultrasound has not been tested for long-term side effects.

With internal monitoring, a catheter is pushed into your vagina and up into your uterus (which increases the risk of infection). The catheter is then filled with water and connected to a pressure sensor, which records the contractions. In addition, an electrode is inserted into your vagina with a thin spiral-wire ending that is screwed into your baby's head, recording his heart activity. Both tubes are strapped to your leg. Often this means rupturing an intact bag of waters just to insert the spiral electrode into the baby's scalp.

Many doctors believe that every woman in labor should be monitored electronically and are doing just that. Most are using the internal monitor, but sometimes a woman is put on the external monitor early in labor and on the internal monitor later.

It looks pretty unappealing. If it made a difference for your baby you would probably put up with it anyway. But the fact is that out of five scientific studies (randomized controlled trials) of fetal monitors, four showed no differences in outcome for the babies whether the fetal monitor was used or not.[5] Only one showed an improved outcome for the babies, and that study has been severely criticized for poor scientific methodology.[6]

Dr. A. D. Haverkamp of Denver told the Central Association of Obstetricians and Gynecologists in 1975 that research showed no difference in the health or survival rate of babies when internal electronic fetal heart monitoring was used to manage deliveries. But the big difference, he said, was in the cesarean-section rate. It was 16.5 percent in the group of women who underwent electronic fetal monitoring but only 6.8 percent in the group whose births were managed by frequent use of the stethoscope to check the baby's well-being.[7]

Clearly, repeated scientific studies show that the baby does not benefit when the mother is electronically monitored. These studies show that the major difference in outcome when the fetal monitor is used is for the mother. *The cesarean surgery rate is as much as tripled!*

More women undergo the trauma and risks of major surgery, the days of pain afterward, the dual difficulties of recovering from a major operation while also trying to learn how to mother a new baby, and for what? When so many studies tell us that we only get more women having major, high-risk surgery, then don't you think it's time to say the risks outweigh the benefits?

Let's take a look at the scenario of the fetal-monitor C-section. This is how it happened for Sharon and Tom with their first baby.

SHARON: When we got to the hospital, I was seven centimeters dilated. I was elated. Tom had to go down for the admittance papers. We had filled out everything we could ahead of time, but it still took about twenty minutes before he returned. We'd looked over the Xeroxed handouts of various studies in our birth classes and, if it didn't make things better for the baby, I didn't want to be attached to a machine and wires. But when I turned the monitor down, they told me that everyone had to have it, it was a rule, and my baby would be much safer with it. I just couldn't argue. When Tom got back I know he was surprised to see me attached to the monitor. He knew how I felt about it. Well, we just kept working and I went really quick to ten centimeters. We'd only been in the hospital for two hours.

TOM: But the doctor didn't like what he saw on the fetal monitor printout. He told us the baby's heart rate was dropping periodically and that he would have to deliver it right away if we wanted to avoid brain damage. Brain damage! I didn't know what to do. Sharon and I both sure didn't want a brain-damaged baby, but I knew she was thinking the same thing I was—all those studies that showed more cesarean sections for nothing. We wished we hadn't allowed the fetal monitor. I kicked myself for not being there to help her refuse it. We would have felt more confident of the decision to do the cesarean if Sharon had only been monitored with a stethoscope.

SHARON: Our baby came out in perfect shape. He breathed right away and was a nice pink. I was relieved, but at the same time it was hard to see what he had been saved from. We had been told the baby was in trouble and we were willing to do whatever was necessary to protect our baby, but neither of us could see that our baby had been saved from anything.

What happened to Sharon and Tom is a daily occurrence, repeated across the country. How can this be? How can the fetal monitor show a "distressed baby" and yet after cutting the mother open the doctor pulls out a baby who is clearly in no trouble?

Some doctors claim that when you see a "nonreassuring pattern, you do a cesarean right away and you prevent a problem from developing." This argument is supposed to explain how they can cut a mother open and find a baby in no trouble after all. But we now know beyond a doubt that this argument is not true. The controlled studies have shown us that mothers who are not monitored do not have more babies in trouble.[8]

The problem is that we have a machine that gives us the beat-to-beat variations of the baby's heart rate. We are getting more information about what's going on with the baby, but the results make it clear that *we don't really understand just what this additional information means.*

"That reliable recording could be done seems to have blinded most observers to the fact that this additional information will not necessarily produce better outcomes," say Drs. Banta and Thacker in their review of EFM. "This is not surprising, given the lack of precision of EFM for the diagnosis of fetal distress, and the general difficulty of separating normal fetal stress during labor from fetal distress."[9]

The studies show us that the stethoscope, tested side by side with EFM, will pick up *sustained* distress of a serious nature—meaningful distress that requires action. The bottom line is this: The stethoscope is a valued diagnostic tool for well-defined fetal distress. It will not miss the baby in real trouble.

So, how to avoid the fetal-monitor cesarean section? Sharon and Tom feel they have the answer. When they have their next baby, they are absolutely not going to be on a fetal monitor. They're convinced that it is essential to *stay off the monitor* if you want to avoid unnecessary cesarean surgery. As Tom says, "What can you say when the doctor says, 'Brain damage if I don't do a C-section'? How can you deal with that? You can't say, 'That's all right, Doc, we'll take the chance.' Who would say that? Once you're

in that situation it's all over, it just isn't possible to deal with it when it happens. The trick, I'm convinced, is to just stay off the fetal monitor in the first place. When we have our next baby we'll certainly allow monitoring with the ordinary stethoscope occasionally. We do want a healthy baby; what we don't want is another unnecessary C-section."

If you go to a doctor who uses the monitor with the idea that you will just refuse the procedure (which, of course, you can do), remember, he really believes that it works and that you are being stubborn by refusing it. The result is you may become the recipient of a lot of ill will. *This is definitely not a good laboring situation.* Bad feelings generated by others can seriously inhibit your labor! My advice is this: Don't put yourself in this situation. Instead, find a doctor who doesn't use the monitor.

There is one other important consideration. Birth is an incredibly safe and successful journey for ninety-nine babies out of a hundred, but there will be about one out of every hundred babies who will die. This inevitable death occurs whether a woman is on the monitor or not. Although these are terrific odds, if you have the one who dies, the experience is 100 percent for *you.* If you go to a doctor who uses the monitor regularly and you refuse it, and if you happen to have that one baby out of a hundred, then you might be told that you caused your baby's death because you wouldn't allow the fetal monitor. Could you really cope with that? Although there are plenty of studies to prove you denied your baby nothing, this is not what you will hear from a doctor who believes otherwise.

When you have found a doctor who does not use the fetal monitor, you have eliminated the risk of an unnecessary fetal monitor C-section. Your physician will listen to the baby's heartbeat regularly with a stethoscope and you are far less likely to get a false alarm.

THE FETAL MONITOR UPDATE FOR THIS THIRD EDITION

Alfirevic and colleagues (2013) reviewed thirteen randomized trials, using the Cochrane Database, involving more than 37,000 women. They concluded that electronic fetal monitoring increased the rate of cesarean and operative vaginal deliveries and yet it produced no improvement in rates of perinatal mortality, neonatal seizures, or cerebral palsy.[10]

A Current Commentary in *Obstetrics and Gynecology* noted that while electronic fetal monitoring was used in 85 percent of almost four million births every year in the United States, it had failed as a public health screening program. Shockingly, the positive predictive value for fetal death in labor or cerebral palsy is near zero when the electronic fetal monitor is used, meaning that "almost every positive test result is wrong."[11]

The *Contemporary OB/GYN*, written by doctors for doctors, in February 2013, carried a commentary by a member of their editorial board, Sarah J. Kilpatrick, MD, PhD. In her article she was discussing a new screening tool that was being proposed. It had nothing to do with electronic fetal monitoring, but her comment at the end of the article did:

> We do not want to have another clinical scenario similar to the rollout of fetal heart rate monitoring in which our testing has resulted only in increased maternal morbidity (i.e., increased cesarean delivery) without a demonstrated improvement in neonatal outcome.[12]

She did not cite any studies; she felt no need to explain what she meant, because at this time every obstetrician knows exactly what she is talking about, without an explanation or a reference to studies to support her statement. They do know that the electronic fetal monitor is causing harm to mothers with no benefit to babies! Yet they continue to subject women to needless risk.

Women taking classes also know this, and yet, when a mother says she doesn't consent to the electronic fetal monitor and would rather be monitored with a stethoscope, she is almost always told she does not have a choice, or she is told, "Well, we'll just do an initial twenty-minute strip [during which time you are exposed to risk without benefit] and then when labor gets going, twenty minutes out of every hour [during which time you will be exposed to risk without benefit], and then when you are close to the pushing stage, it will be used constantly until the baby is born."

The end result is that the fetal monitor cesarean is still going strong.

THE "TOO BIG BABY" CESAREAN

If you're told you need a cesarean for a baby that is too big, or an induction before the baby *gets* too big, and you are not a diabetic, then you will want to know that according to the 2014 edition of *Williams Obstetrics* there are "no current methods to assess fetal size accurately." That's right. Ultrasound does not provide an accurate assessment of a baby's size.

When a woman questions doing a cesarean or an induction for this reason, she is often told about avoiding a brachial plexus injury, which is damage to nerves that af-

fect the baby's shoulder and can cause paralysis in the arm. But almost half of these injuries, when they result in permanent damage, occur during a cesarean surgery.[13]

You might ask your doctor to review *Williams Obstetrics*, pages 885 to 887, about inducing to prevent a big baby, about doing a cesarean to prevent a brachial plexus injury, and about how unreliable this diagnosis is in the first place. Ask your doctor to discuss what *Williams Obstetrics* says to help you come to an informed decision.[14]

THE PUTTERER CESAREAN SECTION

You already know that each woman will produce a baby at her own speed, and that this can vary from the "speedster" to the "textbook" labor to the "putterer." There are two kinds of putterers. One is the on-again-off-again putterer, whose labor actually stops and starts, stops and starts.

My own third birth is a perfect example of a putterer birthing normally, the on-again-off-again variety. I labored from 4:00 p.m. to midnight in light to moderate labor, four nights in a row. Gruesome? Not at all. I wasn't working hard yet. I got a full eight hours sleep each night, had a whole day off from labor, and started again the next evening doing light to moderately hard work. False labor? Hardly. I was dilating a little more each night. On Monday morning when labor had stopped, my husband went to work and I went to the grocery store and stocked up on labor snacks and things I could make and freeze. On Tuesday morning when labor stopped, I baked the "birthday cake." On Wednesday I went to one of my student's births. When labor stopped Thursday morning, I was five centimeters dilated. Thursday night labor took off, and then I labored moderately hard to quite hard. The doctor attending my home birth arrived about midnight, and I began pushing at four in the morning. Then I pushed for two hours of hard work, turning Polly from a posterior position to the more usual one, and birthed her around 6:00 in the morning. There was a lot of work in this labor, not all jammed together but nicely spread out over the week (which I think is precisely the reason the uterus behaved this way). If I had birthed Polly in a hospital, my labor pattern would not have been allowed. The putterer's pattern would not have been allowed. The putterer's pattern is labeled "prolonged labor," "dystocia" (abnormal labor), "uterine inertia" (lazy uterus), "failure to progress," and finally "**CPD.**"

Currently, out of every 2,500 births, at least 100 women have their babies removed surgically due to CPD.[15] **Cephalopelvic disproportion** means the mother's pelvis is too small for the baby's head to fit through. Now the FDA has published a booklet that lets obstetricians know that "the incidence of a truly 'small' pelvis in patients selected for pelvimetry was as low as one or two cases in 2,500. Furthermore . . . the effects of molding of the fetal head and expansion of the maternal pelvis during labor may render pelvic diameter measurements meaningless."[16]

So what have all these women been having caesarean surgery for? These are the putterers. As the term *CPD* becomes largely invalidated, it will become an embarrassment to those obstetricians with high surgery rates, and I have no doubt it will become a worrisome problem for such obstetricians as malpractice suits are filed for this unnecessary surgery. The term *CPD* will not be used much five years from now, as the FDA publication gets around, but putterers will continue to have their babies surgically removed for uterine inertia, failure to progress, dystocia, or prolonged labor.

The woman who has the putterer pattern spread out over a couple of days is most in danger of unnecessary cesarean surgery. *The mere passage of time by itself, without evidence of trouble, is not a medical emergency.*

The second type of putterer is the one whose labor never stops but takes its sweet, slow time all the way up to about six or seven centimeters. She may have nine to twelve hours of mild to moderate contractions before she really gets down to business. So at the end of this time, say twelve hours, she's really just beginning. It is important that you do not fall into the emotional booby trap of getting exasperated as the time goes by; keep it in perspective by looking at the amount of work you are doing, and don't count the work until it begins to demand your utmost concentration. And if, after all is said and done, you still arrive too early at the hospital, be prepared to turn around and go home. Diony Young and Charles Mahan, in their booklet *Unnecessary Caesareans: Ways to Avoid Them*, give a piece of advice that is worth memorizing: "Plan to stay at home until active labor is well established. Return home if you get to the hospital and are less than four centimeters dilated and the baby is well . . ."[17]

If a woman enters the hospital, she is treated as a medical problem if her labor stops or doesn't move fast enough. If the same woman had stayed at home during that time and later mentioned it to her doctor, he would just say, "Oh well, that was just false labor," while everyone waits for the "real thing." In fact, she has experienced the real thing, but it does not have to take off and go all the way on the same day. Once you enter the hospital, though, you have declared yourself to be in labor, and labor must continue according to the hospital's timetable.

The putterer, birthing normally, is the most bungled, mishandled labor pattern in a hospital birth. Since you are in control of the decision on when to enter the hospital, this is one unnecessary cesarean section it is clearly in your power to avoid. This is why we made such a fuss back when we discussed the emotional map of labor about not going to the hospital in the excitement signpost, nor at the beginning of the serious signpost, but instead waiting until you get some of the hours of serious working labor behind you at home. Those doctors who give instructions to come in when contractions are three minutes apart and one minute long are, in my experience, the ones with the healthiest outcomes for mothers and babies. (Second-timers should be going at four minutes apart and a minute long by these doctors' recommendations.) And the emotional signpost you want to see is absolutely dedicated seriousness, aggravation at having to move, and wondering if in fact she even can. (She can, of course—she only thinks she's made of glass.)

If it is your first baby and you think you have nothing to compare contractions with to know what is hard and what is not, call your teacher; she knows, and she will spot your emotional signpost.

The woman having prolonged labor, dystocia, uterine inertia, or failure to progress is too often just the putterer, and no one is allowed to putter in the hospital. In fact, there is a chart that says you are supposed to dilate about a centimeter an hour. Few women dilate in equal increments. Cesarean surgery for puttering accounts for as many as 20 percent of all C-sections.

Remember that the mere passage of time itself does not constitute a medical emergency situation, and that you should have a doctor who is interested in intervening only when there is an indication to do so.

THE "TIME'S UP" C-SECTION

This one takes less time to explain than the putterer, but is no less important. When you get to the pushing stage in a hospital birth, the clock is running. Many doctors will set it for two hours, and then your time's up! You end up with cesarean surgery (or, if the baby is quite low, a forceps or vacuum-extractor delivery). Some doctors set the clock for three hours. This means that many women whose babies are in posterior positions will end up as C-sections or other operative deliveries. Many posterior positions will require a good amount of pushing time. Other women get a rest in the pushing stage, and their contractions will begin again a while later. But their time may have run out before then. Why should it be okay to push for two hours but not two hours and twenty minutes? Why can't you wait for the uterus to begin again when it's ready? An article in the *American Journal of Obstetrics and Gynecology* further questions this two-hour limit: "Elective termination of labor simply because an arbitrary period of time has elapsed in the second stage is clearly not warranted. Rather, the practice of subjecting patients to potentially traumatic operative procedures merely because they have not delivered within two hours after second stage had begun should be decried."[18]

One of the ways not to "run out of time" is to stall the pushing stage as long as you can. I mean back before you begin pushing in the first place. How? Well, if your last exam revealed that you were, say, six or seven centimeters dilated or more, stall the next exam for as long as you can. The clock begins to run in the pushing stage once someone "officially" knows that you are completely dilated, whether you have an urge to push or not. So even if you think you may be in the pushing stage, hold off that exam as long as possible and buy yourself some time. Allow the extra time to let the pushing urge become so well established that you can no longer reasonably hold off.

As we discussed earlier, nurse-midwives who have had home-birth experience have a far better idea of the range of normality here than their counterparts who have been limited to hospital birth experiences only. Two hours is often the hospital time limit for pushing in second stage, and hospital birth attendants do not get to see what happens if it goes longer. In fact, they are scared of it. Barbara Katz Rothman sheds some real light on this in her book, *In Labor: Women and Power in the Birthplace*. She tells us that some nurse-midwives working in a hospital deal with the challenge of not letting the clock get started by a technique known as "not looking for what you do not want to find. They are careful about not examining a woman who might be fully dilated but doesn't have the urge to push for fear of starting up the clock" sooner than necessary.

Some nurse-midwives have taken this a step further and redefined second stage itself. Rather than saying it starts with full dilation—the "objective," medical measure—they measure second stage by the subjective measure of the woman's urge to push. Most women begin to feel a definite urge to push and begin bearing down at just about the time of full dilation.

But not all women have this experience. For some, labor contractions cease after full dilation. These are the "second-stage arrests," which medicine treats by the use of forceps or caesarean section. Some nurse-midwives now think "second-stage arrest" may just be a naturally occurring rest period at the end of labor, instead of a problem requiring medical intervention. . . .

In the medical model, once labor starts, it cannot stop and start again and still be "normal" . . . But a nurse-midwife can call the "hour or so between full dilation and when she starts pushing" as *not* second stage. This is more than just buying time for clients: this is developing an alternative set of definitions, changing the way she sees the birth process.

Midwives who did not know each other, who did not work together, came to the same conclusion.[19]

The Repeat Cesarean Section

The repeat cesarean section requires more information than I can do justice to here. If you had a C-section the first time or have a friend who had a C-section the first time, go straight to *Silent Knife* by Nancy Wainer-Cohen and Lois J. Estner. This is an absolute must for anyone approaching a repeat C-section. "Once a C-section always a C-section" is not necessarily true at all.

SOME NECESSARY C-SECTIONS

Bleeding

This one is pretty commonsense, isn't it? Bleeding can be life-threatening for both mother and baby, and in such an instance a cesarean can be appropriate and lifesaving. I don't know of anyone who has had trouble realizing this at the time.

Cord Prolapse

This is so rare that it is a less-than-1-percent occurrence (.3 to .6 percent). The umbilical cord can slip down before the baby's head, even protrude from the vagina, and the head then presses down on it, cutting off the baby's oxygen supply. Again, when this rare accident has occurred, I have never known of anyone who had difficulty realizing that a cesarean might be in order to save the baby.

Fetal Distress

Yes, of course there is such a thing, and as we have already discussed, the stethoscope or fetoscope will pick up the real thing, sustained, meaningful fetal distress that may require a C-section to save the baby in trouble. What we have objected to here is not the validity of fetal distress as a reason for doing a C-section but the inaccuracy of the electronic fetal monitor in identifying fetal distress.

Herpes

An open lesion in the birth canal at the time of labor is thought to increase the chances of the baby being infected. A C-section will probably be done. Recurrent herpes at-tacks have not been conclusively shown to cause this problem, and studies on this will bear watching.

CPD

Yes, there is also such a thing as CPD, the baby's head not fitting through the pelvis. But it is astoundingly *rare*, as noted—only about one or two cases in 2,500.

How can a doctor know when CPD is for real? There is only one way, a good trial of labor. A second stage in which there is a series of intense contractions and a uterus that stops, gives another thrust forward, and stops with no progress is the only way to be tipped off to this. An arbitrary two-hour limit does not allow time for the many posteriors or putterers to birth. To do cesarean surgery before allowing this to come clearly into focus puts hundreds of women and their babies at the risk of surgical complications.

SOME FREQUENTLY ASKED QUESTIONS ON CESAREANS

I can't understand why there is such a gap between the evidence and the way doctors practice. In spite of the information available on the inefficiency and hazards of fetal monitoring, most women continue to be monitored. In spite of the fact that there are three times as many caesarean sections that do not result in better odds for babies, women are still getting surgery at these increased rates. Why? Dr. Marieskind gives us the answer in her book *An Evaluation of Cesarean Surgery*: "Habits and beliefs are already formed and the specter of suits for past unnecessary interference [is] too great."[20]

My doctor says he just uses the fetal monitor for high-risk pregnancy. If I'm high-risk, will my baby benefit, and am I less likely to have one of those unnecessary cesareans? Two of the five controlled trials *were* with high-risk pregnancies and showed no differences in outcome and triple the C-section rate, so I don't understand the rationale for thinking that it should be used on high-risk mothers.

My doctor tells me that since this book came out newer evidence demonstrates the efficacy of the fetal monitor. The information is outdated. So now, as the book goes into yet another edition, here's the updated information as reported in *The New England Journal of Medicine* in 1990.[21] A new study was set up to see if the electronic monitor helps for riskier deliveries of premature babies. The monitor was used with eighty-two premature infants. An additional ninety-one premature infants were monitored with the stethoscope alone. The expectation was that the study would demonstrate an improved outcome for those eighty-two babies electronically monitored. It didn't. In fact, it showed the *outcome was considerably worse for the electronically monitored group*. The babies were followed up at eighteen months, and 20 percent were diagnosed with cerebral palsy, compared with 8 percent of the infants monitored by stethoscope alone. That's triple the rate of cerebral palsy when the fetal monitor was used with these premature infants. In addition, the electronically monitored infants had lower neurological development scores than those monitored by stethoscope.

This is the first time the electronic monitor failed to *at least* break even with the stethoscope in outcome for the baby. Of course it has never managed to break even in outcome for the woman's health, since the monitor is clearly associated with increased high-risk surgery for mothers, but this time it didn't even come out benignly where the baby is concerned. Why do we continue to use it? *Habit!* Why did we ever start using it before these studies were performed? *Expectation* and *belief* that it would work! Should we accept technology based on habit and belief or should we expect medicine to be based on scientific evidence and practiced like a science?

The *Boston Globe* reported Dr. Benjamin Sachs, chief of obstetrics and gynecology at Boston's Beth Israel Hospital, as saying, "What happened with fetal monitoring is that it came into the standard of care, by osmosis, and everyone believed in it."[22]

A SOLUTION

Every woman *should* be able to easily find out her doctor's C-section rate before she hires him. Unfortunately, it will probably take an act of Congress (or something stronger) to require that obstetricians be accountable to their clients by publishing their annual statistics for C-sections, forceps deliveries, and use of drugs in labor as a ratio of their total births.

Just as the Occupational Safety and Health Administration has businesses post their accident and injury record annually where workers can see it, OBs should be required to post their total births attended and number of C-sections and other procedures performed annually.

Consumers have a right, even a parental responsibility, to get this information. I have worked for a number of doctors and have known their C-section rates firsthand. But I have watched women ask what the doctor's rate is and be given dishonest, "reassuring" answers.

Women should be protected from this misinformatiown and lack of information. Like anyone else selling a service, OBs should be accountable to consumers.

A VBAC BIRTH (VAGINAL BIRTH AFTER CESAREAN)

OUR BIRTH STORY: ELIZABETH AND CRAIG CASWELL

The story of our daughter's birth is remarkable only by today's standards of a typical labor and delivery. From the beginning of the pregnancy, we wanted to have the pregnancy, labor, and birth be as intervention-free as possible. My previous pregnancy resulted in a C-section because our daughter was transverse (lying sidewise in the uterus, making it impossible for the baby to come out, which is uncommon—only 1 in 300 births). Though there was disappointment in that, also there was gratitude. We needed

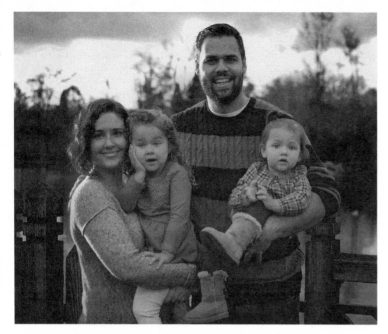

Elizabeth and Craig Caswell

a C-section and were so grateful it was an available option. We both knew that if another pregnancy was in our future we would VBAC, and we suspected it would not be an easy road.

We were excited to be pregnant again. My doctor wasn't as excited or confident as we were, but from the beginning she emphasized that she was VBAC-friendly. Despite the mounting feeling in my gut that I was not being supported in the way I would prefer, it was early in the pregnancy and I didn't want to be overly zealous.

My pregnancy progressed beautifully. I worked hard to stay in healthy parameters lest something be a road-block on my path to VBAC. Then, on a routine prenatal appointment at thirty-seven weeks, a consent form was placed in my hand and I was instructed to sign it. I had to consent to a routine induction at thirty-nine weeks, and if I happened to go into labor before then, on my own, then I had to consent to having my water broken upon arrival at the hospital. I was shocked. I told the doctor I would not be signing the form immediately but would need time to read it over with my husband to make an informed decision. The reply was that our signatures were required to continue care with this doctor. I went home with a heavy heart, knowing that at thirty-seven weeks' pregnant, I would start the scramble to find a new care provider.

Fast-forward to my forty-week appointment. I'd been under the care of nurse-midwives for two weeks and was feeling calm, confident, and respected. I submitted to the blood glucose test and the Group B strep test with favorable results. I was excited to hear my baby's heartbeat, which was perfect. But the head of midwifery met with me for this appointment to inform me that her recommendation was that I head over to the hospital immediately for a C-section. Flabbergasted, I asked why she would recommend that a perfectly healthy mother and healthy baby should be walked into surgery.

Her reasons were things I would be hearing for the next eighteen days: "low amniotic fluid," "old placenta," "pressure on my uterus," "uterine rupture," and I'm sure there were more, but those specifically stood out to me. The reason they stood out was because the previous weekend, my husband and I had a follow-up class with Susan and it was specifically focused on labor and delivery for VBAC. She provided us with scientific, research-based evidence about each of these issues in advance. She said she couldn't tell us what to do about any of these issues; she could not make decisions for us, but she could provide us with evidence-based information, because that's the role of an educator, to provide information. She connected us with excellent resources for the information we might need so that we could make informed decisions.

The result was that the nurse-midwife and I went back and forth for a few minutes. I did my best to listen to her without interruption (a great challenge for me!) and to repeat back what I was hearing to confirm that I was understanding her correctly. She agreed that there was no indication that I was in trouble, there was no indication that my baby was in trouble, but a C-section was the recommended route. Of course, I declined and went home knowing I would be in for a challenge.

The next eighteen days are a blur for me. Primarily because every appointment went the same. I was weighed, vitals taken, measured, baby's heartbeat was listened to, and all these things were fine, but whichever midwife was meeting with me said the same things in different ways. There was great frustration over my declining membrane sweeps to get things started, as well as concern over my "aging placenta." My standard twenty-minute appointment was now forty minutes long as I was told over and over again about the risks of an old placenta and going past my due date. But no one discussed risks of induction or risks that accompany a C-section. I was told the midwives were uncomfortable with my decision to continue my pregnancy, and induction, at the least, was recommended.

Once I reached forty-one weeks, the energy intensified. I received daily calls, messages, and e-mails. I even received a concerned e-mail from the doctor whose care I'd left to be with the midwives. There was never talk of letting me go as a patient, and I am grateful that despite the disagreements we had over how to safely and healthily gestate, labor, and deliver, we were civil and respectful in our dialogue. In the moments, it was stressful; but looking back I can see that they remained very caring despite mounting pressures on them to not have a forty-two-week woman under their care walking around. As a side note, my mom carried me for forty-four weeks and her mother had seven babies all beyond forty weeks, including twins!

At forty-two weeks and three days I had a midwife appointment and a nonstress test. Baby was doing fine. I'd had lots of scattered, light contractions that week. I went to a friend's house after my appointment and she invited me to take a bath in her huge tub. I could actually fit in it. After the bath, my friend made me a smoothie and lunch and I joked with her that I was so relaxed she was going to send me into labor. And that's when I started real contractions!

I called my husband and he came home right away. Contractions were forty-two seconds long and one-and-a-half minutes apart. They were good ones. I labored for an hour standing and swaying while I got our daughter her dinner and I ate ferociously to fuel my labor. Then I told my husband I could no longer labor while standing and talking; I needed to lie down and I needed quiet. I went into the bedroom and labored for another hour. My husband coached. He was instrumental in helping me to let the contractions go once they were over.

Things were going very much like we had been taught. The waves were predictable and timely. Focusing on keeping relaxed, and welcoming the contraction is no joke. I could always tell when I hindered the contraction through tension because they were shorter and weaker, which in the moment I wanted because it felt better than the long, strong ones. But, my husband reminded me I wanted the long, strong contractions because they meant baby, and that helped me to not fight my body.

After a couple of hours the contractions changed. What before was a predictable wave became a double peak. The wave would settle, I would feel the release and then another peak, another tightening. Double peaks soon turned to triple peaks and it was increasingly harder to relax. My contractions were one minute, fifteen seconds long and a minute apart.

My husband told me it was time to go to the hospital, but I didn't want to go. I was concerned we were going too early and I would be pressured with the ticking clock and interventions. After two more triple-peak contractions ending with a dash of nausea, my mother-in-law said, "Get her to the hospital unless you want to have this baby here." It was my ideal situation. I had been saying for weeks I wanted to go in ready to push, and I didn't know it, but that was what was happening.

I continued to labor in the car and did not experience a noticeable stall. When we arrived at the hospital, I expected the triage I had read about, but instead, after the nurses observed one of my contractions in the entryway, I was sent straight to the laboring room. A doula was offered and I was delighted to have the additional help. The midwife on duty came in and introduced herself. Although we had met before, it was very briefly. She was the one midwife in the clinic I had not had an appointment with and so I didn't feel tension or a need to prove myself. I felt free to labor and that was just what I needed. The midwife and doula observed two contractions, which had shortened briefly upon arrival, but wasted no time in reestablishing themselves. The doula suggested the tub and I was surprised this was being offered to me because I was told previously that hospital policy required an internal exam to make sure I'm dilated to a seven centimeters before entering the tub. The doula said, "Oh, I'm quite certain you are ready for the tub. You don't need to be checked. You're ready!" I was relieved and excited that I could get in the tub and that I seemed to be far enough along to "qualify."

Moments after entering the tub the breaks between contractions became brief, and when the OB came in to talk and ask me to accept an IV lock, I couldn't answer back before another contraction began. It was comical. Eventually, I said to him, "I'm not trying to be rude! I just can't talk to you right now with these contract— Hold on, another one!" After that interaction, he chuckled and left.

From there, I labored for about another half hour and then experienced a sensation I can only describe as sensory overload. In an instant I *had* to be out of the tub and not have water, or anything touching my body. For the next few contractions, I tried to find a comfortable laboring position. Frustrated at being unable to do so, I told my husband, "I can't get comfortable. No matter what position I try, I'm uncomfortable."

He helped me into a supported squat position and my next contraction came with a new sensation at the end—pressure. After experiencing another of these contractions, I exclaimed, "I can't do this!" My midwife asked what was going on. What was I feeling? I told her I was feeling pressure, enormous pressure, and it was very uncomfortable. She asked me what I wanted to do when I felt the pressure and I responded, "Push!" She replied, "Then push!" With the next contraction, I pushed when I felt the pressure and it was the strangest sensation of relief and intense, physical work I've ever experienced. I could feel my baby making her way through the cervix and into the birth canal. Some might describe it as painful, I describe it as uncomfortable. An "I-have-a-baby-in-my-birth-canal" uncomfortable.

I reached a series of contractions that felt especially powerful, and primal sounds emerged from my throat that I didn't think I could make. Some people say all self-consciousness goes out the window, but I was incredibly self-conscious about those deep, guttural sounds and I asked ever so demandingly that the door be shut. My midwife and doula cheered at my zoo noises and said I was doing the hard work and my baby would be here soon! In typical self-doubt emotional signpost fashion, I felt disbelief. I never seemed to realize how "far along" I truly was because I'd assumed I would be a putterer, or textbook at best. We hadn't been at the hospital for three hours yet and I labored at home for just five, so it couldn't be time, I told myself! But it was.

She was near crowning and the pressure to push became more intense. I turned to my midwife and asked, "How much longer?! Ten minutes? Fifteen minutes?" I don't remember what she replied, but I know it wasn't, "Why, in the next push she'll be here," so I was mad. I chastised her, saying I couldn't physically sustain this for much longer, and for *some* reason (wink, wink) with those words she sprang into action. She came over with her flashlight and checked and then quickly I saw kits being opened and carts wheeled in. "Oh my gosh!" I thought. "It's finally happening!" My bag of waters was still intact and protruding about an inch out, so my midwife told me to feel the bag of waters. It was extraordinary!

Once the water broke (and I had an ample amount of fluid in spite of all the low-fluid talk) my baby crowned quickly, and I did not experience the "ring of fire" many refer to. It didn't burn or feel fiery. It felt exactly like skin being stretched, which isn't trivial in terms of comfort or ease. It was unusual, but I did not experience it as painful.

This was the moment in my labor where I finally allowed myself to be fully convinced that I was "far along" and she would truly be here soon. I waited uncomfortably, but excitedly, for the perineum to gently stretch over the crest of my baby's head, with no tearing, and resumed pushing. Baby was born just a few pushes later and they placed her on my chest in all her dark-haired perfection.

She took to breast-feeding intuitively and the nurses and doula commented on how mature she seemed, holding herself and feeding; they agreed she needed all forty-two weeks and four days to be ready—and she was! I noticed at this point a lot of people in the room and I asked the nurse why there were additional staff. She replied that not many people get to witness births after forty weeks, especially VBAC and especially medication-free.

I also noticed a gathering at the table where the placenta was. The OB and my midwife came over and said I had a remarkable placenta. It was not only not "old," but it was heart-shaped due to an extra lobe. The OB quipped that I could've been pregnant for months more! They congratulated us and told us how good it was we stuck to our decision to wait until the baby was ready.

She was perfectly healthy, perfectly perfect, and our unremarkable pregnancy became a wonderfully remarkable labor and delivery.

CHAPTER TWENTY-SEVEN

Controversies in Hospital Birthing

RISK. RISK. HOME-BIRTHERS CONFRONT risks; the home-birth dangers must be faced and put into perspective. So the home-birther learns about birthing and plans for good prenatal care, which will screen her out of a home birth for obvious problems. The home-birther finds a skilled birth attendant to watch for problems that are not obvious, and a medical backup to be in readiness. With no drugs used and a mother who will nurse after birth, the home-birth risks are statistically small. The California Department of Health studied 1,146 cases of *planned* home birth and found that the perinatal mortality rate for home birth remained lower than the state average. The key seems to be planning, which means adequate prenatal care, plenty of knowledge, and a good birth attendant. (If you are planning a home birth you will find much useful information in Rahima Baldwin, *Special Delivery* [Berkeley: Celestial Arts, 1979].)

The major risk to the mother in home birthing is unexpectedly heavy bleeding *after* the birth. A midwife or other attendant must know what to do in this most unlikely life-threatening event. Bleeding *before* birth is rarely sudden. In almost every instance there are preliminary signs of bleeding that are not severe enough to threaten life, but are ample warning to go to the hospital. Most other kinds of problems have to do with the baby not coming, and in that event it is always possible to move to the hospital.

Next, the home-birther needs to consider risks to the baby. The attendant should know ordinary resuscitation techniques, but there will be no intensive-care nursery minutes away to help a baby born with severe problems. (Some small hospitals don't have them, either.) There are problems the baby may have that cannot be handled in a home birth. But if you are healthy, have had prenatal care to screen out toxemia or other predictable problems, and have selected an attendant (usually a midwife) who is competent, then you have confronted the risks of home birth and reduced them to a minimum. Still, home birth is not the choice of most people. You should only consider it if you can confront these risks and feel totally comfortable with your decision.

What the home-birther does, the hospital-birther must do also: Get to know the risks; weigh them deliberately, consciously, and knowingly; decide whether or not they are acceptable; and then go about the business of reducing all risk to a minimum. The hospital-birther can be falsely lulled into thinking that the hospital birth is 100 percent safe with a guaranteed perfect outcome because *no one talks about hospital-birth risks* as they do about home-birth risks.

So this chapter is especially for the hospital-birther. It is provided so you, too, will get to know the risks in the hospital birth you are planning and be able to reject those that are not acceptable.

This process of learning the risks so that you can reduce them to the barest minimum is just as necessary for the hospital-birther as it is for home-birther.

INTRAVENOUS DRIP (IV)

What is an intravenous drip? A hollow tube is inserted into a vein in your arm so that fluids can be dripped directly into your bloodstream, and you have taken your first giant step away from birthing normally.

After the nurse hooks up an IV, she will often say, "You may notice your contractions slowing down." Isn't it just common sense that dripping fluid into an open vein is going to dilute the bloodstream that carries oxygen and nutrients around the body, as well as the hormone the body produces to make the uterus contract? No wonder an estimated 30 to 40 percent of women in labor have so-called uterine inertia or dystocia and then need some artificial hormone added to the IV to force the uterus to contract. Having caused the problem with the intervention of a routine IV, it is necessary to solve it with a drug that has numerous known side effects and risks.

Women who are given IVs are often not allowed to eat or drink and are told the IV will replace the food and water they may need in labor. But the denial of food and water can make a woman's contractions weak and ineffectual in a long labor. Her ability to work with pushing contractions may be affected if she has just gone eighteen to twenty hours without anything to eat.

Williams Obstetrics (2014) makes it clear that there is no need for an IV in a normal-birthing mother *UNTIL* drugs are used. Women using epidurals must be on an IV first, since 20 percent of these mothers will suffer a drop in blood pressure, and that is serious. Blood flow to the uterus and to the baby decreases. More drugs are quickly used via the IV to counteract this drug-related complication.

Or she may be told it is necessary to have an open vein in case of bleeding that requires a transfusion. (Not only is this rare, but an IV can be hooked up at that time if needed.)

A harmless procedure? Think again. When almost every woman in labor is declared to be dehydrated, we should begin to be suspicious. There is an important process going on here that we don't know much about. We don't know enough about what constitutes "normal" for the laboring mother to start instituting corrective measures, en masse, for all laboring women.

Dr. Louis Pollack tells us, "At the very least, it would appear that a woman in active labor with an estimated gestation greater than 37 weeks and no associated complications need not be burdened by an unnecessary intervention that has no proved benefits and well-documented potential neonatal complications."

His comment ran in the June 1988 issue of the *Birth Journal* carrying several articles documenting IV hazards to the baby. It is the *routine* use of the IV that I decry here. Our technology needs to be used selectively or rather specifically, in response to a problem. A normal healthy woman in a normal labor is not a problem, but a "routine" IV can create a problem.

POSTMATURITY

Postmaturity is one of the most common reasons parents are given for inducing (forcing) labor. Postmaturity is a theory that assumes that if you go past your "due date" the placenta gets old and starts to deteriorate.

This is supposed to result in a tiny baby who has lost weight in the womb. (It does not mean a baby who was allowed to grow too long and is getting too big, a common misconception women have when their doctors mention postmaturity.)

Dr. Bradley makes it quite clear in *Husband-Coached Childbirth* that he doesn't believe in trying to second-guess nature. Although he has occasionally had to induce a labor for medical reasons, he has never induced any woman merely for going past her so-called due date.

Dr. Bradley says that an obstetrician who thinks he can tell when the baby is ready to be born is fooling himself and will occasionally "pick a green apple."

This has happened to several of my students. One

went four weeks over her calculated due date. She was told her baby would be postmature if they waited any longer. After her forced labor was over, the pediatrician diagnosed her three-pound baby as *pre*mature. The first year of this baby's life was extremely expensive for the parents, both financially and emotionally.

Another student, induced for the same reason, discovered that her labor simply would not get going in spite of the induction. Since her membranes (bag of waters) had been ruptured artificially, in an attempt to force labor to start, she couldn't be sent home from the hospital. Something had to be done, so she had a cesarean section.

This problem is not at all uncommon in induced labors. It is one of the recognized risks of induction: that it might simply not work. A C-section will then be done. Few women realize that once they start this procedure, there is no turning back if it doesn't work.

I will never forget the student who was told her labor would have to be induced because she was so far past her due date that labor would never start on its own. Have you ever heard of a permanently pregnant woman?

I could go on and on. The majority of our students choose not to have a labor induced for postmaturity reasons. They do so with confidence in Dr. Bradley's book. His chapter "When Will the Baby Come?" is a must for any couple past their "due date."

Ultrasound is often used to tell if the baby is ready to be born—if he is mature enough or the right size. But ultrasound is not adequate to the task. It can be off by five to six weeks![1] That is not a reasonable margin of error.

At Dulwich Hospital in London in 1980 a study was done of 142 women who had been pregnant forty-two weeks or longer. In following up the courses of these so-called overdue mothers' deliveries, researchers found that women whose labors were induced ended up with cesarean surgery far more often than the women allowed to start labor normally; in fact, the surgery rate tripled for the forced-labor mothers. Even more significant, the infants born in both induced and noninduced groups showed similar Apgar scores and were evaluated in every way as equally healthy. The induced group of babies had no advantage, and yet their mothers were subjected to the higher risks of surgery without benefit to their babies.[2]

RUPTURING THE MEMBRANES (AMNIOTOMY)

Rupturing the membranes means breaking the bag of waters. This is most commonly done with the idea of speeding up labor. But does it?

After studying the matter, Dr. Robert Caldeyro-Barcia, a past president of the International Federation of

Obstetricians and Gynecologists, has determined that breaking the waters speeds up the average labor, as previously discussed, by thirty to forty minutes. He condemns the practice of rupturing the membranes to speed up labor and also for the sole purpose of using an invasive fetal monitor.

The amniotic sac is filled with fluid that surrounds the baby like a hydraulic cushion. It is protective. When the bag of waters is ruptured, the walls of the baby's house close in on him and he experiences direct pressure on his spine, neck, and head. The bag of waters acts as a buffer for the infant's head. Says Dr. Caldeyro-Barcia, "Premature rupture of these membranes can produce massive tears in brain tissue due to misalignment of the yet unfused bones of the skull."[3]

When the bag of waters remains intact during labor, it serves the mother as well as the infant. Part of it can protrude before the baby's head through the cervix when there is enough dilation. This is called the forewaters. The forewaters acts as an efficient conical dilator of the cervix. It is gentler than the hard head, so the mother is apt to be more comfortable when it is left intact. When the sac is intact, pressure from the forewaters during a contraction helps to spread the cervix back and to dilate it more evenly.

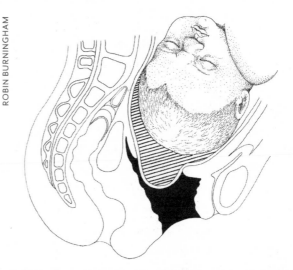

43. Bag of waters intact. The forewaters acts like a wedge to help open the cervix, gently and evenly.

FORCEPS

The forceps is an instrument used to pull the baby out of the woman's vagina. The traction and force required to pull the baby out of you would surprise you. It is not a gentle art.

Your broad ligaments may be torn, and the damage may not be discovered at birth. It may not be diagnosed until you have gone through years of great pain with intercourse. Then, if you are lucky, you might find a doctor who can identify the problem.

Women who suffer this damage are often told they are frigid. Masters and Johnson have seen five cases of women with damaged broad ligaments (not all due to forceps extraction) who went many years being told they were frigid. Finally, they found their way to doctors who knew what was wrong and corrected it with major surgery.

The forceps puts a great deal of traction on the baby's neck and spine and often results in some bruising of the baby's head. Forceps extraction may also be implicated in our cerebral palsy rate. Occasionally, a facial nerve is paralyzed by the use of forceps, and the mother's pelvic tissues can be accidentally torn.

Most doctors will tell you that they only use "low forceps" or "outlet forceps" to control the birth of the head. This is supposed to be easier on the baby's head than the mother pushing.

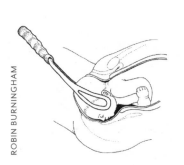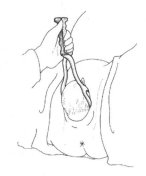

ROBIN BURNINGHAM

44. Forceps delivery

But, obviously, the mother's body parts are soft, and nature intended for the baby to be pushed from behind, not tugged and pulled out by the head and neck with hard metal instruments.

Women tend to think that the forceps is something rarely used, but in 2014 the American College of Obstetricians and the Society for Maternal-Fetal Medicine released new guidelines aimed at reducing the C-section rate. We are returning to forceps. Ironic, isn't it? Forceps were abandoned in favor of the "safe" cesarean. Now, cesareans have increased the maternal mortality rate—so we are returning to forceps.

If you select a doctor who believes in controlling the head this way (instead of simply telling the mother when to stop pushing), then you will probably end up with a forceps extraction of your infant.

I don't think you will be pleased with the experience. Most women describe it as quite painful and requiring some powerful anesthetic. An episiotomy is practically mandated when forceps are used.

Vacuum Extractor

This is something like a vacuum cleaner. A caplike cup is attached to the baby's head and suction pulls part of the scalp into the cup. Then the doctor grasps the handle and

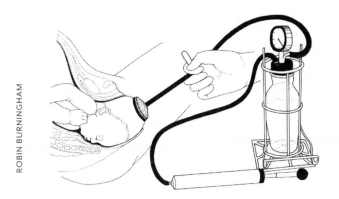

ROBIN BURNINGHAM

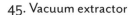

45. Vacuum extractor

pulls and tugs the baby out of you. It can cause severe molding of the cranial bones, and you still risk the traction damage to the broad ligaments.

Like the forceps, it's an experience I think you will be less than pleased with, and it is not without some of the same hazards to you and your baby that were described with forceps delivery.

Stress Test

You're nine months' pregnant. Your doctor suggests that you check into the hospital for the afternoon and he will connect you to an IV with Pitocin in it to force your uterus to contract three or four times, so that he can see on the chart how your baby is going to take contractions. Of course, your baby isn't ready for labor or you'd be in labor, so you are risking recording a baby who is not ready for labor. This is another road to cesarean surgery. There is a high "false positive" rate with this test, as you might expect. In other words, there are a good number of babies who appear as though they are going to have trouble in labor and then don't have trouble.

There is also a *nonstress* test. This one is called nonstress because no drug is used to force a contraction. Instead, the baby's heart is listened to whenever you feel him move during the test. This, too, has a high false positive rate. Both of these tests are far from reliable and yet cesarean surgery may be performed as a result of either.

BREECH BABIES

A breech baby (one who will be born feet or bottom first) does not have to mean automatic cesarean surgery. If your doctor tells you it does, he or she hasn't kept up with the latest on the subject, contained in a 1981 report from the National Institutes of Health, Task Force on Caesarean Childbirth. It recommends that "vaginal delivery of the term breech should remain an acceptable obstetrical choice" under certain conditions, the most important of which to you is that the doctor you choose be experienced in this kind of birth.[4] If your baby is breech, you will need to know more, and the best place to look is Nancy Wainer Cohen and Lois Estner's *Silent Knife*.

INDUCING LABOR WHEN THE WATER BAG BREAKS

Physicians have become extremely aggressive in the last few years about forcing labor to start soon after the water bag breaks, instead of waiting for you to start contractions on your own. They are afraid you and your baby will get an infection if you don't have your baby soon. What is soon? It used to be forty-eight hours, then twenty-four, and recently I have had a few students who were told they would have to come into the hospital and be induced immediately, and if they didn't have their babies in twelve hours, they would have cesarean surgery.

Frankly, infection is most often the result of vaginal exams. It takes only one vaginal exam after the water bag breaks for the examining fingers to carry potentially bad organisms up into the uterus. In fact, one doctor reporting on a study involving women with ruptured membranes tells us that mere time passing is not related to infection rates. As a result of his study, he tells us "there would appear to be no real basis for the stimulation of labor in patients with premature ruptures of the membrane, especially before thirty-two weeks of gestation, since *the risk of infection was unrelated to the duration of membrane rupture*" (italics mine).[5]

He goes on to state that only a "hands-off" policy will reduce the chances of infection. Sometimes a culture is taken and women are put into a state of alarm by being told they have bad organisms in the vagina. In fact, the same experienced researcher says cultures often show such organisms but have very little use in predicting whether or not the woman will get an infection. The mere presence of bad organisms is not the same as succumbing to them. For example, throat cultures often show bad organisms in people who are not sick.

Three women in my last class of ten couples started with the water bag breaking. One of these six birthed within or at forty-eight hours, and two birthed one week later. All of them received good advice from their birth attendant. They were told not to put anything whatsoever in the vagina—no tampons to stop the leaking, no douche—and not to have intercourse, and were asked to take their temperatures regularly and report immediately if there was any rise in temperature. There were no infections. There were also no vaginal exams.

CHAPTER TWENTY-EIGHT

More Questions for Your Doctor or Birth Attendant

NEAR THE BEGINNING OF this book you learned that a lot of decisions about the kind of birth experience you have are made at the time you choose your doctor or other birth attendant. The problem was that at first you did not know just what to ask a prospective doctor or how to interpret his or her answers. Now you know a lot more about the controversies in childbirth. You can decide what is really important to you and what matters less. And you can now ask more specific questions and understand what the answers mean.

This chapter will give you a list of questions you may want to ask a prospective birth attendant. The way you ask them and the way you listen to the answers are important. Try to avoid the questionnaire, clipboard, and pencil routine. If you are checking out a new doctor in a face-to-face interview, you may want to make notes about what to ask, but we advise against bringing in a long list of written questions.

Doctors do not like to feel they are being interrogated. Try not to challenge the doctor on the procedures he or she uses. But do not make it easy for the doctor to just reassure you by answering with what you want to hear. Ask questions that draw out a matter-of-fact explanation of what the doctor thinks is best in birthing, and compare that to what you have come to look for.

As discussed in Chapter Four, if the doctor's or birth attendant's answers are at odds with your ideas on points that are quite important to you, don't think you will be able to convince that person to change later on. Move on to find a birth attendant who already thinks the way you do on the main points and seems at least adaptable on the points that are less critical to you. Now, here are some further questions.

What do you think of the fetal monitor and a routine IV in labor? If the doctor thinks that everyone should be hooked up, you have quickly found out that he or she does *not* support birthing normally. This doctor is not experienced at natural childbirth. His or her cesarean surgery rate will be an unnecessary risk that you should avoid. And you took a shortcut with this question to get directly to this doctor's view of birth.

What would you do if I were nine months' pregnant and my bag of waters broke, but no contractions followed? If the answer is that you must produce your baby within twelve hours, this may not be the doctor for you. A reasonable answer to this would be something like: "Well, I would want you to report immediately if you started running a temperature. In the meantime, no tampons or anything should be put in the vagina and you would probably start labor within the next forty-eight hours. It is rare not to start labor within that time span, so it is highly unlikely you would need to be induced."

As long as everything is normal—I am fine and the baby is fine—how long will you let me push? If the doctor answers two hours (or less), this may not be the doctor for

you. You are looking for a doctor or birth attendant who says something like this: "Well, as long as there are no problems with you or the baby, you can continue pushing as long as you are willing to."

What do you think about episiotomies? "Well, I don't do them routinely but I find most first-time mothers need them or they tear." This answer tells you two things. Either this doctor does a routine episiotomy every time (otherwise he or she would know by experience that most women do not tear), or the doctor hurries the birth by forceps, vacuum extractions, or by holding onto the baby's head so it won't slide back. The hurrying causes tears. The answer you want to hear is rather something like: "I rarely do an episiotomy because most women don't need them. Sometimes there is a small tear but it is usually minor."

How do you feel about women birthing in a labor bed rather than in a delivery room? If the answer is, "We have an alternative birthing room and a lot of women are opting for that," it is a good sign. But you want to go a step further and ask, "Do you leave the bed like it is or do you 'break' it open like a delivery table with stirrups at the time of birth?" If the answer is that the doctor prefers to use the stirrups and you say that *not* using them is quite important to you, this may be a subject for further discussion. If the doctor is adamant about the stirrups, which defeats one of the purposes of staying out of the delivery room, he or she may not be the doctor for you.

Do you have a time limit for producing the placenta before you feel that you must take measures like mashing on the stomach or going into the uterus after it? You want a doctor or attendant who is willing to let you nurse peacefully and wait up to a half an hour or even longer to produce the placenta as long as there are no indications of problems. Patience and a willingness to stay out of the picture are sometimes rare traits in doctors and other birth attendants. You want someone who realizes the importance to you of this special time and has no arbitrary time limits for the placenta to be delivered.

If you have satisfactory answers to the questions so far, it sounds like you are on the right track. If the answers to these important questions have not been satisfactory up to this point, you have probably already left the office, hung up the phone, or started to look for another birth attendant to interview. The questions that follow have more to do with things that are really up to you to handle *during* labor. But it is a good idea for your birth attendant to know that they are important to you so he or she can help you make your choices happen.

How do you feel about routine ultrasound exams when there is no medical indication to have one? If he says he only starts doing them when you're thirty-seven weeks, or thirty-eight, or thirty-nine, or forty, then ask, "What would be the indication though?" Late-pregnancy ultrasounds in the absence of any problem often lead to inductions.

How do you feel about purposely breaking the bag of waters during labor? I really don't want this done. This should be just a simple matter of declining the procedure, but talking about it ahead of time alerts the birth attendant that you do not want to be "surprised" by having the waters broken without being asked.

What if I get to the hospital too early and find that I am less than four centimeters dilated and my labor is just poking along? I would rather go back home and continue to labor normally, rather than being induced or speeded up. Would you support me in this? The best birth attendants know that a hospital is not the best place to pass the early hours of first-stage labor and will encourage the laboring couple to return to the familiar comforts of home if labor has not progressed as far as expected.

Do you know about the pressure episiotomy in the unlikely event that a cut should be necessary? I don't want a little shot of anything in the bottom at the last moment before birth when I am crowning. I understand there is sometimes a misunderstanding about this, so I want to be quite clear. Of course, if I need a few stitches after the birth, then I would be happy to have a shot at

that time. You should already feel that your doctor will help you give birth without an episiotomy if that is important to you, but this question will make it clear that you want no medication before the birth of the baby.

How do you feel about the use of a routine shot of Pitocin after birth to force the uterus to contract after the placenta is out? Your doctor or birth attendant should already know that you expect to nurse immediately so the uterus will contract naturally. A shot of Pitocin can give the woman a painful "double whammy" of artificial contractions on top of natural ones. This is just an unnecessary nuisance that can be avoided.

Finally, if you have made it this far with satisfactory answers and good feelings between you and your prospective birth attendant, you may want to sum up your expectations for this birth ahead of you. You might say something like this: "What I am really asking you is to refrain from anything that is a routine procedure unless you see a situation that requires special treatment."

If you find your prospective birth attendant agreeing wholeheartedly with this statement, you can feel confident you have found the right person. The responsibility for having the kind of birth you want still rests with you and your coach, of course, but you can feel assured that your birth attendant will be a help, not an obstacle to your plans.

Now you know the major birthing issues and the techniques needed to go after the safest and most fulfilling birth experience. Be decisive and don't hesitate to act on your decisions. We have, through these pages, done what we can to help you help yourself to a great birth. Our last word to you is, "Don't give your birth away."

CHAPTER TWENTY-NINE

Breast-Feeding

WHY SHOULD YOU BOTHER to breast-feed when bottle-feeding is just as good, and much easier; you have more freedom and your husband gets to feed the baby, too?

Let's start with easier. With my first baby I breast-fed for three months. I felt like I was feeding the baby *all* the time. It seemed that every time I turned around, I was breast-feeding *again*, so I switched to bottle-feeding, and to my surprise I discovered that I was bottle-feeding all the time. New babies just *feed* all the time, whether breast- or bottle-fed.

Now that I had switched, I had to make sure enough formula was in the house. I envisioned myself as an organized person, but no matter how organized I tried to be, there was always that inevitable time or ten when I had run out of formula or some essential part of the apparatus. Meantime, the baby was screaming while I was getting the bottle together, and my nerves were chorusing right along with the baby's screaming. I longed for the days when all I had to do was just sit down and hook up.

In my experience, bottle-feeding wasn't easier. Of course, it had its entertainment value for my husband, like the time I was boiling the rubber nipples and forgot them. When I went back into the kitchen, I had a very good example of the law of conservation of mass. The rubber nipple mass was now hanging from the ceiling in gooey stalactites of black ash and clinging stickily to the cabinets.

Regrettably, not until I gave up breast-feeding did I become fully aware of the peripheral benefits of nursing my baby. While my husband was a good sport the first night and stumbled out to the kitchen to grope for a bottle for the 2:00 a.m. feeding (and that was the first and last time that I was organized enough to have a bottle ready and waiting), he soon suffered a notable diminishing of noble zeal for this nightly event. You know the saying, "The spirit was willing but the flesh was not." His flesh was the warm mound under the covers while mine shivered in the kitchen.

I missed being able to stay under the covers while he merely lifted the baby out of the bassinet and placed him beside me, the three of us nestling together as I hooked up with the baby and fell promptly back to sleep.

And what about freedom, that implied promise with every purchase of a container of formula? I'm sure you've seen those always beautiful, very together, on-the-go women who are in the bottle-feeding promotional pictures. You know, like the cigarette advertisements that always show a background of nature, peace, and serenity and a person sucking on a cigarette who looks like somebody you want to be.

I had much more freedom breast-feeding than bottle-feeding. I didn't have to double-check my inventory of formula before heading out somewhere. I didn't have to fix anything. I didn't even have to carry anything with me except the baby and a diaper.

I traveled to many conferences, and I particularly remember a time sitting on my suitcase at the airport waiting for a cab with a happily nursing baby. It was so easy!

Well, what about bottle-feeding so your husband can get to feed the baby? How many husbands are home for anything but the evening feeds, and what's the matter with just holding the baby, talking to it, playing with it?

If breast-feeding is easier, what else might keep you from it? What about retaining your figure? Will you lose it if you breast-feed? Will your breasts get saggy? If you're worried about this, then you'll actually want to breast-feed. A part of your body that you don't use gets out of shape, atrophies. It is more likely to stay in shape if you use it. (The breast does tend to enlarge and drop a little due to pregnancy, however, whether you breast- or bottle-feed.)

What about modesty? Will that stop you from breast-feeding? Relax. One doesn't have to display the breast in order to breast-feed. If that's not a concern for you, fine, more power to you, but it was for me. If it's important to you, too, then rest assured that it only takes a little practice to get rather clever at comfortable concealment in plain view of others. I'll never forget going out to dinner with my parents to an elegant restaurant. My very proper Bostonian mother leaned over and said to me, "Just what are you going to do if the baby gets hungry while we're here, dear?" The baby and I were already hooked up, very discreetly, and my mother couldn't tell. I just chuckled and said, "I don't know, Mom."

The trick is to wear two-piece outfits. It's silly to be caught out with a hungry baby and you're in a one-piece dress that zips down the back. Get a bra that opens in the front so that all you have to do is slide your hand up your blouse, lean forward a little and unhook it. Look for a bra that's easy to unhook *one-handed*. Then slide the baby up your tummy and he'll latch on to the nipple. Just let your blouse hang down over his face. He won't smother. He would sputter and let go first. His body covers any bare tummy.

I must admit the first time I tried nursing in public, I was dripping perspiration and very tense. I kept my eyes down, glued to the baby; I was just sure everyone in the restaurant was staring at me. My husband realized my dilemma and told me to look up. When I did, of course, I realized no one was looking at me. If someone had been, what do strangers do when they lock eyes? They look away.

MECHANICS

When I say breast-feeding is easier, I mean in the *long run* it is much easier, and when it comes to feeding a baby that is exactly what you are in for, the long run. But before it's easier, you *do* have to learn the knack of nursing, and that can take a nursing novice two or three weeks. There is a definite front-loaded investment of your time, effort, and frustration level as you launch, or rather lurch, along this path.

Those first three weeks are fraught with difficulties, and it is here that most women give up, but the majority of the difficulties are a consequence of not understanding how the breast/brain and baby mesh together. This is a sensitive feedback system; your brain monitors outflow and immediately moderates production to match demand. Any business executive would envy the rapidity and accuracy of this demand-supply loop. How many commercial enterprises can respond to a fluctuation in demand by moderating supply to match new levels of consumption within a mere twenty-four to forty-eight hours *and* maintain quality?

HERE'S HOW IT WORKS

You have these grapelike sacs that fill with milk inside the breast. They are clustered together, again much like grapes, and have stems (ducts) that radiate toward the nipple (see illustration 46).

A *baby does not suck milk out of the breast.* The baby sucks just enough to draw the nipple into his mouth, and then he *gums* up and down on the nipple. The gumming sends a stimulus, an impulse to the brain, specifically to the pituitary gland. The pituitary then dumps oxytocin into the bloodstream and causes the grapelike sacs to contract and *eject* the milk from the breast. So milk isn't sucked from the breast, it actually sprays or squirts out.

You will see the baby take hold, gum several minutes, and then stop to gulp, gulp, gulp, swallowing like crazy as

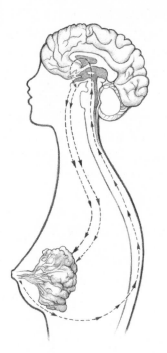

46. How the breast works

the milk is sprayed into his mouth. Gum, gum, gum, gulp, gulp, gulp. If he lets go while the milk is spraying, you may see it spray a surprising foot or two away from the breast, an ejection of liquid in ten or twelve streams.

When he stops swallowing, then the spray has stopped. Now he must gum again to get the next several swallows of milk to eject into his mouth.

This sounds like the makings of a song: The breast is connected to the nerves and the nerves are connected to the brain and the brain is connected to a gland, that makes hormones, that are dumped into the bloodstream, that cause the sacs within the breast to contract and then the milk squirts out. Whew! Amazing intricacy, and we've only talked about the delivery system or *how* to get the milk to the consumer.

At the beginning of a feed, you will notice the gumming is vigorous, with appropriate pauses to gulp down the resulting sprays of milk. Perhaps seven to ten minutes into a feed, the gumming is less frantic, and the baby gums at a more moderate pace, now that the sharp edge of his initial hunger has been assuaged. In another ten minutes or less, his gumming will be slower yet, and when it gets downright lackadaisical, and he is drowsy from the warmth of your body and your milk and from his sweaty little efforts, this is a good time to change a diaper (wakes him up) and then hook up to the other breast.

Again, the gumming will begin at a rapid, eager pace since you've roused him from his drowsy state and given him the other full breast, and after seven to ten minutes (or more), again he slows down to moderate sucking and finally fades away to just hang on—after all, the breast is a nice cozy place to be—but you can be sure the meal is over. If you're enjoying sitting there, fine, but if you want to move on to doing other things, be assured he's finished when the gumming has faded away. Slide a finger into his mouth, break the suction, and disengage (unhook).

Quality control is even more interesting. The mixture of components in the milk will be present in different ratios at different months of the baby's life. The milk you make is actually *age* specific. Imagine that! A newborn with a rapidly developing brain will have different nutritional needs than the bigger six-month-old who will need more fat and carbs. The ratio of different components of milk actually changes constantly to meet the changing needs of your baby, hour by hour, day by day. You realize, of course, infant formulas can't change hour by hour, day by day, to meet the age-specific needs of the baby.

Quantity control is the next truly crucial thing to understand. If a baby takes six ounces of milk from your breast today at ten in the morning, then tomorrow at ten o'clock your breast will have about six ounces of milk in it.

Now, can you imagine what happens if you give the baby a bottle of water at nine o'clock? If you fill his tummy up with water, will he be likely to take as much milk at ten o'clock? Milk is left in the breast and the brain gets the signal: *Make less milk, make less milk!* And *twenty-four hours later, at the ten o'clock feed, the breast is making less milk.* You then have a fussy baby who doesn't get the six ounces of milk he wants at ten o'clock the next day and all because

of a monkey wrench you threw into the system the day before: a water bottle. If the breast didn't respond by making less milk when the baby takes less milk, then the breast would just back up with milk until it burst, so it's a good thing the breast and brain work together this way, but you can see how you derail the system with an unnecessary bottle of water.

What now? Well, you would put the fussy baby to the breast off and on for the next hour or two. He would nurse fitfully at the empty breast. The increased sucking would send a stimulus to the brain that says, *Make more milk at this time of day, make more milk at this time.* Twenty-four to forty-eight hours later, your milk supply at that time of day is back up to par. All that trouble caused by an innocuous bottle of water. But doesn't the baby need water? No—90 percent of breast milk *is* water. If it's exceptionally hot, then there might be a need for extra fluid, but this is the exception, not the norm.

What do you suppose would happen if you gave the baby a bottle of formula? Same problem.

A mother once called me to tell me that her baby didn't like her milk. I asked her how she knew the baby didn't like it and she told me tearfully, "She spits it out." I dropped by to visit her and stayed until the baby woke up crying and mother put her to the breast. I unobtrusively observed a very smooth mother/baby interaction for thirty or forty minutes. The baby did the expected: initially gumming vigorously, then slowing down to moderate midmeal gumming, and finally petering out to a minimal amount of gumming; when that minimal amount produced milk, the baby let it run out of her mouth because she was *stuffed*.

Let's do an instant replay on that one to be sure the picture is as vivid for you as it is for me. Vigorous sucking for seven to ten minutes and an alert baby, moderate sucking for another seven to ten minutes, smooth interaction, not fussy, and finally, very slow sucking. Change diaper, offer other breast, renewed vigorous sucking, moderate sucking, *slow slow slow sucking and dribbling milk out of mouth quite contentedly. Absolutely stuffed!*

Then there is the "fighting at the breast phenomenon," where the baby's face gets all red as he cries and straightens and stiffens his legs, arches his back, and doubles up his little fists, waving them around and struggling.

When do you see this? If you put the baby to breast every time he cries, you must realize that babies cry for reasons other than needing to be fed. They cry when you've kept them up too long and they need to sleep; they cry when they need to have a bowel movement during the first few weeks of life. After all, they didn't have any need to have any of those in the uterus, so they don't know quite how to accomplish it. They only know that they are un-comfortable, and, of course, when they cry they are tightening all the right muscles and soon learn how to do this.

But if you put the baby to breast for every cry, when he is not hungry, he will still grab the nipple vigorously, as if he is starving, so how do you know he's not? You know because he lets go the minute the milk lets down. He doesn't need or want any, and you see the fighting-at-the-breast phenomenon.

If he lets go *as soon as the milk starts to spray*, read this right. He isn't hungry. So obvious, isn't it? So why don't we get it and instead drive ourselves and our babies crazy? Because we live in a culture that has no confidence in breast-feeding, doubts the efficacy of breast over bottle. At least with a bottle, you can see it's empty and know the baby couldn't be hungry. So you look for some other reason for the crying. But with the breast you don't see the milk go in, don't have the empty bottle to document the quantity, yet if milk is refused when let down, and you have lots of wet diapers, then rest assured, the crying is not about hunger.

Let's do a rehearsal. There you are. You've just had your baby. You put him to breast right after birth and he actually nurses a little bit, or at least he nurses sometime during the first hour following the birth. This is great. Your uterus is stimulated to contract, and the baby gets colostrum. Colostrum is loaded with immunity factors that start protecting the baby at once and the sooner the better, because the hospital is a warehouse for some of the most antibiotic-resistant bacteria. Fortunately, however, breast milk provides protection against some of these. Colostrum is also extra concentrated in a variety of nutrients needed by the baby, as well as providing protection from disease. It packs a lot in a little. Think of it as milk concentrate.

Next, you go home after a few hours, having picked a supportive obstetrician and pediatrician who concur, following your uncomplicated, undrugged birth. Your supportive hospital doesn't even offer you the free pack of formula any more than they would offer a box of chocolates to someone who declared an intent to diet.

When you get home, you don't consider dieting or exercising for the first six weeks at least. Your uterus is not yet back to its normal size, and doing exercises that contract the abdomen, thereby compressing the still somewhat enlarged uterus, can dangerously increase or restart bleeding.

Give yourself a break, eat normally. You just had a baby. Your body is doing a lot inside, even though you can't see it. Think of this: Breast-feeding itself will use up a lot of calories.

Most newborns want to nurse about every three or four hours (although there is some variation from one baby to the next). In a twenty-four-hour period, they often have one fussy stretch of a few hours. My babies always did this between 7 and 9 p.m. It almost seemed they were taking a double feed. Following this double feed time, they also took their longest sleep of about six hours. Just relax, sit down and nurse, and give yourself a chance to see the evolving pattern. These first three weeks will be the most demanding. Don't fall into the trap of showing the world that having a baby hasn't changed your life at all. The first few weeks of a newborn, your life is turned upside down. Don't worry. Things will reach a new "normal" state after a while.

POSITIONS

If you're sitting up to breast-feed a newborn, try tailor sitting. Put a pillow or two in your lap, so your arm won't get tired holding the baby to breast. Always get a glass of water before you sit down. Your mouth and throat will dry up like a desert the minute you hook up.

Your baby has a "rooting reflex." When he feels the breast against his cheek, he will turn toward it. His mouth opens like a little bird and he roots around for the nipple. If you are touching his other cheek to push him toward your breast, you will confuse him. He will turn toward your hand on his cheek and away from your breast. Just support the body and put your breast against his cheek, near his mouth. Do not "put" the nipple into the baby's mouth; let him root for it. If you always put the nipple into his mouth, he will lose the rooting reflex, and then it's harder to nurse discreetly.

If your breast is so full it pushes against the baby's nose, he will have to let go to breathe. In that case, just take a finger and press the breast away from his nose. You may also have to remove the baby's fist from his mouth. It's hard to get the nipple in there when his fist is in the way.

If you're lying down to nurse, then angle the baby's feet in toward your tummy. Letting him clutch your finger is one way to keep his fist out of his mouth. Those little feet angled in toward a mother's tummy often make a stepping movement. The mother tightens her abdomen reflexively against these tiny kneading feet. Think of it as nature's own tummy exerciser.

Now let's go back and start our rehearsal again with a different scenario. Perhaps you stay three days but you have rooming in and the baby never goes to the nursery.

Here's a third scenario. Your baby goes to the nursery and you discover how extremely difficult it is in some hospitals to avoid water bottles. Even when your pediatrician leaves orders for no bottles, it is not uncommon for a nurse to give one anyway. She may not want other babies in the nursery to wake up.

You already know how a water bottle can throw off quantity control, but even worse, a newborn only a few hours or days old can be completely confused by being switched back and forth from rubber-nippled bottles to the breast. How so? Taking milk from a bottle is a whole different pattern of oral activity from taking milk from the breast. When a baby takes milk from a bottle, it is purely sucking, but when it takes milk from the breast the baby does a minimum of sucking and a maximum of gumming. A newborn is not thinking at a sophisticated level of "Aha, this is rubber nipple, employ oral activity pattern A; oh, this is Mommy, switch to oral activity pattern B." This leads to a confused baby syndrome and is a nightmare. (See Frequently Asked Questions on page 296 to find out what to do.)

Here's a tip. When frustrated and ready to quit, tell yourself, "Fine, I'll quit if I feel the same way three days from now." Almost all breast-feeding difficulties clear up in that time and you feel differently.

IS BOTTLE-FEEDING JUST AS GOOD AS BREAST-FEEDING?

We now see milk as a living tissue, with almost as many live cells as blood itself.
—MAUREEN MINCHIN, MA, *BIRTH* 14, NO. 1 (MARCH 1987)

Is infant formula really equivalent to human milk?

"Look around," you say. "Look at all the human babies surviving on formula." But here is the caveat: the difference between the words *survive* and *thrive*.

survive: to endure or to live in spite of.
thrive: to grow or develop vigorously; flourish.

There are people who don't want to hear this, who would call this a hard sell, but I concur with Maureen Minchin, medical researcher. She says: "Many also believe that women must be free to choose breast or bottle-feeding, and that any critique of formula (though not of breast-feeding) is an intrusion upon that choice. But to be free, choice must be informed."[1]

Being informed means knowing that chemists have not been able to identify and copy all components of human breast milk, and as a consequence, every few years something new is discovered to be an essential ingredient and added to formulas, which are then touted to be "as good as mother's milk," until another missing ingredient is discovered and added and then the formulas are *now* "as good as mother's milk," until . . .

For example, zinc was added after it was discovered that zinc-deficient infant formulas caused lesions of the skin, suboptimal growth, and sometimes retardation,[2] and biotin was added after a lack of it was associated with sudden infant death syndrome.[3] Up until the 1970s, convulsions in formula-fed infants were common. It turned out this was due to minerals that were added to the formula in excessive amounts.[4]

During 1978–79, one US formula company, Syntex Laboratories, eliminated salt from some of its products (New-Mull-Soy and Cho-Free formulas). The FDA recommended criminal prosecution of Syntex, but in 1984 the Justice Department declined. (You see, the FDA had not required a specific amount of sodium chloride in infant formulas.)

According to the National Institutes of Health, however, more than 20,000 infants had been exposed to these two deficient soy-based formulas, and health problems were documented in at least 247 infants who used them.[5] The problems ranged from "consistently delayed speech, slow gross motor development, increased convulsion rates, rotting teeth, kidney defects, mild retardation and cerebral palsy."[6]

On a lighter note, breast-feeding triggers the release of a hormone called relaxin into the mother's bloodstream that does what it sounds like it does; I know I've experienced the effect of this hormone. Babies don't always pick a convenient time to nurse. Actually, they almost *never* pick a convenient time to nurse. Mine could be counted on to wake up and want to be fed just as I was putting dinner on the table. Being human and not the supermom we would all like to be, I would sit down to nurse feeling frustrated and frantic. But this feeling evaporated as soon as the milk let down. I would relax and figure dinner would eventually make it to the table, and I'm sure that was the effect of relaxin. Mothering is a hard job, and I'm all for anything that makes it easier.

Milk is not just age specific; it is species specific. Seal milk is designed to put blubber on a baby seal, about 160 pounds in forty days. Cow milk is designed for an animal with a small brain and a big body. Human milk is designed specifically for the human blueprint: *species specific*. For optimal development of the human to reach maximum potential, *to thrive*, pick one of the above.

FREQUENTLY ASKED QUESTIONS

How can I avoid sore nipples? Nurse as soon after birth as the baby will cooperate, and as frequently as the baby wants thereafter. The worst nipple problems occur when babies and mothers are separated at birth and the first feed is delayed. If the first feed is delayed too long, the breast tends to become excessively distended, the nipple pulls flat, and the baby then gums just the tip, because he can't get the overly swollen, flattened nipple into his mouth. This damages the nipple and can greatly increase soreness. Reduce this problem to a minimum by not delaying the first feed and by keeping the baby with you, so you can nurse on demand.

How do I know if my milk is too thin or too thick? Any farmer could tell you. Your milk is not homogenized. The foremilk *is* thin, like skim milk, and it is high in protein. The hind milk is thick and creamy, containing more carbohydrates. Dinner before dessert.

What can I do if I know my baby had bottles in the nursery and I'm pretty sure I'm seeing the "fighting at the breast phenomenon"? If the baby goes home confused after three days of this, he may well use the wrong pattern at the breast and not get any milk, which is definitely not healthy. In this case you see the "fighting at the breast phenomenon," but signaling something very different from what we discussed before.

In this case, you're not letting down milk because he's using the wrong oral activity pattern. There is no spray of milk when he lets go; there's a paucity of wet diapers. Now what? Call La Leche League, your birth teacher, and your pediatrician. You may need to run the baby back and forth for a checkup by someone who knows what dehydration looks like, until you get the breast-feeding reestablished.

Actually, all mothers need to know something about dehydration. We live in a culture where many girls grow up seeing little of newborns. So as women, having our own first babies, we don't have much experience to make comparisons with. A dehydrated baby has saggy, baggy elephant skin. When you pinch it, it crinkles up in folds instead of feeling like firm flesh. The soft spot on his head can become depressed; that is, the skin over it looks kind of concave. Such a baby is lethargic. Lethargy is alarming.

Bottle-feeding mothers need to know these signs, too, as should any woman who has had drugs during labor. Whether breast- or bottle-feeding, her baby may not be vigorous enough to feed well during the first week.

What should I do if I'm really not sure, but I think something isn't going right? If in doubt or needing reassurance, whether breast- or bottle-feeding, I wouldn't hesitate to call the pediatrician and ask if your husband can run the baby by for a quick checkup. If you picked a supportive pediatrician, he understands you just want reassurance. It should be a quick trip. I am not comfortable with a pediatrician who tells a worried mother over the phone to just keep breast-feeding or bottle-feeding and don't worry.

I just can't believe my body can make milk for my baby. How can you think that suddenly, because the baby is on the outside, your bloodstream can't get appropriate nutrients to the breast and the breast make milk, when, in fact, your body supported this child perfectly well for nine months via the same bloodstream carrying nutrients to it?

Why shouldn't your body be able to continue to supply the necessary nutrients now that the baby's on the outside? It just takes the nutrients to a different place, to the breast instead of to the placenta. Why would it suddenly stop working unless you throw a monkey wrench into the system by a lack of knowledge of how it works?

CAUTION

If you have had any breast surgery, biopsies, or implants, or have cysts in the breast, then you need to work in close collaboration with your pediatrician.

FINALLY

This is a *chapter* about breast-feeding, not a book. My intent is to provide enough information to help you through the first three weeks in normal circumstances.

Notice that I haven't dealt with anything beyond the third week. Can you work and continue to breast-feed? When should you introduce solid food and how much and what kind? Can you breast-feed after a cesarean? When and how to wean or not to wean and much more. I urge you to read a *book* on breast-feeding. La Leche League's *The Womanly Art of Breastfeeding* is excellent. I hope you attend some of their meetings. You should also check with your birth teacher. Many of them have special training in breast-feeding and can be enormously helpful.

References

CHAPTER TWO: How Is the Bradley Method® Unique?
1. Feldman, Silvia, *Choices in Childbirth* (New York: Grosset & Dunlap, 1979), pp. 108, 109.

CHAPTER THREE: How to Choose Your Childbirth Teacher
1. Feldman, *Choices in Childbirth*, p. 103.

CHAPTER FOUR: Choosing Your Doctor or Your Midwife
1. Kozhimannil, B., et al., "Cesarean Delivery Rates Vary Tenfold Among US Hospitals: Reducing Variation May Address Quality and Cost Issues," *Health Affairs* 32, no. 3 (March 2013), 527–35.

CHAPTER FIVE: Nutrition: How Does Your Garden Grow?
1. Burke, B.S., et al., "Nutritional Studies During Pregnancy," *Amer J of Obstet and Gynecol* 46 (1943), p. 38; and Montagu, A., Life Before Birth (New York: New American Library, 1977), p. 25.

2. Ebbs, J. H., et al., "The Influence of Prenatal Diet on the Mother and Child," *Jour of Nutr* 22 (1941), p. 515.

3. Shneour, E. A., "Nurture Needs of the Unborn Baby," in *Expecting*, a special enclosure in *Parents Magazine* (Fall 1974), pp. 12, 26; and Dubos, R., "Progress in Prevention of Birth Defects," *Leaders Alert Bulletin,* no. 27 (New York: National Foundation/March of Dimes), p. 1.

4. Brewer, Gail S., and Brewer, Tom, *The Brewer Medical Diet for Normal and High-Risk Pregnancy* (New York: Simon & Schuster, 1983), p. 220.

5. Cunningham, F. G., et al., *William's Obstetrics*, 24th ed. (New York: McGraw Hill, 2014), p. 877.

6. John Dobbing of the University of Manchester, England, quoted in "Crucial Time for Brain Growth," *Woman's Day,* November 1970, p. 44.

CHAPTER SIX: Drugs During Pregnancy

1. Okuda, S., "Yale Researchers Establish Link Between Drug, Birth Defect," AP domestic wire, AM Cycle, December 16, 1982; also printed as "Anti-Nausea Drug, Birth Defect Linked," Honolulu *Star-Bulletin*, December 24, 1982, p. A-10.

2. "Stuart, M. J., et al., "Effects of Acetylsalicylic Acid Ingestion on Maternal and Neonatal Hemostasis," *New England J of Med* 307, no. 15 (October 7, 1982), pp. 909–12. Also reported as "Aspirin Use During Pregnancy Linked to Birth Complications," *Los Angeles Times,* September 5, 1975, Part I, p. 25; and "Physician Warns: Aspirin Can Be Harmful," *Health Insurance News,* Washington, D.C., Health Ins. Assoc. of America (April 30, 1983), p. 1.

3. Ibid.

4. Hazell, L. D., *Commonsense Childbirth* (New York: G. P. Putnam's Sons, 1969), p. 129.

5. Bracken, M. B., et al., "Exposure to Prescribed Drugs in Pregnancy and Association with Congenital Malformations," *Obstetrics and Gynecology* 58, no. 3 (September 1981), pp. 336–43.

6. Yaffe, Sumner J., et al., American Journal of Pediatrics Committee on Drugs, "Stilbestrol and Adenocarcinoma of the Vagina," *Pediatrics* 51, no. 2 (February 1973), pp. 297–99.

7. Brody, Jane E., "Shadow of Doubt Wipes Out Bendectin," *New York Times,* June 19, 1983, p. 7, sec. 4.

8. Ibid.

9. Bracken, "Exposure to Prescribed Drugs," pp. 336–43.

10. Ang, E. S. Jr, et al., "Prenatal Exposure to Ultrasound Waves Impacts Neuronal Migration in Mice," *Proc Natl Acad Sci USA* 103, no. 34 (August 22, 2006), pp. 12903–10. Epub August 10, 2006.

11. http://www.acog.org/About-ACOG/News-Releases/2013/Study-Finds-Adverse-Effects-of-Pitocin-in-Newborns.

CHAPTER SEVEN: Weighing Evidence

1. Dawber, T. R., Nickerson, R. J., Brand, F. N., and Pool, J., "Eggs, Serum Cholesterol, and Coronary Heart Disease," *Am J Clin Nutr* 36, no. 4 (October 1982), pp. 617–25. Pub Med PMID:7124663.

2. Song, W., and Kerver, J. M., "Nutritional Contribution of Eggs to American Diets," *J Am Coll Nutr* 19, suppl. 5 (October 2000), pp. 556S–62S.

3. Powell, A., Harvard Staff Writer, "The Entire Egg: Willett Welcomes Shift on Cholesterol, Stresses Whole-Food Approach," in an interview with Walter Willett, chair of the Harvard T. H. Chan School of Public Health's Nutrition Department, *Harvard Gazette, Science & Health. Health & Medicine,* February 24, 2015.

CHAPTER EIGHT: Sexuality and Birthing

1. Haire, D., and Haire, J., *Implementing Family-Centered Maternity Care with a Central Nursery* (Milwaukee: International Childbirth Education Association, 1971), pp. III-1–III-25.

2. McDonald, S. J., Middleton, P., Dowswell, T., and Morris, P. S., "Effect of Timing of Umbilical Cord Clamping of Term Infants on Maternal and Neonatal Outcomes," *Cochrane Database of Syst Rev,* issue 7 (2013), Art. No.: CD004074. DOI:10.1002/1465f1858.CD004074.pub3.

3. Weeks, A., "Umbilical Cord Clamping After Birth," *BMJ* 335 (August 18, 2007), p. 312.

4. Fogelson, N. A. P., Department of Obstetrics and Gynecology, USC School of Medicine, January 30, 2011, https://academicobgyn.com/2011/01/30delayed-cord-clamping-grand-rounds.

5. Hutton, E. K., Hassan, E. S., "Late vs. Early Clamping of the Umbilical Cord in Full-Term Neonates: Systematic Review and Meta-Analysis of Controlled Trials," *JAMA* 297, no. 11 (March 21, 2007), pp. 1241–252.

6. Andersson, O., et al., "Effect of Delayed Cord Clamping on Neurodevelopment at 4 Years of Age: A Randomized Clinical Trial," *JAMA Pediatr* 169, no. 7 (2015), pp. 631–38. DOI:10.1001/*jamapediatrics.*2015.0358.

7. Nelson, H., "Decreased Drug Use in Pregnancy Urged," *Los Angeles Times,* March 15, 1973, Part II, p. 5.

CHAPTER NINE: The Mechanics of Labor and Birthing

1. Harman, T., and Wakeford, A., *Microbirth,* a documentary film, subtitled "www.oneworldbirth.net" (2014), Alto Films Ltd., interview with Martin Glazer, director of the Human Microbiome Program at NYU and author of *Missing Microbes.*

2. Ibid., interview with Rodney Dietert, professor of Immunotoxicology at Cornell University.

CHAPTER TEN: Exercises: Getting Your Body Ready for Birthing

1. U.S. Department of Health and Human Services, Public Health Service-FDA, "The Selection of Patients for X-Ray Examinations: The Pelvimetry-Examination" (July 1980), pp. 3, 25.

2. Ibid., 24.

3. Dumoulin, C., Hay-Smith, J., "Pelvic-Floor Muscle Training Versus No Treatment, or Inactive Control Treatments, for Urinary Incontinence in Women," *Cochrane Database of Syst Rev* (2010), issue 1, Art. No.: CD005654 DOI:10.1002/14651858.CD005654.pub2.

CHAPTER FIFTEEN: The Emotional Map of Labor

1. Cunningham, et al., *Williams Obstetrics,* 24th ed., p. 448.

2. Huhn, K. A., Brost, B. C., "Accuracy of Simulated Cervical Dilation and Effacement Measurements Among Practitioners," *Am J Obstet Gynecol* 191, no. 5 (2004), pp. 1797–99.

CHAPTER SIXTEEN: First-Stage Labor

1. Cunningham, et al., *Williams Obstetrics,* 24th ed., p. 448.

2. Bailit, J. L., et al., "Outcomes of Women Presenting in Active Versus Latent Phase of Spontaneous Labor," *Obstet Gynecol* 105 (2005), p. 77.

CHAPTER SEVENTEEN: Pushing: The Second Stage of Labor

1. Cunningham, et al., *Williams Obstetrics,* 23rd ed. (2010), p. 143.

2. Ibid., 108, 393.

3. Department of Health, "Patients for X-Ray Examinations," p. 24.

4. Cunningham, et al., *Williams Obstetrics,* 24th ed., p. 439.

CHAPTER EIGHTEEN: Completing the Pushing Stage

1. Cunningham, et al., *Williams Obstetrics,* 23rd ed., pp. 511–12.

2. Ibid., 382.

3. Cunningham, et al., *Williams Obstetrics,* 24th ed., p. 460.

4. Menticoglou, S. M., et al. "Perinatal Outcomes in Relation to Second-Stage Duration," *Am J Obstet Gynecol* 173, pp. 906, 1995a.

5. Eagleman, D. M., *Incognito* (New York: Pantheon Books, 2011), p. 83.

CHAPTER NINETEEN: Drugs During Labor

1. Brackbill, Y., et al., "Obstetric Premedication and Infant Outcome," *Obstet/Gynec* 118 (1974), p. 377; and Kron, R. E., et al., "Newborn Sucking Behavior Affected by Obstetric Sedation," *Pediatr* 37 (1966), p. 1012.

2. Bernal, J., and Richards, M., "Effects of Obstetric Medication on Mother-Infant Interactions on Infant Development," paper presented at the Third International Congress of Psychology of Medicine in *Obst/Gynec* (London), April 1971.

3. Cunningham, et al., *Williams Obstetrics,* 23rd ed., p. 456.

4. Thorpe, J. A., and Breedlove, G., "Epidural Analgesia in Labor: An Evaluation of Risks and Benefits," *Birth* 23 (1996), p. 63.

5. Caldwell, J., et al., "Determination of Bupivacaine in Human Fetal and Neonatal Blood Samples by Quantitative Single-Ion Monitoring": "Bupivacaine . . . is known to enter the maternal blood stream rapidly from the epidural space, and from there cross the placenta so that a measurable concentration is present in the fetal circulation within ten minutes of epidural injection," *Biomed Mass Spectrom* 4 (1977), pp. 322–25.

6. Dr. Avis Erickson: nationally recognized author, speaker, educator, and administrator in the field of pharmacy.

7. Kaminski, H. M., et al., "The Effects of Epidural Analgesia on the Frequency of Instrumental Obstetric Delivery," *Obstet/Gynec* 69 (1987), p. 770.

CHAPTER TWENTY: Evidence-Based Medicine versus Belief-Based Medicine

1. Department of Health, "Patients for X-Ray Examinations," p. 3.

2. Heffernan, Margaret, "Dare to Disagree," TedGlobal 2012, 12:56, filmed June 2012.

CHAPTER TWENTY-ONE: Inductions (Early Inductions)

1. Cunningham, et al., *Williams Obstetrics,* 23rd ed., p. 500.

2. Cunningham, et al., *Williams Obstetrics,* 24th ed., p. 524.

3. Lozoff, Betsy, professor of Pediatrics and Communicable Diseases, and research professor at University of Michigan, Ann Arbor; Diaz-Barbosa, Magaly, medical director of Neonatology at Miami Children's Hospital, "Babies Born Even Slightly Early May Lag Behind," *Pediatr* (May 2013).

4. Brody, J., "A Campaign to Carry Pregnancies to Term," *New York Times,* August 8, 2011. Interview with Dr. Eve Lackritz, Chief of the Maternal and Infant Health Branch of the National Centers for Disease Control and Prevention.

5. Ibid. Interview with Dr. Uma Reddy, National Institute of Child Health and Human Development.

CHAPTER TWENTY-TWO: What to Expect with an Induction

1. Boulvain, M., Stan, C., and Irion, O., "Membrane Sweeping for Induction of Labour," *Cochrane Database Syst Rev* (2005), issue 1, Art. No.: CD000451.

2. Esakoff, T. F., and Kispatrick, S. J., "The Transcervical Foley Balloon," *Contemporary OB/GYN* (November 2013), p. 39.

3. Maslovitz, S., Lessing, J. B., and Many, A., "Complications of Trans-Cervical Foley Catheter for Labor Induction Among 1,083 Women," *Arch Gynecol Obstet* 281, no. 3 (2010), pp. 473–77.

4. Cunningham, et al., *Williams Obstetrics,* 24th ed., p. 524.

5. Cunningham, et al., *Williams Obstetrics,* 23rd ed., p. 547.

6. Collins, D., J. D., "Did Standing Order Fail?," *Contemporary OB/GYN* 60, no. 10 (October 2015), p. 64.

CHAPTER TWENTY-THREE: Late Inductions

1. Cunningham, et al., *Williams Obstetrics,* 24th ed., p. 862.

2. Gulmezoglu, A.M., et al., "Induction of Labour for Improving Birth Outcomes for Women At or Beyond Term," *Cochrane Database of Syst Rev* (2012), issue 6, Art. No.: CD00494a5. DOI:10.1002/14651858.CD004945.pub3.

3. Cunningham, et al., *Williams Obstetrics,* 24th ed., p. 865.

CHAPTER TWENTY-FOUR: The Mother's Dilemma and the Doctor's Dilemma

1. Heffernan, Margaret, *Willful Blindness* (New York: Walker & Co., 2011), pp. 246–47.

2. Ibid., 247.

3. Cunningham, et al., *Williams Obstetrics,* 24th ed., p. 335.

4. Lalor, J. G., et al., "Biophysical Profile for Fetal Assessment in High-Risk Pregnancies," *Cochrane Database Syst Rev* (2008), issue 1. DOI:10,1002/14651858.CD000038.pub2.

5. Enkin, M., et al., *A Guide to Effective Care in Pregnancy and Childbirth,* 3rd ed. (New York: Oxford University Press, 2000), p. 225.

6. Conway, D. L., et al., "Isolated Oligohydramnios in the Term Pregnancy: Is It a Clinical Entity?," *J Matern Fetal Med* 7, no. 4 (July/August 1998), pp. 197–200.

7. Larsen, T., Larsen, J. F., Petersen, S., and Greisen, G., "Detection of Small-for-Gestational-Age Fetuses by Ultrasound Screening in a High-Risk Population: A Randomized Controlled Study," *BJOG* 99, pp. 469–74. DOI:10.1111/j.1471-0528.1992.tb13783.x.

CHAPTER TWENTY-FIVE: The Episiotomy

1. Cunningham, et al., *Williams Obstetrics,* 24th ed., p. 550.

2. Wessel, H. S., *Natural Childbirth and the Christian Family* (New York: Harper and Row, 1963), p. 196.

3. Banta, D., and Thacker, S. B., "The Risks and Benefits of Episiotomy: A Review," *Birth* 9, no.1 (Spring 1982), p. 26.

4. Kegel, Dr. A., Untitled film on the pubococcygeal muscle, documenting the permanent damage often caused by the me-

diolateral episiotomy; a copy was given to the American Academy of Husband-Coached Childbirth for teaching purposes.

5. Banta and Thacker, "Risks and Benefits," p. 27.

6. Cunningham, et al., *Williams Obstetrics,* 24th ed., p. 550.

7. Banta and Thacker, "Risks and Benefits," p. 27.

CHAPTER TWENTY-SIX: Cesarean Surgery

1. Kozhimannil, K. B., et al., "Cesarean Delivery Rates," pp. 527–35.

2. Hibbard, L. T., "Changing Trends in Caesarean Section," *Amer J of Obstet and Gynecol* 125 (July 1976), p. 798.

3. Enkin, M. W., "Having a Section Is Having a Baby," *Birth and the Family Journal* 4, no. 3 (Fall 1977), pp. 99–105.

4. Beasley, D., "U.S. Birth Data Underscores Higher C-Section Risks, CDC Says," *Health* (May 20, 2015).

5. Haverkamp, A. D., et al., "The Evaluation of Continuous Fetal Heart Rate Monitoring in High-Risk Pregnancy," *Amer J of Obstet and Gynecol* 125, no. 3 (June 1976), pp. 310–20; and Haverkamp, A. D., et al., "A Controlled Trial of the Differential Effects of Intrapartum Fetal Monitoring," *Amer J of Obstet and Gynecol* 134, no.4 (June 15, 1979), pp. 399–412; and Kelso, I. M., et al., "An Assessment of Continuous Fetal Heart Rate Monitoring in Labor—A Randomized Trial," *Amer J of Obstet and Gynecol* 131, no.5 (July 1978), pp. 525–32; and Renou, P., et al., "Controlled Trial of Fetal Intensive Care," *Amer J of Obstet and Gynecol* 126, no. 4 (October 1976), pp. 470–76.

6. Marieskind, H. I., *An Evaluation of Caesarean Surgery in the United States* (Washington, D.C.: U.S. Dept of Health, Education and Welfare, 1979), p. 14.

7. Haverkamp, A. D., quoted in, "Criticism of Electronic Monitoring," *Ob Gyn News* 10, no. 24 (December 15, 1975), p. 1.

8. Murphy, J. R., et al., "The Relation of EFM to Infant Outcome," *Amer J of Epidemiol* 114, no.4 (October 1981), pp. 539–48.

9. Banta, D., and Thacker, S., "Costs and Benefits of Electronic Fetal Monitoring: A Review of the Literature," U.S. Department of Health, Education and Welfare, Office of Health Research, Statistics, and Technology, National Center for Health Services Research, DHEW Pub. No. (PHS) 79-3245 (April 1975), p. 18.

10. Alifrevic, Z., Devane, D., and Gye, G. M., "Continuous Cardiotography (CTG) as a Form of Electronic Fetal Monitoring (EFM) for Fetal Assessment During Labor," *Cochrane Database Syst Rev* (2013), issue 5, Art. No.: CD006066.

11. Grimes, D. A., and Peipert, J. F., "Electronic Fetal Monitoring as a Public Health Screening Program," *Obstet Gynecol* 116 (2010), p. 1397.

12. Kilpatrick, S. J., "Prediction and Prevention of Preterm Birth: What Have We Learned Since 2001?," *Contemp OB/GYN* 58, no. 2 (February 2013), pp. 47–49.

13. Cunningham, et al., *Williams Obstetrics,* 23rd ed., pp. 854–55.

14. Ibid., 855.

15. Banta and Thacker, "Costs and Benefits of Electronic Fetal Monitoring: A Review of the Literature," NCHSR report #79–91, p. 7.

16. Department of Health, "Patients for X-Ray Examinations," p. 3.

17. Young, D., and Mahan C., *Unnecessary Caesareans: Ways to Avoid Them* (Minneapolis: International Childbirth Education Assoc., 1980), p. 10.

18. Cohen, W. R., "Influence of the Duration of Second-Stage Labor on Perinatal Outcome and Puerperal Morbidity," *Obstet and Gynecol* 49, no. 3 (March 1977), pp. 266-69.

19. Rothman, B. K., *In Labor: Women and Power in the Birthplace* (New York: W.W. Norton, 1982), p. 268.

20. Marieskind, *Caesarean Surgery,* p. 19.

21. Shy, K. K., et al., "Effect of Electronic Fetal-Heart-Rate Monitoring, as Compared with Periodic Auscultation on the Neurologic Development of Premature Infants," *New England J of Medi* 332 (1990), pp. 588–93.

22. Kong, D., "Benefits of Electronic Fetal Monitoring Are Questioned," *Boston Globe,* February 1990. Interview with Dr. Benjamin Sachs, Chief of Obstetrics and Gynecology at Boston's Beth Israel Hospital.

CHAPTER TWENTY-SEVEN: Controversies in Hospital Birthing

1. Marieskind, *Cesarean Surgery,* p. 15.

2. Gibbs, D. M. F., et al., "Prolonged Pregnancy: Is Induction of

Labour Indicated?," *British Journal of Obstetrics and Gynecology* 89, no. 4 (April 1982), pp. 292–95.

3. Caldeyro-Barcia, R., quoted in Anderson, Sandra F., "Childbirth as a Pathological Process: An American Perspective," *Amer J Matern Child Nursing* 2, no. 4 (July/August 1977), pp. 240–44.

4. "Caesarean Childbirth: The Final Report of the Consensus Development Conference," (Bethesda, MD: National Institutes of Health Office of Research and Reporting), 1981, p. 14.

5. Kaminetzky, H., and Iffy, L., eds., *New Techniques and Concepts in Maternal and Fetal Medicine* (New York: Van Nostrand Reinhold Company, 1979), p. 198.

CHAPTER TWENTY-NINE: Breast-Feeding

1. Minchin, M., "Infant Formula: A Mass, Uncontrolled Trial in Perinatal Care," *Birth* 14, no. 1 (March 1987), p. 25.

2. Moynahan, E. M., "Acrodermatitis Enteropathica: A Lethal Inherited Zinc Deficiency," *Lancet* (1974), pp. 399–400.

3. Hood, R. L., and Johnson, A. R., "Supplementation of Infant Formulations with Biotin," *Nutr Rep Int* 21 (1980), pp. 727–31.

4. Minchin, "Infant Formula," p. 28.

5. "News," *Birth* 12, no. 4 (Winter 1985), p. 245.

6. Minchin, "Infant Formula," p. 28.

Further Reading

Every student in our classes borrows these essential books from our lending library.

Husband-Coached Childbirth by Dr. Robert A. Bradley (New York: Harper & Row, 1981)

This is a classic. Pay particular attention to the chapter entitled "It's Not Nice to Fool Mother Nature." And Dr. Bradley's chapter "When Will the Baby Come?" is essential reading for all birthing parents.

Immaculate Deception by Suzanne Arms (Boston: Houghton Mifflin, 1975)

Writer and photographer Suzanne Arms gives you a close-up view of what birth is like when you pick an unhelpful birth attendant or passively approach the experience expecting others to take care of things for you. She alerts you to the experience of mechanized, high-tech, depersonalized childbirth. Through her interviews you will be able to pick up on attitudes that tell you whether a birth attendant will be helpful or not. This will help tune your ear for when you are interviewing your own prospective attendant.

The Brewer Medical Diet for Normal and High-Risk Pregnancy by Gail Sforza Brewer with Tom Brewer, MD (New York: Simon & Schuster, 1983)

There is no book equal to this one on nutrition in pregnancy. If you think it is a boring subject, this book will pleasantly surprise you. Reading chapters like "Forty Weeks, Forty Problems: Situations Most Likely to Interfere with Your Diet," you will find yourself thinking, "How do they know so much about me?"

Children at Birth by Marjie and Jay Hathaway (Sherman Oaks, Calif.: Academy Pubns., 1978—can be ordered through your Bradley teacher)

If you are planning to have your other children with you at the birth, this book is an essential part of the preparation for you and your children. It is full of practical advice in chapters such as "How to Decide If Your Child

Should Be at a Birth" and "How to Prepare Your Child." The book includes the experience of birth through the eyes of children who have been there.

How to Relax and Have Your Baby by Edmund Jacobson, MD (New York: McGraw-Hill, 1965)

> This book is dated in many ways, and Jacobson thinks women should be totally obedient to the physician. It is also enormously aggravating that he believes women do not need to know anything about labor and birth, only relaxation. Still, he is an expert on relaxation, which is of major importance in labor, and his great wisdom is his understanding of how to acquire the ability to relax as a skillful tool. Ignore his idiosyncrasies and read this small book to get that wisdom.

The Womanly Art of Breastfeeding by La Leche League (local chapters are listed in phone books)

> This is one of the first and still one of the best books on nursing. It is a fast read, completely practical and to the point. I recommend purchasing a copy (that way you also support a worthwhile organization) to read before the birth and to have on hand for quick reference after.

Nursing Your Baby by Karen Pryor (New York: Simon & Schuster, 1976)

> This is THE BEST book on breast-feeding. Though not as quick and easy to use as La Leche League's book,

it contains all of the practical information and much more. If you want your reading detailed and referenced, this is the one, but both these breast-feeding books are valuable to read and have.

For the avid reader who wants more, we recommend:

Childbirth Without Fear by Grantly Dick-Read, MD (New York: Harper & Row, 1978)

> This is an oldie-but-a-goodie by the "father" of modern natural childbirth, and which always offers some valuable insight that has been temporarily lost in the art of birthing.

Silent Knife by Nancy Wainer Cohen and Lois J. Estner (South Hadley, Mass.: Bergin & Garvey, 1983)

> This book is the latest word on caesarean surgery and is especially useful to the mother who has had a C-section but wants a vaginal birth the next time around.

In Labor: Women and Power in the Birthplace by Barbara Katz Rothman (New York: W. W. Norton, 1982)

> A book that looks at the sociology of childbirth and especially at the reemergence of the midwife.

A Woman in Residence by Michelle Harrison, MD (New York: Random House, 1982)

> This is a personal account by a woman doctor who tried to buck the medical birth establishment from the inside.

Appendix: *Protein Counter*

FOOD	QUANTITY	GRAMS
DAIRY PRODUCTS		
Cow's milk, whole	1 cup	8
Cow's milk, skim	1 cup	9
Milk, powdered,		
whole	1 cup powder	27
skim, instant	1⅓ cup powder	30
skim, non-instant	⅔ cup powder	30
Yogurt (of partially skim milk)	1 cup	8
Custard, baked	1 cup	13
Ice cream	1 cup	6
Ice milk	1 cup	9
Cream, light (or half-and-half)	½ cup	4
heavy or whipping	½ cup	2
Cottage cheese		
creamed	1 cup	30
uncreamed	1 cup	38

FOOD	QUANTITY	GRAMS
Cheddar (or American cheese)	1 in. cube	4
Cheddar, grated	½ cup	14
Cream cheese	1 oz.	2
Processed cheese	1 oz.	7
Swiss cheese	1 oz.	7
Eggs		
yolks only	1	3
whole	1	6
MEAT AND POULTRY		
Bacon	1 slice	2
Beef (chuck or pot roasted)	3 oz.	23
Hamburger (ground lean)	3 oz.	24
Roast beef	3 oz.	16
Steak, sirloin	3 oz.	20

FOOD	QUANTITY	GRAMS
Chicken,		
(thigh, leg, or breast)	3 oz.	25
Chicken liver	3 oz.	22
Turkey	3 oz.	27
Lamb, chop	4 oz.	24
leg	3 oz.	20
shoulder	3 oz.	18
Pork chop	3 oz.	18
Ham, cured	3 oz.	16
Pork roast	3 oz.	21
Pork sausage, bulk	3 oz.	18
Veal cutlet	3 oz.	23
Chili con carne (with beans)	1 cup	19
without beans	1 cup	16
Sausage, bologna	2 slices	7
Frankfurter	1	7

FOOD	QUANTITY	GRAMS
FISH AND SEAFOODS		
Clams (steamed or canned)	3 oz.	12
Cod	3½ oz.	28
Crabmeat	3 oz.	14
Fish sticks	2	7
Flounder	3 oz.	30
Haddock	3 oz.	15
Halibut	3 oz.	26
Salmon (canned)	3 oz.	17
Sardines	3 oz.	12
Scallops	3½ oz.	18
Shrimp	3 oz.	23
Swordfish	1 steak	17
Tuna, canned	3 oz.	25
VEGETABLES		
Artichoke	1	2
Asparagus	6 spears	1
Beans (green snap)	1 cup	1
lima, green	½ cup	4
lima, dry, cooked	½ cup	8
navy, with pork	¾ cup	11

FOOD	QUANTITY	GRAMS
kidney, canned	1 cup	15
Bean sprouts	1 cup	15
Broccoli	½ cup	1
Brussels sprouts	1 cup	1
Cabbage (as coleslaw)	1 cup	1
steamed	1 cup	2
Carrots	1 cup	1
Celery	1 cup	1
Corn	1 ear	3
Cucumbers	6	0
Eggplant	1 cup	0
Lentils	½ cup	7
Lettuce	¼ head	1
Mushrooms	½ cup	2
Onions	½ cup	1
Parsley	1 T.	1
Peas	1 cup	5
Peppers (pimientos)	1 pod	0
raw, green	1	1
stuffed with beef (and bread crumbs)	1 med.	9
Potato chips	10	1
Potatoes, baked	1 med.	2
french fried		0

FOOD	QUANTITY	GRAMS
Soybeans	½ cup	11
Spinach	1 cup	3
Squash, summer	1 cup	1
Sweet potatoes	1 med.	2
FRUITS		
They have 0 to 1 or 2 grams.		
BREADS, CEREALS, AND GRAINS		
Biscuit	1	3
Bran flakes	1 cup	3
Bread (cracked wheat)	1 slice	2
rye	1 slice	2
whole wheat	1 slice	2
Cornbread	1 serving	3
Cornflakes	1 cup	2
Cornmeal (yellow)	1 cup	9
Crackers (graham)	2 med.	1
soda	2	1
Flour, soy, full fat	1 cup	39
wheat, all purpose	1 cup	12
wheat, whole	1 cup	13

FOOD	QUANTITY	GRAMS
Macaroni	1 cup	5
Noodles	1 cup	7
Oatmeal (or rolled oats)	1 cup	5
Popcorn	2 cups	3
Puffed rice	1 cup	0
Puffed wheat	1 cup	1
Rice, brown	1 cup	15
white	1 cup	14
Rolls, breakfast	1 large	3
Shredded wheat	1 biscuit	3
Spaghetti (with meat sauce)	1 cup	13
Wheat germ	1 cup	26
Wheat germ cereal	1 cup	20

SOUPS, CANNED AND DILUTED

FOOD	QUANTITY	GRAMS
Bean	1 cup	9
Beef and vegetable	1 cup	6
Bouillon, broth	1 cup	5
Chicken or turkey	1 cup	4
Clam chowder (without milk)	1 cup	5
Cream soups	1 cup	7
Noodle (rice and barley)	1 cup	6
Split pea	1 cup	8
Tomato with milk	1 cup	6
Vegetable	1 cup	6

DESSERTS AND SWEETS

FOOD	QUANTITY	GRAMS
Candy, caramels	5	0
plain fudge	2 pieces	0
Chocolate syrup	2 T.	0
Cupcake	1	3
Doughnuts (cake type)	1	2
Hard candies	1 oz.	0
Honey, strained	2 T.	0
Jams and jellies	1 T.	0
Marshmallows	5	0
Milk chocolate	2 oz. bar	2
Molasses	1 T.	0
Pie, apple	1 slice	3
cherry	1 slice	3
Sugar, white	1 cup	0
brown	1 cup	0
Syrup, maple	2 T.	0
Tapioca pudding	1 cup	10

NUTS AND SEEDS

FOOD	QUANTITY	GRAMS
Almonds	½ cup	13
Cashews	½ cup	13
Peanut butter	⅓ cup	12
Peanuts	⅓ cup	13
Pecans	½ cup	5
Sesame seeds (dried)	½ cup	9
Sunflower seeds	½ cup	12
Walnuts	½ cup	7

BEVERAGES

FOOD	QUANTITY	GRAMS
Alcoholic drinks		0
Carbonated drinks		0
Coffee, black	1 cup	0
Tea, black	1 cup	0

SUPPLEMENTARY FOODS

FOOD	QUANTITY	GRAMS
Desiccated liver	½ cup	28
Brewer's yeast (powdered)	½ cup	13

SOURCE: Department of Health, State of Hawaii, plus additional nutritional information.

Index

Afterword by Marjie Hathaway

IT IS WITH GREAT excitement that I write an afterword to this outstanding book. We hope it will increase everyone's understanding of the Bradley Method® and will help inform many mothers-to-be that natural childbirth is not dead but is alive and well in their local Bradley classes.

Our interest in natural childbirth started in 1965. After having three extremely difficult deliveries, I was pregnant with our fourth child, and my husband, Jay, and I felt there had to be a better way. We learned (the hard way) that medication does not take away the pain. In most cases it just postpones it. Each time I recovered in great pain, while trying to take care of our new baby. We just knew there must be a better way than the "normal" delivery.

Instead, we wanted to have natural childbirth with Jay in the delivery room. After much searching, we could not find any doctors or hospitals in Southern California that would allow this radical "new" idea in 1965. Therefore,

at last, we flew to Denver, Colorado, where Dr. Robert A. Bradley practices medicine, to give birth to our fourth baby, using the techniques he had perfected and practiced. We were so delighted with our birth that we started teaching and developing the Bradley Method® ourselves for the first time outside of Denver. It took literally years of writing and testing and traveling to confer with Dr. Bradley before we developed the system of childbirth education that now extends throughout the United States: The American Academy of Husband-Coached Childbirth®.

One of the major tasks the AAHCC® undertook was to train other Bradley Method® teachers. The demand for Bradley teachers grew so fast, we soon began holding training workshops all over the country. Susan McCutcheon was one of the first people to take our training, and over the years she has been a guest speaker at many of our workshops, helping us train many other fine Bradley teachers. Her application of the principles of the Bradley

Method® is an inspiration to anyone looking for a truly natural way to have a baby. Today you can find Bradley teachers in every state who are trained professionals, ready to teach others and share the wonder of the Bradley Method®.

We have found that it is essential to educate yourself as much as possible during your pregnancy. Read as many books as you can and attend Bradley classes in your area. This book was not intended as a substitute for classes taught by affiliated Bradley teachers; attending classes is important preparation, and no book can fill that need.

Bradley classes are longer than other childbirth classes because we include information on the entire experience of pregnancy, birthing, and becoming a family. There are twelve units of instruction and free weekly reviews until birth. Certified Bradley instructors are also required to keep classes small enough for individual attention. Ask to see your instructor's current Certificate of Affiliation, which will assure you of a trained, up-to-date, nationally affiliated instructor who is well qualified. You should also ask what percentage of students in her class actually are able to have unmedicated births. Our teachers are ready and willing to give you this information. Our teachers are chosen because of their experience with natural childbirth (most of them are experienced Bradley mothers themselves), and through AAHCC® they have completed one of the most extensive childbirth training programs in the United States. After you have successfully used the Bradley Method®, you might consider the impact you could have in your community if you took the AAHCC® training and became a Bradley teacher yourself. Because of the growing enthusiasm and demand for the Bradley Method®, we need many new teachers in all parts of the country.

We are really excited about the impact *Natural Childbirth the Bradley® Way* will have on the general public, and about the possibility of reaching couples interested in the Bradley Method® who were not previously aware of this positive alternative in childbirth. After you have your Bradley birth, we ask your help in compiling statistics that we hope will help others. Please fill out the feedback form at the back of this book. This information will be entered into our computer to help update and improve ourselves and benefit others. And do have a happy birth day!

—MARJIE HATHAWAY
AMERICAN ACADEMY OF HUSBAND-COACHED CHILDBIRTH®

The Bradley Method® FEEDBACK FORM

Please help us serve the unborn by communicating and sharing with the American Academy of Husband-Coached Childbirth®.

Name _____

Address_____

City, State, Zip_____

Baby's name_____

☐ I want to share the following information, so you can update the statistics in your computer.

FOLLOW-UP REPORT

BIRTH:

☐ I pushed the baby out

☐ They pulled the baby out (forceps)

☐ Caesarean surgery

☐ Vaginal birth after previous caesarean (VBAC)

DRUGS:

☐ None

☐ Local anesthetic for episiotomy only

☐ Analgesic (pain reliever): Demerol, Nistetil, Vistaril, Valium, Phenergan, etc.

☐ Anesthesia (pudendal block, epidural/spinal/saddleblock, gas)

ATTENDANT:

☐ MD ☐ DO ☐ DC ☐ CNM ☐ Midwife ☐ None

BABY/MOM:

☐ Boy   ☐ Girl   ☐ First baby

☐ Second baby   ☐ Third or more   ☐ Twins

Baby's weight____lbs____ozs

Mom's weight gain____lbs

Mom's daily average protein intake____grams

CLASSES:

☐ Bradley®   ☐ Lamaze   ☐ Other_____

Number of classes:

☐ Four ☐ Six ☐ Eight ☐ Ten ☐ Twelve ☐ More

ULTRASOUND:

☐ Scan   ☐ Doptone used in office or in labor

☐ External fetal monitor

Total radiation time:_____hours

DOCTOR/MIDWIFE   HOSPITAL/BIRTH CENTER   TEACHER

NAME_____

ADDRESS_____

CITY/ST/ZIP_____

Send to: American Academy of Husband-Coached Childbirth®
THE BRADLEY METHOD®
Box 5224-R, Sherman Oaks, CA 91413-5224
(800) 423-2397 or (818) 788-6662 (California)